Sitaraman and Friedman's
Essentials of Gastroenterology

Sitaraman and Friedman's Essentials of Gastroenterology

Edited by

Shanthi Srinivasan, MD

Professor of Medicine, Division of Digestive Diseases, Emory University School of Medicine;
Chief of Gastroenterology, Atlanta Veterans Affairs Medical Center, Atlanta, GA, USA

Lawrence S. Friedman, MD

Professor of Medicine, Harvard Medical School, Boston;
Professor of Medicine, Tufts University School of Medicine, Boston;
The Anton R. Fried, MD, Chair, Department of Medicine, Newton-Wellesley Hospital, Newton;
Assistant Chief of Medicine, Massachusetts General Hospital, Boston, MA, USA

Foreword by

Frank A. Anania, MD, FACP, AGAF, FAASLD

R. Bruce Logue Chair and Professor of Medicine, Director, Division of Digestive Diseases, Emory University Department of Medicine, Atlanta, GA, USA

Second Edition

WILEY Blackwell

Registered Office(s)
John Wiley & Sons, Inc., 111 River Street, Hoboken, NJ 07030, USA
John Wiley & Sons Ltd, The Atrium, Southern Gate, Chichester, West Sussex, PO19 8SQ, UK

Editorial Office
9600 Garsington Road, Oxford, OX4 2DQ, UK
For details of our global editorial offices, customer services, and more information about Wiley products visit us at www.wiley.com.

Wiley also publishes its books in a variety of electronic formats and by print-on-demand. Some content that appears in standard print versions of this book may not be available in other formats.

Library of Congress Cataloging-in-Publication Data

Names: Srinivasan, Shanthi, editor. | Friedman, Lawrence S. (Lawrence
    Samuel), 1953– editor.
Title: Sitaraman and Friedman's essentials of gastroenterology / edited by
    Shanthi Srinivasan, Lawrence S. Friedman.
Other titles: Essentials of gastroenterology. | Essentials of gastroenterology
Description: Second edition. | Hoboken, NJ : John Wiley & Sons, 2017. | Preceded by
    Essentials of gastroenterology / edited by Shanthi V. Sitaraman, Lawrence S. Friedman. 2012 |
    Includes bibliographical references and index. |
Identifiers: LCCN 2017034316 (print) | LCCN 2017035044 (ebook) |
    ISBN 9781119235194 (pdf) | ISBN 9781119235187 (epub) | ISBN 9781119235224 (pbk.)
Subjects: | MESH: Gastrointestinal Diseases | Handbooks | Case Reports
Classification: LCC RC801 (ebook) | LCC RC801 (print) | NLM WI 39 |
    DDC 616.3/3–dc23
LC record available at https://lccn.loc.gov/2017034316

Cover Design: Wiley
Cover Image: © Science Photo Library - PASIEKA/Gettyimages

Set in 10/12pt Warnock by SPi Global, Pondicherry, India

Printed in the UK

In Memory of Shanthi V. Sitaraman, MD, PhD

Contents

Contributor List

Frank A. Anania, MD, FACP, AGAF, FAASLD
R. Bruce Logue Chair and Professor
of Medicine
Director, Division of Digestive
Diseases, Department of Medicine
Emory University School of
Medicine
Atlanta, GA, USA

Stephen H. Berger, MD
Physician
Huron Gastroenterology Associates
Ypsilanti, MI, USA

Qiang Cai, MD, PhD
Professor of Medicine
Director, Advanced Endoscopy
Fellowship
Division of Digestive Diseases
Emory University School of
Medicine
Atlanta, GA, USA

Lisa Cassani, MD
Assistant Professor of Medicine
Division of Digestive Diseases
Emory University School of
Medicine
Atlanta Veterans Administration
Medical Center
Atlanta, GA, USA

Saurabh Chawla, MD
Assistant Professor of Medicine
Division of Gastroenterology
Emory University School of
Medicine
Grady Memorial Hospital
Atlanta, GA, USA

Jennifer Christie, MD, FASGE
Associate Professor of Medicine
Clinical Director
Division of Digestive Diseases
Emory University School of
Medicine
Atlanta, GA, USA

Nader Dbouk, MD
Physician
Atlanta Gastroenterology Associates
Conyers, GA, USA

Tanvi Dhere, MD
Associate Professor
Division of Digestive Diseases
Emory University School of
Medicine
Atlanta, GA, USA

Sujaata R. Dwadasi, MD
Gastroenterology Fellow
University of Chicago
Chicago, IL, USA

Mary M. Flynn, MD
Gastroenterology Fellow
Emory University School of
Medicine
Atlanta, GA, USA

Ryan M. Ford, MD
Assistant Professor of Medicine
Division of Digestive Diseases
Emory University School of
Medicine
Atlanta, GA, USA

Lawrence S. Friedman, MD
Professor of Medicine,
Harvard Medical School;
Professor of Medicine, Tufts
University School of Medicine,
Boston, MA, USA

and

The Anton R. Fried, MD,
Chair, Department of Medicine
Newton-Wellesley Hospital
Newton;
Assistant Chief of Medicine
Massachusetts General Hospital
Boston MA, USA

Anthony M. Gamboa, MD
Assistant Professor of Medicine
Division of Gastroenterology
Vanderbilt University School of
Medicine
Nashville, TN, USA

Stephan Goebel, MD
Assistant Professor of Medicine
Division of Digestive Diseases
Emory University School of
Medicine;
Atlanta Veterans Administration
Medical Center
Atlanta, GA, USA

Nicole M. Griglione, MD
GI Associates, LLC
Brookfield, WI, USA

Melanie S. Harrison, MD
Assistant Professor of Medicine
Division of Digestive Diseases
Emory University School of
Medicine;
Atlanta Veterans Administration
Medical Center
Atlanta, GA, USA

Steven Keilin, MD, FASGE
Associate Professor of Medicine
Director, Pancreaticobiliary Service
Associate Director, Advanced
Endoscopy Fellowship
Division of Digestive Diseases
Emory University School of
Medicine
Atlanta, GA, USA

Jan-Michael A. Klapproth, MD
Associate Professor of Medicine
Division of Gastroenterology
University of Pennsylvania
Philadelphia, PA, USA

Stephen K. Lau, MD
Assistant Professor
Department of Pathology
Emory University School of
Medicine
Atlanta, GA, USA

Edward Lin, DO, MBA, FACS
Associate Professor of Surgery
Department of Surgery
Emory University School of
Medicine
Atlanta, GA, USA

Rebecca G. Lopez, MD
Children's Healthcare of Atlanta at
Egleston
Atlanta, GA, USA

Julia Massaad, MD
Assistant Professor of Medicine
Division of Digestive Diseases
Emory University School of
Medicine
Atlanta, GA, USA

Pardeep K. Mittal, MD
Associate Professor
Department of Radiology and
Imaging Sciences
Emory University School of
Medicine
Atlanta, GA, USA

Courtney C. Moreno, MD
Associate Professor
of Radiology
Department of Abdominal
Radiology
Emory University School
of Medicine
Atlanta, GA, USA

JP Norvell, MD
Assistant Professor of Medicine
Division of Digestive Diseases
Emory University School of
Medicine
Atlanta, GA, USA

Kamil Obideen, MD
Atlanta Gastroenterology Associates
Northside Forsyth Hospital
Cumming, GA, USA

Samir Parekh, MD
Assistant Professor of Medicine
Division of Digestive Diseases
Emory University School of
Medicine
Atlanta, GA, USA

Pruthvi Patel, MD, MPH
Assistant Professor of Medicine
Division of Gastroenterology
Stony Brook University School
of Medicine
Stony Brook, NY, USA

Anjana A. Pillai, MD
Associate Professor of Medicine
University of Chicago Medical Center
Chicago, IL, USA

Meena A. Prasad, MD
Assistant Professor of Medicine
Division of Digestive Diseases
Emory University School
of Medicine;
Atlanta Veterans Administration
Medical Center
Atlanta, GA, USA

Emad Qayed, MD, MPH
Assistant Professor of Medicine
Division of Gastroenterology
Emory University School of
Medicine;
Grady Memorial Hospital
Atlanta, GA, USA

Shreya Raja, MD
Assistant Professor of Medicine
Division of Digestive Diseases
Emory University School of Medicine;
Atlanta Veterans Administration
Medical Center
Atlanta, GA, USA

Preeti A. Reshamwala, MD
Assistant Professor of Medicine
Division of Digestive Diseases
Emory University School of
Medicine
Atlanta, GA, USA

Zakiya P. Rice, MD
Assistant Professor
Department of Dermatology
Emory University School of Medicine
Atlanta, GA, USA

Robin E. Rutherford, MD
Emeritus Professor of Medicine
Emory University School of Medicine
Atlanta, GA, USA

Sonali S. Sakaria, MD
Assistant Professor of Medicine
Division of Gastroenterology
Emory University School of Medicine
Atlanta, GA, USA

Kavya M. Sebastian, MD
Assistant Professor of Medicine
Division of Digestive Diseases
Emory University School of Medicine
Atlanta, GA, USA

William C. Small, MD, PhD
Professor
Department of Abdominal Radiology
Emory University School of Medicine
Atlanta, GA, USA

Shanthi Srinivasan, MD
Professor of Medicine
Division of Digestive Diseases
Emory University School of Medicine;
Chief of Gastroenterology
Atlanta Veterans Affairs
Medical Center
Atlanta, GA, USA

Robert A. Swerlick, MD
Professor
Department of Dermatology
Emory University School of Medicine
Atlanta, GA, USA

Joel P. Wedd, MD
Assistant Professor of Medicine
Division of Digestive Diseases
Emory University School of Medicine
Atlanta, GA, USA

Field F. Willingham, MD, MPH
Associate Professor of Medicine
Director of Endoscopy
Division of Digestive Diseases
Emory University School of
Medicine
Atlanta, GA, USA

Shani Woolard, MD
Gastroenterology Fellow
Emory University School of Medicine
Atlanta, GA, USA

Vincent W. Yang, MD, PhD
Professor and Chair
Department of Medicine
Stony Brook University School
of Medicine
Stony Brook, NY, USA

Foreword

The practice of gastroenterology and hepatology continues to evolve at a seemingly revolutionary pace. Since the First Edition of *Essentials of Gastroenterology* was published in 2012, we have witnessed the advent of powerful new biologic agents for the treatment of inflammatory bowel disease. And who could have imagined then that we could cure over 90% of patients with chronic hepatitis C virus infection with direct-acting antiviral therapies? Despite these (and other) important advances, the clinical foundation of the field of gastroenterology that has been the basis of such important treatment strategies remains the same. Understanding the pathophysiology and clinical features of gastrointestinal and liver diseases is a critical aspect of every medical student's education in human diseases.

The First Edition of this textbook was developed and co-edited by the late Shanthi V. Sitaraman, MD, PhD, Professor of Medicine and Pathology at Emory University School of Medicine who, sadly, did not live to see her work published. Shanthi was an exceptional teacher, physician and scientist who died far too young in April 2011. Lawrence S. Friedman, MD, Professor of Medicine at Harvard Medical School and Tufts University School of Medicine, co-edited the first edition with Shanthi and suggested to me that we update the text as a Second Edition, and I am truly grateful that Shanthi Srinivasan, MD, Professor of Medicine and Chief of Gastroenterology at the Atlanta Veterans' Affairs Medical Center and a colleague and close friend of Shanthi Sitaraman, agreed to serve as co-editor with Dr Friedman of this Second Edition.

As in the First Edition of *Essentials of Gastroenterology*, each chapter of the Second Edition begins with a clinical vignette after which the fundamental aspects of pathophysiology, clinical features, and approach to treatment are presented. This technique in education is used in many medical schools, including Emory University School of Medicine, in which first-year medical students are immersed in patient-related case histories when studying each organ system. The chapters are written concisely to give the trainee the ability to take away key points ('Pearls') that are critical to the development of skills in differential diagnosis, assessment, and treatment planning. Furthermore, easy-to-understand diagrams and tables, as well as exceptionally clear illustrations, endoscopic photographs, and radiologic images, make this book particularly useful not only as a guidebook for medical students, but also as a quick reference for medical house officers who are confronted with patients with gastrointestinal and liver disease.

The success of the First Edition of this textbook and its design is not fortuitous. Dr Friedman, one of the foremost master clinicians of gastroenterology and hepatology in Boston – and a former mentor of the late Dr Sitaraman – has once again, along with Dr Srinivasan, devoted a great amount of time to carefully editing each chapter. The result is a brilliantly crafted, concise, and enjoyable book to read. The questions and answers presented at the end of each chapter are timely and integrative in design, giving trainees the ability to sharpen the depth of their conceptual knowledge about the approach to the natural history of diseases seen in the practice of gastroenterology. Impressively, Drs Srinivasan, Friedman, and the contributing authors of the updated text provide new information on treatment approaches for the major diseases covered in this book.

Finally, the editors and authors owe a tremendous debt of gratitude to Carla Fairclough and Alison Sholock, who incorporated the numerous editorial changes made by Drs Srinivasan and Friedman. They meticulously transformed handwritten edits sent to them on the original and revised manuscripts into polished final versions. Their organization has made the work of the editors immensely easier. I am also deeply grateful to our faculty (including some former faculty) in the Division of Digestive Diseases at Emory University School of Medicine who wrote and revised all of the chapters in this text. Many of them are teachers in the first-year medical student curriculum 'Foundations of Medicine' course, which was initially organized by Dr Sitaraman. To paraphrase a sentiment expressed by Dr Daniel K. Podolsky in the Foreword to the First Edition of *Essentials of Gastroenterology*, "...though we have been deprived of Shanthi Sitaraman's distinguished career as a teacher, mentor, physician, and investigator," the Second Edition of this textbook "...once again serves as an important hallmark of Shanthi's enduring legacy" to our discipline.

Frank A. Anania, MD, FACP, AGAF, FAASLD
Emory University School of Medicine

Preface

This Second Edition of *Essentials of Gastroenterology* is the first for which Shanthi V. Sitaraman has not served as a co-editor, because of her untimely death as the First Edition was published in 2012. A tribute to Shanthi Sitaraman follows this Preface and the Acknowledgments. Succeeding Shanthi Sitaraman as co-editor is her colleague and friend, Shanthi Srinivasan, an accomplished editor, gastroenterologist, and professor at the Emory University School of Medicine with an interest in basic enteric neuroscience and gastrointestinal motility. The title of the book has been revised to include Shanthi Sitaraman's name to reflect her enduring contribution.

The field of gastroenterology and hepatology has progressed at a rapid pace, and *Sitaraman and Friedman's Essentials of Gastroenterology, Second Edition*, reflects this progress with an updated content five years after the First Edition of the book was published. In editing this book, we have kept the format similar to that of the First Edition, which was well received, but have updated the content. Throughout the book, we have continued to emphasize fundamental clinical points in a clear, organized, and concise manner. Our goal remains for the book to provide up-to-date, foundational knowledge of gastrointestinal medicine and of the most important and common clinical problems encountered in the field. Among the areas in which remarkable changes have occurred since publication of the First Edition are new treatment regimens for hepatitis C, improved management of portal hypertension, and expanded drug therapy for inflammatory bowel disease. Primary biliary cirrhosis is now called primary biliary cholangitis. In the chapter on peptic ulcer disease, treatment protocols for *Helicobacter pylori* and the indications for confirming the eradication of *H. pylori* have been updated. Other major changes include updated methodology for the diagnosis of motility disorders, including the wireless motility capsule and three-dimensional high-resolution manometry, a new section on eosinophilic esophagitis, and updated criteria for the diagnosis of irritable bowel syndrome.

The book represents contributions from faculty and fellows in the Division of Digestive Diseases and the Departments of Pathology, Radiology, and Surgery at the Emory University School of Medicine, and is geared toward medical students studying gastroenterology in an introductory course on clinical medicine or on a clinical rotation in medicine or gastroenterology. Many of the contributors have been recipients of awards for outstanding contributions to medical education. New authors include faculty who have recently come to Emory. Each has helped to revitalize and refresh the book.

The format of the Second Edition remains unchanged. The book has 28 chapters that are organized into five sections. Each chapter covers a key clinical issue in the practice of gastroenterology, and the Picture Gallery provides the proverbial 'textbook' examples of dermatology, radiology, and pathology findings in gastroenterology. The chapters are written in an easy-to-read outline format that covers the basics of pathophysiology, clinical features, diagnosis, natural history, prognosis, and treatment of the common disorders seen in the practice of gastroenterology. Figures and tables illustrate and highlight key information. Shaded boxes draw attention to important practice points, and a concluding segment in each chapter in the first four sections provides a list of 'pearls' useful in clinical practice. Illustrative cases begin each chapter in the first four sections, and multiple-choice questions pertaining to these clinical vignettes and to the content of the chapter provide an opportunity for the reader to test his or her knowledge of the subject matter after reading a chapter. A few key references and web links are provided. The aim is to make the information as clear, concise, and 'digestible' as possible. Medical students will find the information relevant and readily understandable, while more senior trainees can use the book to obtain a quick and practical review of the field in a short amount of time. Readers should find the book useful and focused, without being overwhelming.

We are excited to present this Second Edition and hope that it will continue to be an enduring tribute to Shanthi Sitaraman's dream of fostering excellence in medical education.

Shanthi Srinivasan, MD
and Lawrence S. Friedman, MD

Acknowledgments

We are grateful for the invaluable assistance and support of the faculty and fellows at the Emory University School of Medicine, and particularly of members of the Division of Digestive Diseases. Their adherence to deadlines, attention to detail, and commitment to excellence were essential to the successful completion of this book. We are particularly grateful to Dr. Frank A. Anania, Chief of the Division of Digestive Diseases at Emory, for his extraordinary support of this project and for his gracious preparation of the Foreword to this book. Each contributor to this book deserves acknowledgment for his or her effort. We are also grateful for the support of our families, including parents Anbukili and V.K. Chetty, husband Muthayyah, and children Karthik, Arjun, and Anand (S.S) and wife Mary Jo Cappuccilli, son Matthew Friedman, and grandson Christopher Friedman (L.S.F.).

The support of the staff of our publisher, Wiley, including Oliver Walter and Priyanka Gibbons (Publishers, Clinical Medicine), Alice Wheeler (Editorial assistant), Thaatcher Missier-Glen (Project Editor), Arabella Talbot (Editorial assistant), Yogalakshmi Mohanakrishnan (Project Editor), William Down (Copyeditor), and Sandeep Kumar (Production Editor) was phenomenal, and we cannot thank them enough. We also acknowledge the remarkable efforts of our Assistants, Carla Fairclough (S.S.) and Alison Sholock (L.S.F), who served as surrogate editors for the book.

Shanthi Srinivasan, MD
and Lawrence S. Friedman, MD

Tribute to Shanthi V. Sitaraman

Essentials of Gastroenterology, First Edition, was conceived, developed, and co-edited by Shanthi V. Sitaraman, MD, PhD, who tragically passed away after a long illness as the book was nearing completion. The book reflects Shanthi's dream and vision to create a textbook of gastroenterology targeted specifically to medical students but useful as well to residents rotating on a gastroenterology service and fellows and practitioners preparing for certification examinations and desiring a quick, focused review of the state-of-the-art of the field.

The opportunity to work with Shanthi Sitaraman on the First Edition of this book was a once-in-a-lifetime experience that we will always treasure. We have both had the privilege and honor of working with Shanthi. To Shanthi Srinivasan, Shanthi was a best friend, mentor, colleague, and confidante. To Lawrence Friedman, Shanthi was a star trainee, superb clinician, and accomplished researcher. As we edited each chapter, we remember the discussions we had with Shanthi about the book and the passion she infused in us to make it as perfect as possible. She loved students, and the book was her long-lasting gift to them and an enduring legacy to the field of gastroenterology. Her love of gastroenterology and passion for teaching were evident throughout the entire project, and shine in this book.

Shanthi was a brilliant and dedicated physician-scientist who, as a faculty member at Emory, made numerous contributions to education, research, and clinical practice. Her work in inflammatory bowel diseases resulted in over 200 publications that advanced our understanding of basic mechanisms of inflammation and led to novel approaches to therapy. Her devotion to patients was legendary, and in 2011 she received the Crohn's and Colitis Foundation of America Premier Physician Award in Georgia. She mentored and taught countless medical students, residents, fellows, and junior faculty, and her humanitarian service to the greater Atlanta community was inspiring.

Essentials of Gastroenterology is both a fitting tribute to, and a wonderful legacy of, an exceptional educator, colleague, and friend. Shanthi herself was an award-winning teacher who was beloved by the students, residents, fellows, and faculty at Emory. She was a recipient of the Silver Pear Mentoring Award from the Department of Medicine, the Student Association Teaching Award and Dean's Teaching Award from the School of Medicine, and the Attending of the Year designation and the Mentor Award from the Division of Digestive Diseases at Emory, among numerous other honors. She is sorely missed, and we are proud to dedicate the Second Edition of the retitled *Sitaraman and Friedman's Essentials of Gastroenterology* to her.

Shanthi Srinivasan, MD
and Lawrence S. Friedman, MD

Luminal Gastrointestinal Tract

Shreya Raja and Melanie S. Harrison

1

Gastroesophageal Reflux Disease

Shani Woolard and Jennifer Christie

Clinical Vignette

A 50-year-old man with a history of hypertension and hyperlipidemia presents with a 4-month history of chest discomfort. He describes the discomfort as a burning and occasionally a pressure sensation in the mid-sternal area. The discomfort often occurs 45 minutes after eating a meal and lasts for about 3 hours, gradually improving thereafter. He occasionally awakens in the morning with a sore throat, cough, and bitter taste in his mouth. He has tried over-the-counter ranitidine, with only minimal relief. He was recently seen in the emergency department for an episode of severe chest pain. A cardiac work-up, including an electrocardiogram, cardiac enzymes, and a stress echocardiogram, was negative. Physical examination reveals a well-built, well-nourished man in no apparent distress. The blood pressure is 137/84 mmHg, pulse rate 72 per minute, respiratory rate 14 per minute, and body mass index 30. The physical examination is otherwise unremarkable.

General

- Gastroesophageal reflux disease (GERD) is defined as symptoms or tissue damage caused by the reflux of gastric contents into the esophagus.
- GERD is a common disorder, affecting almost half of the US population, with varying severity. Some 40% of the US population experiences reflux symptoms about once per month, 20% complain of symptoms once per week, and 7–10% report daily symptoms.
- GERD affects 10–20% of western populations. It is less common in Asian and African countries.
- It is estimated that GERD costs the US nearly $2 billion each week in lost productivity.

Sitaraman and Friedman's Essentials of Gastroenterology, Second Edition.
Edited by Shanthi Srinivasan and Lawrence S. Friedman.
© 2018 John Wiley & Sons Ltd. Published 2018 by John Wiley & Sons Ltd.

> The most common symptoms of GERD are heartburn and regurgitation. GERD is the most common cause of noncardiac chest pain.

Risk Factors

- Advancing age (>65 years)
- Obesity
- Genetic factors
- Alcohol use
- Pregnancy
- Smoking

Spectrum of GERD

- The clinical spectrum of GERD ranges from nonerosive reflux disease (NERD) to erosive esophagitis (Figure 1.1). NERD is defined as symptoms of acid reflux without evidence of esophageal damage, such as mucosal erosions or breaks on esophagogastroduodenoscopy (EGD) in patients who are not on acid-suppressive therapy.
- A small proportion of patients will develop metaplasia of the squamous esophageal epithelium to columnar epithelium (Barrett's esophagus). Barrett's esophagus is a risk factor for adenocarcinoma.
- Some patients who present with heartburn have 'functional' heartburn. This is defined as a burning retrosternal discomfort in the absence of

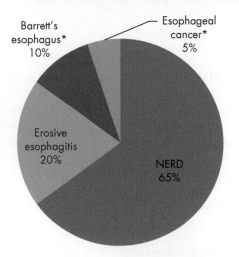

Barrett's esophagus* 10%

Esophageal cancer* 5%

Erosive esophagitis 20%

NERD 65%

Figure 1.1 Clinical spectrum of GERD. (*May be associated with erosive esophagitis; NERD, nonerosive esophageal reflux disease.)

gastroesophageal reflux or an esophageal motor disorder. Ambulatory pH testing may be useful to differentiate NERD from functional heartburn.

Pathophysiology

- Transient lower esophageal sphincter relaxations (TLESRs):
  - The etiology of GERD is multifactorial; however, 'aberrant' TLESRs are the major pathophysiologic factors in many patients with GERD.
  - A TLESR is defined as relaxation of the lower esophageal sphincter in response to gastric distension. In healthy persons, TLESRs occur in the absence of a swallow, last 10–30 seconds, and result in physiologic gastroesophageal reflux.
  - TLESRs are regulated by the neurotransmitter γ-aminobutyric acid (GABA) acting on GABA type B receptors located in the peripheral nervous system, as well as in the brainstem.
  - In many cases, GERD is thought to be caused by an increased number or a prolonged duration of TLESRs.
- Gastric factors:
  - Increased gastric acid production as well as delayed gastric emptying with distention may trigger TLESRs.
- Diminished esophageal clearance:
  - Poor esophageal clearance due to defects in primary or secondary esophageal peristalsis allows prolonged exposure of the esophageal mucosa to acid.
- Diet and medications:
  - Dietary factors such as acidic foods, caffeine, alcohol, peppermint, and chocolate may reduce lower esophageal sphincter (LES) tone or increase gastric acid production.
  - Medications such as calcium channel blockers, hormones (e.g., progesterone, cholecystokinins, secretin), beta-adrenergic agonists (albuterol), nitrates, and barbiturates can decrease LES tone, thereby predisposing to gastroesophageal reflux.
  - Smoking has also been associated with a predisposition to gastroesophageal reflux.
- Hiatal hernia:
  - A hiatal hernia usually occurs when there is a defect in the diaphragmatic hiatus that allows the proximal stomach to herniate above the diaphragm and into the thorax. It is unclear how this predisposes to gastroesophageal reflux. The barrier function of the LES to prevent the reflux of gastric contents into the esophagus is thought to be disrupted. Large hiatal hernias also lead to increased acid dwell times in the distal esophagus.

Clinical Features

- Thorough history-taking detailing the onset and duration of symptoms and the association of symptoms with meals and diet should be conducted. 'Alarm symptoms' such as vomiting, gastrointestinal bleeding, weight loss, dysphagia, early satiety, and symptoms of cardiac disease should be elicited.
- Patients may present with typical (classic) or atypical symptoms.
- Typical symptoms:
  - **Heartburn** is described as a burning sensation in the substernal area that may radiate to the neck and/or back.
  - **Regurgitation** is the feeling of stomach contents traveling retrograde from the stomach up to the chest and often into the mouth.
  - **Dysphagia** (difficulty swallowing) is reported in about 30% of patients with GERD, even in the absence of esophageal inflammation or a stricture.
  - Less common symptoms associated with GERD include water brash, burping, hiccups, nausea, and vomiting. Water brash is the sudden appearance of a sour or salty fluid in the mouth, and represents secretions from the salivary glands in response to acid reflux. Odynophagia (painful swallowing) occurs when there is severe esophagitis.
  - The sensitivity of typical symptoms for detecting GERD is poor.
- Atypical symptoms:
  - Patients may present with chest pain, chronic cough, difficult-to-treat asthma, and laryngeal symptoms such as hoarseness, throat clearing, or throat pain.
  - Patients with atypical symptoms are less likely than patients with typical symptoms to have endoscopic evidence of esophagitis or Barrett's esophagus. They also have a less predictable response to therapy. Ambulatory esophageal pH testing (see later) is not as sensitive for diagnosing GERD in patients with atypical symptoms as it is in patients with typical symptoms.
- In uncomplicated GERD, physical findings are minimal or absent.

> GERD as the etiology of chest pain should be pursued only after potentially life-threatening cardiac etiologies have been excluded.

Diagnosis

Trial of Proton Pump Inhibitor (PPI) Therapy

- A PPI trial is the simplest approach for diagnosing GERD and evaluating symptom response to treatment.

- A 30-day trial of a PPI (omeprazole, lansoprazole, rabeprazole, pantoprazole, esomeprazole, dexlansoprazole) once daily (taken 1 hour before breakfast) is recommended. If the patient has GERD, symptoms will usually improve within 1–2 weeks.
- The pooled sensitivity of a PPI trial for diagnosing GERD is 78% with a specificity of 54% when compared with 24-hour pH testing.

> A PPI trial is recommended as the initial diagnostic and therapeutic intervention in patients with uncomplicated GERD. In patients who fail a PPI trial, additional testing is recommended.

Barium Swallow

- This is a radiographic test that can detect reflux of barium contrast into the esophagus after the patient drinks the contrast solution (see Chapter 27).
- A barium swallow can evaluate other potential mechanical causes for the symptoms (e.g., stricture, neoplasm); however, the test lacks sensitivity (20–30%) to assess mucosal damage. Therefore, barium swallow studies should not be used to diagnose GERD.

Upper Endoscopy

- Upper endoscopy (esophagogastroduodenoscopy, EGD) allows direct visualization of the esophageal mucosa.
- The test has a high sensitivity (90–95%) for diagnosing GERD, but the specificity is only 50%.
- The spectrum of findings on upper endoscopy in persons with GERD includes normal mucosa and esophageal inflammation characterized by erythema, erosions, mucosal breaks, bleeding, and ulceration of the esophageal mucosa.
- Upper endoscopy is recommended for all patients with alarm symptoms such as weight loss, dysphagia, hematemesis, and bleeding.
- Upper endoscopy is used to detect complications of GERD such as stricture or Barrett's esophagus and other upper gastrointestinal disorders (e.g., peptic ulcer).
- Los Angeles classification of erosive esophagitis:
  - grade A: greater than 1 mucosal break, ≤5 mm long;
  - grade B: greater than 1 mucosal break, >5 mm long;
  - grade C: greater than 1 mucosal break, bridging tops of folds but <75% of the circumference of the esophagus;
  - grade D: greater than 1 mucosal break, bridging tops of folds but ≥75% of the circumference of the esophagus;
  - Most patients have mild (LA grade A–B) esophagitis.

> Endoscopic mucosal biopsies should be obtained in all patients with dysphagia to exclude eosinophilic esophagitis (see Chapter 2).

Ambulatory Esophageal pH Testing

- If an upper endoscopy is normal in a patient with GERD symptoms, esophageal pH testing should be performed next.
- pH monitoring is the 'gold standard' for detecting acid reflux and correlation of reflux with the patient's symptoms.
- A pressure catheter is inserted transnasally and advanced to 5 cm above the manometrically determined LES. The catheter is attached to a data logger that records pH values of the distal esophagus for 24 hours. The patient records his/her meals, position (upright/supine), and symptoms. The patient returns the data logger, and the pH data are downloaded onto a computer that transforms the data into a 24-hour tracing.
- The sensitivity of pH monitoring ranges from 79–96%, with a specificity of 85–100%, in patients with typical symptoms of gastroesophageal reflux.
- A wireless ambulatory pH capsule (Bravo) placed endoscopically allows for 48 hours of pH data recording. The sensitivity of this technique is greater than that of conventional pH monitoring.
- Ambulatory esophageal reflux monitoring should be performed before consideration of endoscopic or surgical therapy in patients with NERD. It is also part of the evaluation of patients refractory to PPI therapy, and should additionally be used in situations when the diagnosis of GERD is questionable.
- Many patients (25–60%) with noncardiac chest pain will have an abnormal ambulatory pH study result.
- Clinical indications for pH monitoring include:
  - refractory gastroesophageal reflux symptoms;
  - atypical symptoms;
  - typical symptoms and a normal upper endoscopy;
  - preoperatively before a fundoplication;
  - follow up of antireflux therapy (see later).
- The most sensitive parameter used to determine pathologic acid reflux includes the percentage of time the pH remains <4 and the correlation with symptoms. A pH <4 suggests that active pepsin may be a part of the refluxate, leading to erosion of the esophageal mucosa and symptoms.
- Some patients continue to have reflux symptoms despite documentation of a negative 24-hour pH test. Weakly acidic (pH = 4–7) as well as nonacidic (pH >7) reflux can produce reflux symptoms. **Multichannel impedance testing** combined with pH testing can be used to assess acidic, weakly acidic, and nonacidic reflux and the relationship of reflux events to symptom events.

Complications

Esophageal Stricture

- The frequency of esophageal strictures (also called peptic strictures) in patients with GERD is 0.1%.
- Esophageal strictures are generally smooth, scarred, circumferential narrowings usually in the distal esophagus (see Chapter 2).
- Patients typically present with progressive dysphagia for solids that usually is not associated with weight loss, as occurs with malignant strictures (see Chapter 2).
- Esophageal peptic strictures are treated with per-endoscopic dilation. Dysphagia improves once the esophageal luminal diameter reaches 15 mm or above.

Barrett's Esophagus

- Prolonged esophageal acid exposure can result in damage to the esophageal mucosa, leading to metaplasia of the squamous epithelium of the distal mucosa to specialized columnar mucosa with goblet cells; this is referred to as **intestinal metaplasia**.
- The diagnosis of GERD is associated with a 10–15% risk of Barrett's esophagus.
- In some persons, intestinal metaplasia may progress to dysplasia and esophageal adenocarcinoma. The risk of progression to adenocarcinoma is estimated to be 0.5–1.0% per year.
- The frequency of Barrett's esophagus is highest in Caucasian men over 50 years of age.
- The diagnosis of Barrett's esophagus is suspected on upper endoscopy by the detection of salmon-colored mucosa extending above the gastroesophageal junction (Z-line) (Figure 1.2). The diagnosis is confirmed by histologic examination (see Chapter 28).
- Endoscopic surveillance should utilize high-resolution/high-definition white-light endoscopy.
- Virtually all patients with Barrett's esophagus are treated with a PPI once daily, indefinitely.
- For Barrett's esophagus patients without dysplasia, endoscopic surveillance should take place at intervals of 3–5 years.
- Endoscopic ablative therapies should not be performed routinely in patients with nondysplastic Barrett's esophagus because of their low risk of progression to esophageal adenocarcinoma.
- In patients with dysplasia, radiofrequency ablation (RFA) is currently the preferred endoscopic ablative therapy, with the goal of removing all neoplasia and Barrett's mucosa. RFA is used to perform circumferential and then focal ablation of dysplasia.

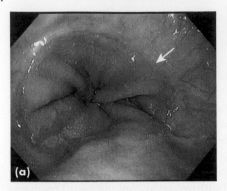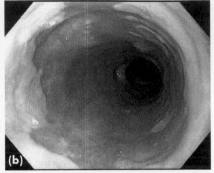

Figure 1.2 Endoscopic images of the normal esophagus and complications of GERD. (a) Normal esophagus showing the squamocolumnar junction (arrow); (b) Barrett's esophagus: intestinal metaplasia is seen as salmon-colored mucosa that extends above the gastroesophageal junction.

- Cryotherapy is a newer method of treating dysplasia, in which liquid nitrogen or carbon dioxide is applied under endoscopic visualization. Studies suggest it eradicates dysplasia in 85–90% of patients.
- Photodynamic therapy uses a photosensitizing agent and laser light to cause cytotoxicity in Barrett's mucosa. It is not used as often as RFA and cryotherapy.
- Endoscopic resection is a technique in which the excision of a large segment of mucosa down to the submucosa is performed. It can be combined with other ablative therapies to eradicate Barrett's esophagus
- After complete elimination of intestinal metaplasia, endoscopic surveillance should be continued to detect recurrent metaplasia or dysplasia.

Treatment

Treatment of GERD depends on the severity of symptoms. Therapy includes lifestyle modification, medication, surgery, or a combination of these.

Lifestyle Modifications

- In patients with mild and infrequent symptoms, lifestyle modifications can decrease the frequency and severity of symptoms, and are considered first-line therapy.
- Recommended changes include weight loss, avoidance of late-night meals, elevation of the head of the bed to at least a 30° angle in an attempt to minimize acid reflux, the avoidance of spicy and greasy foods, acidic foods (such as tomato-based products, and citrus juices), cessation of smoking, and a reduction in alcohol consumption and caffeinated products such as chocolate and carbonated beverages.

- Weight loss and elevation of the head of the bed seem to be the most beneficial lifestyle interventions.

Antacids

- Antacids neutralize gastric acid, thereby raising the pH above 4 and decreasing reflux symptoms.
- The onset of action is approximately 5 minutes after ingestion, and the effect lasts for 90 minutes.
- Over-the-counter antacids and alginates have been found to be helpful in patients with mild, infrequent symptoms of GERD.
- Side effects include diarrhea with magnesium-containing products, and constipation with aluminum-containing formulations.

Histamine H2 Receptor Antagonists (H2RAs)

- H2RAs block histamine H2 receptors on parietal cells of the stomach, thereby inhibiting histamine binding to the cell and decreasing gastric acid production.
- They have a rapid onset of action with a duration of effect from 6–10 hours.
- The healing rate for esophagitis is 50% compared with 24% for placebo.
- These drugs are effective in patients with mild, infrequent symptoms of GERD.

PPIs

- PPIs bind covalently and irreversibly with the hydrogen/potassium adenosine triphosphatase (H+/K + -ATPase) pump on the apical surface of parietal cells in the stomach.
- PPI therapy is the mainstay of treatment for moderate to severe GERD and is used as maintenance therapy.
- Usually, once-a-day dosing is effective. PPIs have been shown to maintain intra-gastric pH above 4 for 15–21 hours. Occasionally, twice-daily dosing is necessary for patients with severe symptoms or those with erosive esophagitis.
- PPIs have been shown to be superior to H2RAs in healing esophagitis at 8 weeks (83–96% for PPIs versus 50% for H2RAs).
- Reasons for a failure to respond to a PPI include poor adherence, inadequate acid suppression with breakthrough acid secretion, weakly acidic reflux as the cause of symptoms, duodenogastroesophageal reflux, delayed gastric emptying, and functional heartburn.
- The most common side effects of PPIs include diarrhea, headache, and abdominal pain. Chronic PPI use has been associated with a slightly increased susceptibility to enteric infections, including *Clostridium difficile* colitis, small intestinal bacterial overgrowth, electrolyte abnormalities, hip fractures, chronic kidney disease, and dementia, although conclusive evidence for most of these complications is lacking.

- Although there may be slight differences among the various PPIs with respect to potency, the choice of PPI is best made on the basis of prescription plan coverage and a history of adverse side effects.

Additional Medications

- Prokinetic agents such as metoclopramide, a dopamine antagonist, may be effective as an adjunct to PPIs in persons with delayed gastric emptying. Prokinetic agents have no effect in improving esophageal clearance. Side effects include tremors, Parkinson-like symptoms, and tardive dyskinesia. The US Food and Drug Administration (FDA) has not approved metoclopramide for GERD.
- Two GABA-B agonists, baclofen and lesogaberan, have been studied in the treatment of GERD in patients who have not responded to PPIs. They act by inhibiting TLESRs and reflux episodes. Side effects include drowsiness, nausea, and an increased risk of seizures. Neither drug is approved by the FDA for the treatment of GERD.

Endoscopic Therapy

- Endoscopic approaches to the treatment of GERD are considered experimental and are not recommended for its routine treatment.
- The goals of endoscopic therapy are to reduce reflux, alter neural response to acid, and improve symptoms.
- Endoscopic approaches include the delivery of radiofrequency energy to the gastroesophageal junction, the injection of bulking agents in the LES, and the implantation of a prosthetic device into the LES.
- Following such therapy, patients often must continue acid-suppression therapy because of persistent, although often less severe, symptoms.
- Endoscopic gastroplication is a technique in which sutures are placed immediately below the LES to strengthen the LES and reduce reflux. This method has been shown to improve symptoms and quality of life.

Surgical Therapy

- Antireflux surgery corrects the mechanical factors that contribute to GERD. The most common surgical procedure performed is the Nissen fundoplication. The technique involves a 360° wrap of the upper portion of the stomach (fundus) around the distal esophagus to enhance the integrity of the LES (see Chapter 4). This prevents gastric contents from flowing in a retrograde manner into the esophagus, thereby reducing GERD symptoms and allowing the esophageal mucosa to heal. In a patient with a hiatal hernia, the hernia is reduced back into the abdomen during surgery.
- A partial wrap (Toupet fundoplication) is performed in patients who have poor esophageal motility.

- These procedures are most often done laparoscopically to reduce the length of hospital stay and operative morbidity.
- Surgery does not appear to reduce the rate of progression of Barrett's esophagus to adenocarcinoma.
- Surgery is as effective as PPIs in controlling symptoms in the short term (5 years).
- Common adverse effects of a fundoplication include dysphagia (20%) due to too tight a wrap at the LES, and so-called 'gas–bloat syndrome' due to difficulty in expelling air from the stomach. Half of all patients who undergo fundoplication still require acid-suppression medication.
- Surgical fundoplication is a good alternative to PPI treatment in patients who:
  - respond to PPI therapy but want a more permanent treatment or do not tolerate PPIs;
  - respond to PPIs in terms of a decrease in heartburn but continue to have regurgitation;
  - develop recurrent complications of GERD such as a stricture or respiratory complications.

An algorithm for the management of GERD is shown in Figure 1.3.

Pearls

- GERD is a common chronic gastrointestinal disorder. Most patients have mild or moderate symptoms that respond to lifestyle modifications and antacid therapy. However, some patients have severe daily, as well as night-time, symptoms that can significantly reduce their quality of life.
- In patients with typical symptoms (heartburn and regurgitation), a PPI is the mainstay of therapy.
- In patients with atypical or refractory symptoms, ambulatory pH testing and, in some cases, impedance testing are helpful in determining whether the symptoms are truly related to gastroesophageal reflux.
- Early recognition of GERD can result in a reduction in both symptoms and complications of GERD and an improved quality of life.
- GERD can lead to Barrett's esophagus, which can occasionally progress to esophageal adenocarcinoma. Therefore, early diagnosis and treatment of GERD are key.
- There are various methods of treating GERD and its complications.
- Surgical treatment is appropriate in patients who do not wish to be on long-term medical therapy or who continue to have complications of GERD.

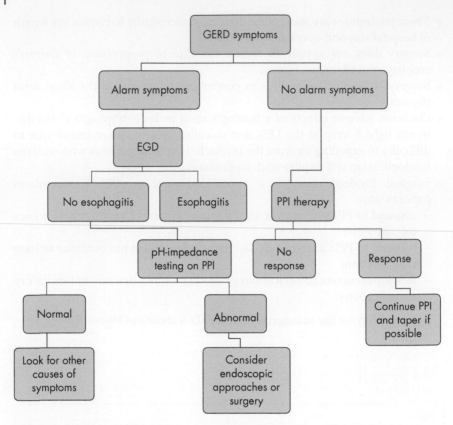

Figure 1.3 Algorithm for the management of GERD. EGD, esophagogastroduodenoscopy; GERD, gastroesophageal reflux disease; PPI, proton pump inhibitor.

Questions

Questions 1 and 2 relate to the clinical vignette discussed at the beginning of this chapter.

1 Which of the following management strategies would you recommend for this patient?
   A Schedule an EGD.
   B Continue ranitidine as needed.
   C Start a PPI.
   D Order a barium swallow.
   E Order a 24-hour pH study.

2 Six months later, the patient reports intermittent difficulty swallowing solid food such as bread or rice. He denies odynophagia, weight loss, vomiting, or other symptoms. Which of the following is the most likely cause of dysphagia?

A Achalasia.
B Benign esophageal stricture.
C Esophageal cancer.
D Barrett's esophagus.
E Hiatal hernia.

3 Which of the following is considered to be the major pathophysiologic factor in GERD?

A Hiatal hernia.
B Smoking.
C Poor esophageal motility.
D TLESRs.
E Obesity.

4 Long-standing GERD is a risk factor for which of the following?

A Squamous cell cancer of the esophagus.
B Adenocarcinoma of the esophagus.
C Peptic ulcer disease.
D Gastric adenocarcinoma.
E Achalasia.

5 Surgical fundoplication for GERD has been shown to result in which of the following?

A Greater improvement in symptoms of GERD compared with therapy with a PPI.
B Greater improvement in symptoms of GERD in patients with persistent regurgitation despite therapy with a PPI.
C Improvement in esophageal clearance.
D Reduction in the frequency of adenocarcinoma in patients with Barrett's esophagus.
E Reduction in gastric acid production.

6 Which of the following does NOT reduce the symptoms of GERD?

A Weight loss.
B Avoidance of caffeine.
C Alcohol cessation.
D Gluten-free diet.
E Tobacco cessation.

7 Which of the following medications does NOT provide symptomatic improvement in GERD?

A GABA-B agonists.

B PPIs.

C Benzodiazepines.

D H2RAs.

E Antacids.

Answers

1 C

The patient presents with symptoms of GERD, including heartburn, chest discomfort, a sore throat, and a bitter taste in the mouth. GERD may cause chest pain that can be indistinguishable from ischemic cardiac pain, and the first priority often is to rule out heart disease as the etiology. In this patient, a cardiac work-up was negative. An upper endoscopy may be a reasonable choice if the patient is >50 years of age (the risks of Barrett's esophagus and adenocarcinoma increase with age), has alarm symptoms such as unintentional weight loss, gastrointestinal bleeding, vomiting, or dysphagia, or does not respond to a trial of a PPI. The most cost-effective diagnostic test for GERD in a younger person is a trial of a PPI. A barium swallow is not sensitive to diagnose GERD. A 24-hour pH study may be obtained if the patient does not respond to a trial of a PPI.

2 B

The most common complication of GERD is a benign esophageal stricture, which occurs in 0.1% of patients with GERD. Esophageal cancer (adenocarcinoma) is a possibility in a patient with long-standing GERD, but is less likely in the absence of alarm symptoms. Patients with Barrett's esophagus are often asymptomatic or have typical symptoms of GERD. A hiatal hernia contributes to GERD but generally does not cause dysphagia. Achalasia is a motility disorder of the esophagus that presents with progressive dysphagia for both solids and liquids.

3 D

The etiology of GERD is multifactorial; smoking, poor esophageal motility, obesity, and hiatal hernia may contribute to GERD. TLESRs are the major etiologic factors in most patients with GERD.

4 B

5 B

Surgical fundoplication (wrapping or plicating of the stomach around the esophagus) is as effective as PPI therapy in controlling symptoms in the short term (5 years). It is a good alternative to PPI treatment in patients who have persistent regurgitation or develop complications of GERD, such as a benign stricture or respiratory complications. Surgical fundoplication does not decrease the rate of progression of Barrett's esophagus to adenocarcinoma and does not affect gastric acid secretion.

6   D

All of the approaches listed have been shown to improve GERD symptoms except for a gluten-free diet. Gluten intake has not been shown to have any effect on GERD.

7   C

Benzodiazepines have not been shown to alleviate GERD symptoms. GABA-B agonists, PPIs, H2RAs, and antacids have all been shown to provide symptomatic improvement in GERD.

Further Reading

Katz, P., Gerson, L., and Vela, M. (2013) ACG Guidelines for the Diagnosis and Management of Gastroesophageal Reflux Disease. *American Journal of Gastroenterology*, **108**, 308–328.

Ness-Jensen, E., Lindam, A., Lagergren, J., and Hveem, K. (2013) Weight loss and reduction in gastroesophageal reflux. A prospective population-based cohort study: the HUNT study. *American Journal of Gastroenterology*, **108**, 376–382.

Richter, J.E. and Friedenberg, F.K. (2016) Gastroesophageal reflux disease, in Sleisenger and Fordtran's Gastrointestinal and Liver Disease: Pathophysiology/Diagnosis/Management, 10th edition, (eds M. Feldman, L.S. Friedman, and L.J. Brandt), Saunders Elsevier, Philadelphia, pp. 733–754.

Shaheen, N., Falk, G., Gerson, L., *et al.* (2016) ACG Clinical Guideline: Diagnosis and Management of Barrett's Esophagus. *American Journal of Gastroenterology*, **111**, 30–50.

Singh, S., Garg, S.K., and Singh, P. (2014) Acid-suppressive medications and risk of oesophageal adenocarcinoma in patients with Barrett's oesophagus: a systematic review and meta-analysis. *Gut*, **63**, 1229–1237.

Weblinks

http://www.nlm.nih.gov/medlineplus/gerd.html
http://www.acg.gi.org/physicians/guidelines/GERDTreatment.pdf
http://www.gastrojournal.org/article/S0016-5085(08)01605-3/fulltext

2

Dysphagia

Emad Qayed and Shanthi Srinivasan

Clinical Vignette

A 55-year-old man is seen in the office for difficulty swallowing for the past 6 months. He says that food 'sticks' in the middle of his chest in the mid-sternal area. This sensation has been worsening over the past several months. For the past 5 years he has had occasional heartburn. He has no difficulty swallowing liquids, and denies odynophagia, choking, cough, or shortness of breath. He denies nausea, vomiting, or abdominal pain. His weight has been stable. His past medical and surgical history is unremarkable. He takes ranitidine as needed for his heartburn, but no other medications. His family history is unremarkable. He works as a consultant in a computer software company. He is married and has three children, all of whom are healthy. He drinks a few beers on the weekends and does not smoke cigarettes. He has no history of illicit drug use. A colonoscopy done 4 years ago was unremarkable. Physical examination reveals a well-nourished, middle-aged man with a blood pressure of 128/88 mmHg, pulse rate 72 per minute, temperature 98.5 °F (37 °C), and body mass index 29. Examination of the oral cavity reveals no lesions, and there are no palpable lymph nodes or swelling in his neck. The chest, cardiac, and abdominal examinations are unremarkable. The neurologic examination is normal. When asked to swallow a sip of water, he swallows normally without choking or coughing. Routine laboratory tests show a normal complete blood count and comprehensive metabolic panel.

Sitaraman and Friedman's Essentials of Gastroenterology, Second Edition.
Edited by Shanthi Srinivasan and Lawrence S. Friedman.
© 2018 John Wiley & Sons Ltd. Published 2018 by John Wiley & Sons Ltd.

General

- **Dysphagia** refers to difficulty swallowing. The condition results from impeded transport of liquids, solids, or both, from the pharynx to the stomach.
- **Odynophagia** refers to pain during swallowing and is frequently associated with dysphagia.
- Swallowing disorders can occur in all age groups, but the frequency of dysphagia is higher in the elderly. From 7–10% of adults older than 50 years of age, up to 25% of hospitalized patients, and 30–40% of nursing home residents experience problems with swallowing.
- Although dysphagia is more common in the elderly, it is not a normal consequence of aging and should be investigated
- Dysphagia is classified as oropharyngeal and esophageal dysphagia. **Oropharyngeal** dysphagia, or transfer dysphagia, refers to difficulty transferring food (solids, liquids, or both) from the oropharynx to the esophagus. **Esophageal** dysphagia refers to difficulty passing food through the esophagus into the stomach.

Physiology of Swallowing

- Normal swallowing is a smooth, coordinated process that involves a complex series of voluntary and involuntary neuromuscular contractions (Figure 2.1). The process of swallowing typically is divided into three distinct phases: oral; pharyngeal; and esophageal. Impairment of any of these phases results in dysphagia.
- The **oral** phase involves preparing and propelling the food from the anterior oral cavity into the oropharynx, where an involuntary swallowing reflex is initiated.

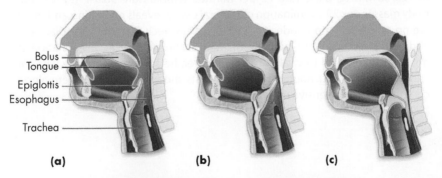

Bolus
Tongue
Epiglottis
Esophagus
Trachea

(a)   (b)   (c)

Figure 2.1 Oral and pharyngeal phases of swallowing. The diagram shows the transfer of a bolus of food from the mouth (a) to the oropharynx (b) to the upper esophagus (c).

The oral phase is the only voluntary phase of swallowing and requires coordinated contractions of the tongue and striated muscles of mastication.

- The **pharyngeal** phase involves overlapping events that are critical to protect the airway while allowing the bolus to transfer to the esophagus. The food bolus is propelled into the pharyngeal cavity, while the soft palate elevates and closes the nasal aperture and the larynx begins to elevate. The food bolus is then propelled into the hypopharynx by pharyngeal contractions. The larynx closes and the soft palate and the posterior pharyngeal wall oppose the posterior aspect of the tongue to prevent reflux of food into the oral cavity. The last step involves opening of the upper esophageal sphincter to allow the passage of food to the esophageal lumen.
  - Alteration of any step of the oral or pharyngeal phases of swallowing, due to mechanical obstruction or a neuromuscular condition, results in oropharyngeal dysphagia.
- In the **esophageal** phase, the food bolus is propelled down the esophagus by peristaltic contractions.
  - Once the food reaches the esophageal lumen, primary peristaltic contractions propel the food bolus down the length of the esophagus to the distal esophagus. This is accompanied by a relaxation of the lower esophageal sphincter and emptying of the esophageal contents into the gastric lumen.
  - Residual food in the esophagus causes local distension and triggers secondary peristaltic contractions that clear the esophagus of remaining food in the lumen.
  - Altered esophageal peristaltic contractions or failure of the lower esophageal sphincter to relax can result in esophageal dysphagia.
  - Another important mechanism of esophageal dysphagia is mechanical obstruction of the esophagus. This can be secondary to intraluminal obstruction or extrinsic compression.

Etiology

Oropharyngeal Dysphagia

Oropharyngeal dysphagia can be caused by mechanical obstruction or neuromuscular disease (Table 2.1). Stroke is the most common cause of oropharyngeal dysphagia in the inpatient setting.

Esophageal Dysphagia

Esophageal dysphagia can be caused by mechanical obstruction of the esophageal lumen, or can be secondary to dysmotility of the esophagus or lower esophageal sphincter (Figure 2.2).

Table 2.1 Causes of oropharyngeal dysphagia.

Category	Etiologies
Structural lesions	Benign or malignant tumors
	Candidal infection (thrush)
	Caustic ingestion
	Cervical spondylosis
	Peritonsillar abscess
	Radiation
	Retropharyngeal abscess or mass
	Thyromegaly
	Zenker's diverticulum
Neuromuscular causes	Diseases of the cerebral cortex and cranial nerves:
	• Alzheimer's disease
	• Bulbar and pseudobulbar palsy
	• Cerebral palsy
	• CNS tumors (benign or malignant)
	• Multiple sclerosis
	• Metabolic encephalopathy
	• Parkinson's disease
	• Stroke
	• Vascular dementias
	Neuromuscular disorders:
	• Botulism
	• Myositis (polymyositis, dermatomyositis)
	• Myasthenia gravis
	• Primary myopathies (myotonic dystrophy, oculopharyngeal myopathy)

CNS, central nervous system.

Mechanical Obstruction

The most common cause of esophageal dysphagia is mechanical obstruction of the esophageal lumen (Table 2.2) due to intraluminal (intrinsic) lesions or extrinsic compression. Dysphagia usually occurs when the diameter of the esophageal lumen is 13 mm or less. The symptoms depend on the degree of obstruction. For example, mild narrowing of the esophageal lumen causes symptoms only with large boluses of food, whereas more complete obstruction

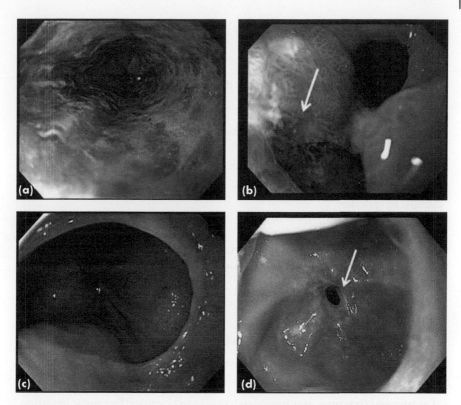

Figure 2.2 Endoscopic images of various disorders that cause esophageal dysphagia. (a) Reflux esophagitis: superficial ulcerations, edema, and erythema are seen in a continuous fashion from the gastroesophageal junction to proximal esophagus in a patient with chronic gastroesophageal reflux; (b) Pill-induced esophagitis: a discrete deep ulcer with sharply demarcated edges and necrotic center (arrow) is seen in a patient with a history of tetracycline use; (c) Esophageal ring: a fibrotic circumferential ring is seen in the lower esophagus; (d) Esophageal stricture: severe narrowing of the esophageal lumen (arrow) with dilatation of the proximal esophagus is seen in a patient with history of lye ingestion.

results in dysphagia for both solids and liquids. Intraluminal causes of dysphagia include the following:

- **Esophageal cancer**: patients with esophageal cancer present with dysphagia that is progressive, from solids to liquids, and associated with constitutional symptoms such as weight loss and anorexia. Patients may have risk factors such as smoking and alcohol use in the case of squamous cell carcinoma, or longstanding gastroesophageal reflux disease in the case of adenocarcimona.

Table 2.2 Causes of esophageal dysphagia.

Mechanical obstruction

Intrinsic narrowing:
- Benign strictures: gastroesophageal reflux disease, caustic substances, medications, postsurgical, radiation therapy
- Cricopharyngeal hyperplasia/bar
- Esophagitis: infectious, eosinophilic, pill-induced; gastroesophageal reflux disease
- Esophageal rings and webs
- Esophageal diverticula
- Tumors: benign or malignant

Extrinsic compression:
- Anterior mediastinal mass
- Vascular lesions:
  - Congenital: aberrant right subclavian artery (dysphagia lusoria), right-sided aorta
  - Acquired: aortic aneurysm, left atrial enlargement, right-sided aorta

Esophageal motility disorders
- Achalasia
- Distal esophageal spasm
- Hypertensive peristalsis (jackhammer esophagus)
- Hypotensive peristalsis (scleroderma)

- **Esophageal stricture**: esophageal strictures can be caused by caustic ingestion, certain medications, gastroesophageal reflux disease, and radiation therapy.
- **Esophageal rings and webs**: rings or webs typically cause intermittent nonprogressive dysphagia.
- **Esophagitis**: dysphagia caused by esophagitis is usually accompanied by odynophagia. Medications known to cause esophagitis include aspirin and other nonsteroidal anti-inflammatory drugs, doxycycline or tetracycline, bisphosphonates, and potassium preparations.
- **Eosinophilic esophagitis** is an increasingly recognized cause of dysphagia.

Eosinophilic esophagitis is a condition in which the esophageal mucosa is abnormally infiltrated with eosinophils. It usually affects males aged younger than 45 years. It is important to rule out eosinophilic esophagitis in patients with dysphagia and a normal upper endoscopy; therefore, an esophageal biopsy is always recommended in such patients, and typically results in intermittent dysphagia and food bolus impactions. Although eosinophilic esophagitis can present without endoscopic changes, most patients will have one or more of the following endoscopic findings: esophageal strictures; rings; longitudinal mucosal furrows; or white specks that mimic the appearance of candidal esophagitis. Some cases respond to treatment with acid suppression using a proton pump inhibitor (PPI) and are referred to as PPI-responsive esophageal eosinophilia. The diagnosis is confirmed by esophageal mucosal biopsies showing eosinophils (>15 per high-power field). For patients who do not respond to a PPI, the dietary elimination of common allergens, including milk, egg, soy, wheat, nuts and shellfish, or treatment with swallowed topical steroids is considered.

Motility Disorders

Esophageal motility disorders are a less common cause of dysphagia than are mechanical causes. Dysphagia due to esophageal dysmotility typically results in difficulty swallowing both solids and liquids. The diagnosis of esophageal motility disorders is frequently made using esophageal manometry, which assesses motor function of the upper and lower esophageal sphincters and the presence or absence of peristalsis of the esophageal body.

- **Achalasia**: characteristic manometric features of achalasia include an absence of esophageal peristalsis and failure of the lower esophageal sphincter to relax with swallowing. The etiology of achalasia is unknown. A selective loss of postganglionic inhibitory neurons innervating the smooth muscle of the esophagus is typically seen, and is thought to result in a hypertensive lower esophageal sphincter that fails to relax with swallowing and leads to a functional obstruction.
- Certain diseases mimic clinical, radiologic, and manometric features of achalasia. Such conditions are termed **pseudoachalasia**. An example of pseudoachalasia is gastric adenocarcinoma of the cardia. Paraneoplastic syndromes can also cause pseudoachalasia.
- Spastic motility disorders have been termed distal (or diffuse) **esophageal spasm** and **jackhammer esophagus**. Patients with these disorders usually present with chest pain in addition to dysphagia
- Systemic diseases such as **scleroderma** can present with dysphagia. Scleroderma causes hypomotility of the esophagus along with a hypotensive lower esophageal sphincter and aperistalsis. Patients often present with gastroesophageal reflux in addition to dysphagia.

Clinical Features

- The clinical history is extremely important in evaluating the cause of dysphagia. In addition to dysphagia, a history of odynophagia should be elicited. Dysphagia should be distinguished from **globus sensation**, which refers to the constant feeling of a lump or tightness in the throat without any demonstrable abnormality in swallowing. Important questions to ask the patient with dysphagia include the time of onset of symptoms, progression, severity, and pattern (intermittent or constant) of symptoms, presence of heartburn, type of food that induces symptoms (liquids or solids, or both), history of head and neck malignancy or surgery, and associated neurologic disorders. A medication history should be obtained.

- Typical symptoms of oropharyngeal dysphagia include choking, cough, or shortness of breath with swallowing. Patients often have difficulty initiating a swallow, and point to the throat as the location where the food is stuck. In some patients, liquids are regurgitated through the nose. Other associated symptoms include dysarthria, nasal speech, hoarseness, weight loss, and recurrent pulmonary infections.
- Symptoms of esophageal dysphagia include a sensation that food is stuck in the chest or throat. Most patients will point to the lower or mid sternum as the location of their symptoms; however, this localization often does not correlate with the anatomic level of the abnormality. Other associated symptoms include heartburn, odynophagia, hematemesis, chest pain, sensitivity to hot or cold liquids, and weight loss.
- Esophageal dysphagia to both solids and liquids initially suggests a motility disorder of the esophagus, whereas dysphagia to solids that progresses over time to involve liquids suggests a mechanical obstruction. Odynophagia suggests esophagitis.
- Physical examination:
  - Important elements of the physical examination include the patient's general appearance and nutritional status, and an assessment of the patient's respiratory distress as well as a mental status examination.
  - Examination of the cranial nerves (especially V and VII–XII) should be performed.
  - Systemic examination should focus on skin and nail, respiratory, and abdominal findings. **Tylosis** is a genetic syndrome characterized by hyperkeratosis of the palm and soles associated with a high frequency of squamous cell carcinoma of the esophagus.
  - It is often helpful to ask the patient to take a sip of water while being observed for symptoms of oropharyngeal dysphagia.

Diagnosis

- In most patients the distinction between oropharyngeal and esophageal dysphagia, as well as among mechanical, motility and neuromuscular causes, can be made by careful history-taking and physical examination. An approach to the diagnosis of esophageal dysphagia is shown in Figure 2.3.
- **Video-radiographic studies (video fluoroscopy).** If the clinical history and physical examination suggest oropharyngeal dysphagia, especially with a risk of aspiration (e.g., neurologic impairment), video-radiographic studies

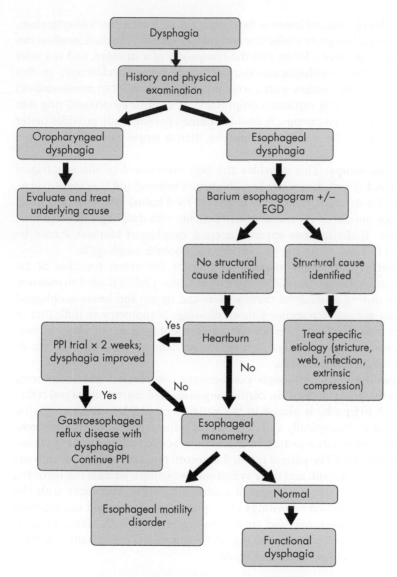

Figure 2.3 Algorithm for the diagnostic evaluation of esophageal dysphagia. EGD, esophagogastroduodenoscopy; PPI, proton pump inhibitor.

are performed to identify the presence, nature and severity of oropharyngeal swallowing dysfunction. This test is performed by a team composed of a radiologist, otolaryngologist, and speech pathologist.

• **Barium studies**. A barium swallow (barium esophagogram) is often recommended as the initial test for esophageal dysphagia. It can help to identify a structural or obstructive lesion of the esophagus, such as Zenker's diverticulum, caustic injury, benign or malignant stricture, or tumor. A barium swallow can show the location of a lesion and the complexity of a stricture, and is a safer initial test than esophagogastroduodenoscopy (upper endoscopy) in this setting. A barium swallow with a solid bolus (barium tablet or marshmallow) is useful in detecting extrinsic compression or a subtle esophageal ring that can be missed by endoscopy. A double-contrast barium study provides better visualization of the esophageal mucosa than a single-contrast study (see Chapter 27).

- **Upper endoscopy**. This provides the best assessment of the esophageal mucosa and allows diagnostic (e.g., biopsy of lesions) and therapeutic (e.g., dilation of a stricture, removal of impacted food bolus) intervention. Upper endoscopy should be the initial test in patients with dysphagia due to a food impaction. If the mucosa appears normal, esophageal biopsies should be obtained to evaluate for the presence of eosinophilic esophagitis.

- **Manometry**. Esophageal manometry assesses the motor function of the esophagus. A nasogastric catheter with electronic probes is used to measure pressure during esophageal contractions and upper and lower esophageal body and sphincter responses to swallowing. Manometry is indicated in patients with dysphagia in whom a barium esophagogram or upper endoscopy reveals no abnormality. High-resolution manometry is the 'gold standard' for diagnosing achalasia.

- **pH measurements**. Although cumbersome, esophageal pH monitoring remains the 'gold standard' for confirming suspected gastroesophageal reflux disease. A pH probe is placed in the patient's esophagus via a nasogastric catheter or endoscopically and detects acid reflux. (pH testing can be combined with impedance testing to assess both acidic and nonacidic gastroesophageal reflux.) The patient is asked to record the occurrence of symptoms over a 24-hour period, and their symptoms are compared with the recorded pH measurements to determine if gastric acid reflux correlates with the symptoms. Combined recordings of esophageal pH levels and intraluminal esophageal pressure may aid in diagnosing patients with reflux-induced esophageal spasm. pH monitoring and manometry are usually available through referral to gastroenterologists.

A barium swallow is the first step in evaluating patients with symptoms of esophageal dysphagia especially if an obstructive lesion is suspected. Upper endoscopy is the recommended initial study with acute obstruction such as an impacted food bolus.

Treatment

See also Chapters 1 and 4.

Oropharyngeal Dysphagia

The goals of management in oropharyngeal dysphagia are to provide adequate nutrition, improve the patient's ability to eat and swallow, and prevent tracheobronchial aspiration. Therapy is individualized based on the functional and structural abnormalities and the initial response to treatment observed at the patient's bedside or during a video-radiographic study.

Esophageal Dysphagia

Mechanical obstruction can be relieved by surgery (e.g., tumors or diverticula) or by endoscopic dilation (e.g., strictures, rings, webs).

If the results of a barium esophagogram and upper endoscopy are normal, and the patient has heartburn or regurgitation associated with dysphagia, a therapeutic trial of a PPI taken twice daily for 2 weeks is recommended. Improvement in symptoms suggests that the dysphagia is related to the presence of gastroesophageal reflux (see Table 2.1).

Achalasia and Other Esophageal Motility Disorders

Definitive treatment of achalasia is surgical cardiomyotomy with partial fundoplication (Heller myotomy; see Chapter 4). Per-oral endoscopic myotomy (POEM) has been developed as an alternative to traditional Heller myotomy. Early outcomes show similar efficacy, although the long-term durability and consequences of endoscopic myotomy continue to be investigated. A trial of nitrates, calcium channel blockers or phosphodiesterase inhibitors may be useful in patients with spastic esophageal disorders.

Pearls

- A detailed history can help identify the cause of dysphagia in approximately 80% of patients.
- Intermittent symptoms and dysphagia to both liquids and solid food are features that most strongly suggest a motility disorder.
- A trial of therapy for reflux symptoms should be undertaken before further diagnostic evaluation of dysphagia in patients who are thought to have gastroesophageal reflux disease.

Questions

Questions 1–3 relate to the clinical vignette at the beginning of this chapter.

1   The differential diagnosis of the patient's dysphagia includes all of the following EXCEPT:
   A Esophageal stricture.
   B Esophageal adenocarcinoma.
   C Achalasia.
   D Eosinophilic esophagitis.
   E Gastroesophageal reflux disease.

2   Which of the following is the usual next step in the management of this patient?
   A Upper endoscopy.
   B Computed tomography of the chest.
   C Barium esophagogram.
   D A trial of a proton pump inhibitor for 8 weeks.
   E Reassurance and follow-up.

3   A barium esophagogram does not reveal any abnormalities. The patient undergoes upper endoscopy, which is completely normal. A biopsy is performed and does not reveal esophageal eosinophilia. The next step in the management of this patient is which of the following?
   A Test and treat for *Helicobacter pylori* infection.
   B A trial of a proton pump inhibitor for 2 weeks.
   C Video-radiographic study.
   D Upper endoscopy.
   E Esophageal manometry.

4   Which of the following neurons is selectively lost in achalasia?
   A Preganglionic neurons containing nitric oxide.
   B Postganglionic neurons containing nitric oxide.
   C Preganglionic neurons containing acetylcholine.
   D Postganglionic neurons containing acetylcholine.

5   An 80-year-old man presents with progressive dysphagia for solid food over the past 3 months. He reports a weight loss of 20 lb (9 kg). He has had gastroesophageal reflux symptoms for the past 15 years. The differential diagnosis of his dysphagia includes all of the following EXCEPT:

A Benign esophageal ('peptic') stricture.
B Adenocarcinoma of the esophagus.
C Squamous cell carcinoma of the esophagus.
D Parkinson's disease.

6 A 65-year-old man presents with progressive dysphagia for liquids and
   solids over the past few weeks. He has episodes of choking when he swallows liquids. His symptoms are intermittent and have not resulted in
   weight loss. He does not take any medications. In addition to dysphagia,
   he notes mild weakness of his left arm and leg. The most likely cause of
   dysphagia in this patient is which of the following?
   A Reflux esophagitis.
   B Neurologic dysfunction.
   C Squamous cell carcinoma of the esophagus.
   D Adenocarcinoma of the esophagus.

7 The best test to establish the diagnosis in the patient presented in Question
   6 is which of the following?
   A Upper endoscopy.
   B Barium swallow.
   C Esophageal pH testing.
   D Video-radiographic study.

8 The best diagnostic test to establish the diagnosis of achalasia is which of
   the following?
   A Upper endoscopy.
   B Esophageal manometry.
   C Esophageal pH testing.
   D Video-radiographic study.

9 A 65-year-old man with intermittent dysphagia is noted to have an
   esophageal ring on upper endoscopy. The patient denies any symptoms of
   gastroesophageal reflux. Which of the following is the best treatment
   option for his dysphagia?
   A Endoscopic dilation.
   B Proton pump inhibitor.
   C Surgical resection.
   D Dietary modification.

10 A 21-year-old man is seen in the clinic for the evaluation of painful swallowing and dysphagia for the past 2 weeks. He describes an intermittent

pain sensation in the mid-sternal area, with inability to eat solid food due to severe pain and dysphagia. His medications include a steroid inhaler for asthma and doxycycline to treat moderately severe acne. He has occasional heartburn (less than twice per month) and takes ranitidine as needed. The family history includes gastric cancer in his father. His physical examination is within normal limits.

Which of the following is the most likely diagnosis?

A Achalasia
B Esophageal cancer
C Erosive esophagitis
D Pill-induced esophagitis
E *Candida* esophagitis

Answers

1 C

2 C

3 B

The patient has classic symptoms of esophageal dysphagia, likely due to mechanical obstruction. In the setting of a prior long-term history of heartburn, the differential diagnosis includes reflux esophagitis, peptic stricture, or adenocarcinoma of the esophagus. Barium swallow with a tablet is generally the first test of choice. If the test is normal, the next step is to perform upper endoscopy. If upper endoscopy, with mucosal biopsies to evaluate for eosinophilic esophagitis, is normal, the patient should be treated empirically for gastroesophageal reflux disease with a PPI twice daily for 2 weeks. If the patient does not respond to a trial of a PPI, esophageal manometry should be performed to rule out an esophageal motor disorder.

4 B

In achalasia, the postganglionic nitric oxide-containing neurons are lost, thereby resulting in failure of relaxation of the lower esophageal sphincter.

5 D

The patient has symptoms of esophageal dysphagia. His recent weight loss raises concern about esophageal cancer. His symptoms are also consistent with a benign stricture, given his longstanding reflux symptoms. Parkinson's disease is usually associated with oropharyngeal dysphagia, and patients complain of cough, choking, or neurologic symptoms.

6   B

The patient has symptoms of oropharyngeal dysphagia including coughing and a choking sensation after eating. This presentation could be secondary to stroke, particularly in light of the weakness on his left side. Esophageal cancer is usually associated with weight loss and progressive dysphagia for solid food. Reflux esophagitis is typically associated with heartburn and odynophagia. Dysphagia for solids and liquids is uncommon in patients with reflux esophagitis.

7   D

A video-radiographic study is used to observe the process of deglutition. Abnormalities in oropharyngeal dysphagia can be detected using this test. When esophageal dysphagia is suspected, one should perform a barium esophagogram with or without an upper endoscopy. In a patient in whom gastroesophageal reflux is a suspected cause of dysphagia, pH testing may be performed.

8   B

Achalasia is a motility disorder characterized by loss of myenteric ganglion inhibitory neurons leading to a loss of relaxation of the lower esophageal sphincter. Manometry is the best test to establish this diagnosis. Upper endoscopy may reveal a tight lower esophageal sphincter, but is not diagnostic for achalasia. A video-radiographic study is useful for the evaluation of oropharyngeal dysphagia. Upper endoscopy is useful for the detection of a structural lesion causing dysphagia. Esophageal pH testing can help in establishing the role of gastroesophageal reflux as a cause of dysphagia.

9   A

The best treatment option for an esophageal ring is to perform an endoscopic dilation. In the absence of reflux symptoms, a trial of a PPI is not recommended. Surgical resection is not a treatment option for an esophageal ring. Dietary modification is generally not beneficial for an esophageal ring.

10   D

This patient likely has pill-induced esophagitis secondary to doxycycline use. Other medications that can lead to pill-induced esophagitis include aspirin, nonsteroidal anti-inflammatory drugs, potassium and iron supplements, and bisphosphonates. Achalasia is unlikely to present acutely with dysphagia and odynophagia, and is not likely in this patient. Esophageal cancer is rare at this age and should not be considered as a possible cause. Although erosive esophagitis is a possibility, this patient has infrequent reflux symptoms, and erosive esophagitis is a less likely cause than pill-induced esophagitis. Candida esophagitis is unlikely in immunocompetent hosts.

Further Reading

Aziz, Q, Fass, R, Gyawali CP, *et al.* (2016) Functional esophageal disorders. *Gastroenterology*, pii: S0016-5085(16)00178-5. doi: 10.1053/j.gastro.2016.02.012.

DeVault, K.D. (2016) Symptoms of esophageal disease, in *Sleisenger and Fordtran's Gastrointestinal and Liver Disease: Pathophysiology/Diagnosis/Management*, 10th edition, (eds M. Feldman, L.S. Friedman, and L.J. Brandt), Saunders Elsevier, Philadelphia, pp. 185–193.

Kahrilas, P.J. and Smout, A.J.P.M. (2010) Esophageal disorders. *American Journal of Gastroenterology*, **105**, 747–756.

Weblinks

http://www.merckmanuals.com/professional/sec02/ch012/ch012b.html?qt=dysphagia&alt=sh
http://emedicine.medscape.com/article/324096-overview

3

Peptic Ulcer Disease

Meena A. Prasad and Lawrence S. Friedman

Clinical Vignette

A 43-year-old woman is seen in the office for epigastric discomfort of 8 months' duration. She describes the discomfort as a constant dull ache that usually occurs postprandially and is associated with nausea, but not vomiting. The pain abates spontaneously after a few hours. She has no nocturnal pain, diarrhea, rectal bleeding, or weight loss. At age 40, she had a colonoscopy for rectal bleeding, which was unremarkable except for hemorrhoids. Her past medical and surgical history is unremarkable except for seasonal allergies. She takes antihistamines for seasonal allergies and ibuprofen 1–2 tablets several times a month for headaches. She does not take any prescription medications. Her parents are alive and well, and her two siblings are healthy. Her paternal grandfather died of colon cancer at age 80. She works as an administrative assistant, is married, and has two children. She drinks a glass of wine with dinner and does not smoke. She has no history of illicit drug use. Physical examination reveals a blood pressure of 114/80 mmHg, pulse rate 67 per minute, and body mass index 22. She is afebrile. The remainder of the examination, including an abdominal examination, is unremarkable. Rectal examination reveals brown stool that is negative for occult blood. A complete blood count is normal.

General

- The lifetime prevalence of peptic ulcer disease (PUD) is approximately 10%.
- PUD affects approximately 4.5 million people in the US annually.

Sitaraman and Friedman's Essentials of Gastroenterology, Second Edition.
Edited by Shanthi Srinivasan and Lawrence S. Friedman.
© 2018 John Wiley & Sons Ltd. Published 2018 by John Wiley & Sons Ltd.

Etiology and Pathogenesis

The majority (95%) of gastric and duodenal ulcers are caused by *Helicobacter pylori* or nonsteroidal anti-inflammatory drugs (NSAIDs).

- ● *Helicobacter pylori:*
  - – Some 70% of gastric ulcers and 80–95% of duodenal ulcers are attributed to *H. pylori* infection.
  - – Approximately 15% of *H. pylori*-infected persons will develop PUD.
  - – In the US, the estimated prevalence of *H. pylori* infection is 20% in persons younger than 30 years, and 50% of those older than 60 years. The prevalence is higher in African-American and Hispanic people.
  - – The majority of affected people acquire *H. pylori* during childhood.
  - – *H. pylori* is a Gram-negative microaerophilic bacterium that colonizes the surface of epithelial cells of the gastric antrum. If found in the duodenum, *H. pylori* is associated with metaplastic gastric epithelium. The bacterium produces urease, which breaks down urea to ammonia and carbon dioxide and is required for the survival of *H. pylori* in an acidic environment (and is the basis of diagnostic tests; see later).
  - – Duodenal and gastric ulcers result as a consequence of both the destruction of antral epithelial cells by *H. pylori* and the production of gastric acid, induced by the bacteria, that overwhelms the intrinsic defense mechanisms in the stomach and duodenum. The inflammatory response to *H. pylori* colonization induces hyperplasia of antral G cells, which in turn secrete gastrin, thereby causing a further increase in gastric acid production.
- ● **NSAIDs:**
  - – Account for 10% of duodenal ulcers and 15–30% of gastric ulcers.
  - – NSAIDs (including aspirin) inhibit cyclooxygenase-1, the enzyme that catalyzes the synthesis of prostaglandins (which act as mucosal protectants). NSAIDs are also weak acids that, when protonated by gastric acid, penetrate the epithelial cell membrane and cause rapid epithelial cell death and mucosal erosion.

Risk factors for developing NSAID-induced ulcers include age >60 years, concomitant use of glucocorticoids, use of multiple or high doses (≥2× normal) of NSAIDs, prior history of PUD, and anticoagulant use.

- ● **Other causes of ulcers:**
  - – Malignancy: adenocarcinoma, lymphoma, gastrointestinal stromal tumor (GIST).

- Less-common causes: gastrin hypersecretory states such as gastrinoma (Zollinger–Ellison syndrome), mastocytosis, antral G cell hyperplasia.
- Rare causes: Crohn's disease, eosinophilic gastroenteritis, viruses (cytomegalovirus, herpes virus).

> In many patients with ulcer-like symptoms (dyspepsia), no ulcer (or other 'organic' disorder) is identified. Such patients are considered to have functional (or non-ulcer) dyspepsia.

Clinical Features

- **Typical symptoms**: these occur in <20% of patients and include dyspepsia (epigastric pain, fullness, or bloating, often with nausea and eructation). The discomfort is often described as gnawing or burning in nature. With duodenal ulcer, the discomfort often occurs 1–3 hours after a meal and is relieved by food or antacids. With gastric ulcer, the discomfort is often exacerbated by food. Symptoms may occur nocturnally. In many patients, symptoms are nonspecific and vague.
- **Physical examination**: in uncomplicated PUD, physical findings are minimal or absent. When present, findings include epigastric tenderness and occult blood in the stool, or melena (black or maroon stools resulting from gastrointestinal bleeding). Peritoneal signs (rebound abdominal tenderness, guarding, and rigidity) signify a perforated ulcer, and a succussion splash is seen with partial or complete gastric outlet obstruction.

Diagnosis

- In most patients with uncomplicated PUD, routine laboratory tests are not usually helpful.
- Confirmation of PUD is best made by an upper endoscopy (esophagogastroduodenoscopy [EGD]) (Figure 3.1). Guidelines for the approach to patients presenting with dyspepsia are shown in Figure 3.2.

Tests for *H. pylori*

- Established indications to test for *H. pylori* include:
  - Active PUD (gastric or duodenal ulcer).
  - Confirmed history of PUD not previously treated for *H. pylori*.
  - Gastric mucosa-associated lymphoid tissue (MALT) lymphoma.
  - After endoscopic resection of early gastric cancer.
  - Uninvestigated dyspepsia (depending on *H. pylori* prevalence).

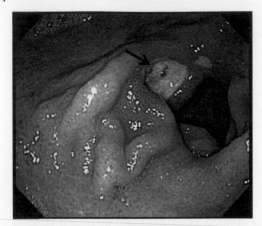

Figure 3.1 Endoscopic image of a pyloric channel ulcer (arrow).

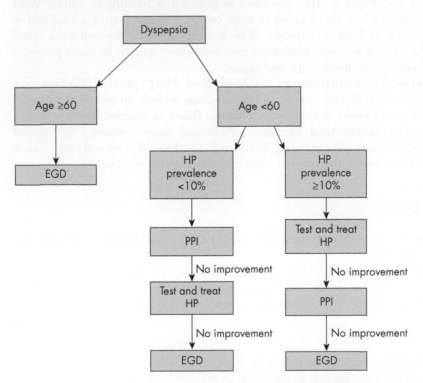

Figure 3.2 Algorithm for the approach to the patient with dyspepsia (American College of Gastroenterology and Canadian Association of Gastroenterology, 2017). (EGD, esophagogastroduodenoscopy; HP, *Helicobacter pylori*; NSAID, nonsteroidal anti-inflammatory drug; PPI, trial of proton pump inhibitor; Test and treat indicates testing for *H. pylori* and treating the infection, if present.)

The decision regarding which test to use depends on whether a patient requires evaluation with upper endoscopy. The advantages and disadvantages of each test must also be taken into consideration (Table 3.1). No single test is considered to be a 'gold standard'.

Table 3.1 Advantages and disadvantages of various diagnostic tests for *H. pylori*.

	Advantages	Disadvantages
Invasive tests		
1. Histology*	Excellent sensitivity and specificity	Expensive and requires infrastructure and trained personnel
2. Rapid urease test*	Inexpensive and provides rapid results. Excellent specificity and very good sensitivity in properly selected patients	Sensitivity significantly reduced in the posttreatment setting
3. Culture*	Excellent specificity. Allows determination of antibiotic sensitivities	Expensive, difficult to perform, and not widely available. Only marginal sensitivity
4. Polymerase chain reaction*	Excellent sensitivity and specificity. Allows determination of antibiotic sensitivities	Methodology not standardized across laboratories and not widely available
Noninvasive tests		
1. Antibody test (quantitative and qualitative)	Inexpensive, widely available, very good NPV	PPV dependent upon background *H. pylori* prevalence. Not recommended after *H. pylori* therapy
2. Urea breath tests (^{13}C and ^{14}C)*	Identifies active *H. pylori* infection. Excellent PPV and NPV regardless of *H. pylori* prevalence. Useful before and after *H. pylori* therapy	Reimbursement and availability are inconsistent
3. Fecal antigen test*	Identifies active *H. pylori* infection. Excellent positive and negative predictive values regardless of *H. pylori* prevalence. Useful before and after *H. pylori* therapy	Polyclonal test less well validated than the urea breath test in the posttreatment setting. Monoclonal test appears reliable before and after antibiotic therapy. Unpleasantness associated with collecting stool

* The sensitivity of all invasive and noninvasive tests that identify active *H. pylori* infection is reduced by the recent use of PPIs, bismuth, or antibiotics.
PPI, proton pump inhibitor; PPV, positive predictive value; NPV, negative predictive value; UBT, urea breath test.
Adapted from Chey, W.D. and Wong, B.C.Y. (2007) American College of Gastroenterology guideline on the management of *Helicobacter pylori* infection. *American Journal of Gastroenterology*, **102**, 1808–1825.

- Invasive (require endoscopy):
  - **Rapid urease test**: this is done on a mucosal biopsy specimen from the antrum, body, or incisura angularis of the stomach (95% sensitive and specific).
  - **Histology**: organisms can be visualized on histologic examination of the surface of epithelial cells in gastric mucosal biopsy specimens. The absence of chronic gastritis (inflammation) on histologic examination of a gastric mucosal biopsy specimen is good evidence of the absence of *H. pylori*.
  - **Culture and sensitivity**: seldom performed, but useful for the treatment-refractory patient to determine antibiotic sensitivities.
- Noninvasive (do not require endoscopy):
  - **Serology**: antibodies to *H. pylori* (sensitivity 90%, specificity 70–80%). Serology is used for the diagnosis of *H. pylori* in previously untreated persons. It is not as useful in confirming eradication of *H. pylori* following treatment because the test can remain positive for years after successful treatment.
  - **Urea breath test**: radiolabeled urea is ingested by the patient, and isotope-labeled carbon dioxide generated by the bacterial urease is measured in exhaled breath (sensitivity and specificity >95%). This test may be used as an initial diagnostic test or to confirm eradication.
  - **Stool antigen**: the test is based on the amplification of *H. pylori* RNA shed in stool (sensitivity >90%, specificity 80–90%). The test may be used as an initial diagnostic test or to confirm eradication.

Tests based on urease activity of the bacteria may yield false-negative results in the setting of recent antibiotic use or treatment with a PPI, histamine H2 receptor antagonist (H2RA), or a bismuth-containing compound. If repeat testing to confirm eradication of *H. pylori* is necessary, it should be done 4 weeks after discontinuation of antibiotics or bismuth and 2 weeks after discontinuation of a PPI or H2RA.

- In the setting of active GI bleeding, the sensitivity of urease-based tests and even histology may be reduced.
- In the setting of GI bleeding from PUD, a positive *H. pylori* result should be treated; however, a negative result could be falsely negative and should be confirmed with another test such as an antibody test or, alternatively, a urease breath test or stool antigen test at a later date after medications that can negatively affect the sensitivities of these tests have been discontinued.

Serum Gastrin Level

- Usually measured if gastrinoma (Zollinger–Ellison syndrome) is suspected (on the basis of recurrent peptic ulcer, severe and multiple ulcers, and concomitant diarrhea).
- Other conditions associated with an elevated serum gastrin level include use of a PPI and atrophic gastritis. *H. pylori* infection may raise the serum gastrin level slightly.
- A serum gastrin level $\geq 1000\,\mathrm{pg\,ml}^{-1}$ is highly suggestive of gastrinoma. If the level is elevated but $<1000\,\mathrm{pg\,ml}^{-1}$, gastric pH measurement may be performed (pH measurement is done on gastric fluid obtained via endoscopy or insertion of a nasogastric tube). A gastric pH <3.0 is consistent with a gastrinoma or antral *H. pylori* infection. A secretin stimulation test will confirm gastrinoma if the rise in serum gastrin after intravenous administration of secretin is $>200\,\mathrm{pg\,ml}^{-1}$. A gastric pH ≥ 3.0 is seen with the use of a PPI or in atrophic gastritis.

Treatment

- Antisecretory agents: administered orally (8 weeks for duodenal ulcer and 8–12 weeks for gastric ulcer). The drugs used to treat PUD are the following:
  - **H2RAs**: block H2 receptors on parietal cells of the stomach; can heal 90% of ulcers in 8 weeks; can be given as a single nighttime dose.
  - **PPIs**: bind covalently and irreversibly with the hydrogen/potassium-adenosine triphosphatase enzyme (H^+/K^+-ATPase pump) on parietal cells in the stomach; more potent acid-suppressing agents than H2RAs; heal >95% of ulcers. Side effects include headache, diarrhea, constipation, nausea, and acid 'rebound' on withdrawal.
- Mucosal protectants (not used as first-line therapy for PUD):
  - **Sucralfate**: after oral ingestion, forms a crosslinking, viscous, paste-like material that coats the ulcer bed; in an acidic environment, binds to proteins such as albumin, pepsin, and fibrinogen to form stable insoluble complexes on the surface of an ulcer.
  - **Misoprostol**: stimulates gastric mucus and bicarbonate secretion after oral ingestion; its primary use is in ulcer prevention, for example, in a patient taking an NSAID who has a high risk of developing PUD; side effects include diarrhea; the drug is contraindicated in pregnancy.
  - **Antacids**: neutralize gastric acid after oral ingestion; multiple daily doses are required to heal ulcers. Side effects depend on the formulation: magnesium-containing, diarrhea; aluminum-containing, constipation; calcium-containing, gastric acid 'rebound' when antacid is discontinued.

- Discontinue NSAIDs:
  - If an NSAID is required despite PUD, consider prophylactic PPI treatment concomitantly. Alternatively, consider administration of a more selective cyclooxygenase-2 (COX-2) inhibitor instead of a nonselective NSAID.
- Discontinue smoking.
- *H. pylori* eradication (Table 3.2):
  - *H. pylori* eradication reduces the recurrence of PUD and decreases recurrent bleeding when compared with ulcer-healing treatment alone or ulcer-healing treatment followed by maintenance therapy with a gastric acid suppressant (ranitidine 150–300 mg at bedtime or omeprazole 20 mg daily × 12–24 months).
  - Triple therapy with PPI plus clarithromycin and either amoxicillin or metronidazole for 7–10 days was previously recommended as first-line therapy, but has become increasingly ineffective, with eradication in less than 50% of cases. Sequential quadruple therapy is also no longer recommended.

Table 3.2 First-line treatment regimens for *H. pylori* eradication.

Concomitant nonbismuth quadruple therapy 14 days	
PPI	BID
Amoxicillin	1000 mg BID
Clarithromycin	500 mg BID
Metronidazole or tinidazole	500 mg BID
Bismuth-containing regimen 14 days	
PPI	BID
Bismuth subsalicylate	2 tablets QID
Metronidazole or tinidazole	500 mg TID or 400 mg QID
Tetracycline	500 mg QID
PPI triple therapy 14 days (restricted to areas with a low rate of clarithromycin resistance or high rate of eradication)	
PPI	BID
Amoxicillin	1000 mg BID
Clarithromycin	500 mg BID on days 5–10
Metronidazole or tinidazole	500 mg TID or 400 mg QID on days 5–10

PPI, proton pump inhibitor, e.g., esomeprazole 20 mg, lansoprazole 30 mg, omeprazole 20 mg, pantoprazole 40 mg, rabeprazole 20 mg; BID, twice daily; TID, three times a day; QID, four times a day.

- Due to increasing rates of treatment failures, all *H. pylori* eradication regimens should be given for 14 days. Either triple therapy, a four-drug concomitant quadruple therapy, or a bismuth quadruple therapy regimen is recommended.
- Triple therapy with a PPI, clarithromycin, and either amoxicillin or metronidazole is restricted to areas known to be associated with a low rate of clarithromycin resistance or high rate of eradication.
- Quadruple therapy consists of a PPI, amoxicillin, clarithromycin, and a nitroimidazole (metronidazole or tinidazole) or bismuth-based quadruple therapy with a PPI, bismuth, metronidazole, and tetracycline. These regimens are associated with *H. pylori* eradication rates of >90%.
- For prior treatment failures, bismuth quadruple therapy or levofloxacin-containing therapy (PPI, amoxicillin, and levofloxacin) is recommended. Rifabutin-containing therapy (PPI, amoxicillin, and rifabutin) is indicated after at least three recommended options have failed.
- Indications for confirming eradication of *H. pylori*:
  - *H. pylori*-associated ulcer.
  - Persistent dyspeptic symptoms despite the test-and-treat strategy.
  - *H. pylori*-associated MALT lymphoma.
  - Following resection of early gastric cancer.
- *H. pylori* eradication and NSAID use:
  - *H. pylori* eradication in chronic NSAID users is insufficient to prevent NSAID-related ulcer disease. Continued prophylactic treatment with a PPI is recommended in high-risk patients.
  - Patients taking an NSAID in whom bleeding from PUD develops should be tested for *H. pylori* and treated for the infection, if present. If such patients require long-term NSAID use, a PPI should also be administered long term.

Complications

- The most common (15–20%) complication is bleeding (see Chapter 22). Others include perforation or penetration into the pancreas (5–7%) and gastric outlet obstruction (<5%).
- Persons with *H. pylori* infection have a 3- to 6-fold increased incidence of gastric adenocarcinoma.
- MALT lymphoma is associated with *H. pylori* infection. Treatment of *H. pylori* infection results in regression or cure of 90% of MALT lymphomas diagnosed at an early stage.
- Gastroesophageal reflux disease may increase in frequency or severity after the eradication of *H. pylori* (see Chapter 1).

Prognosis

The majority of peptic ulcers heal with antisecretory therapy in combination with treatment of *H. pylori* infection and discontinuation of NSAIDs. The frequency of recurrence of an *H. pylori*-related ulcer is 4–10%.

Pearls

- Because a small percentage of gastric ulcers are actually ulcerated gastric carcinomas, all gastric ulcers must be assessed carefully to distinguish a benign from a malignant ulcer.
- Endoscopy should be repeated to ensure that a gastric ulcer (not related to NSAID use), particularly if it is >2 cm, has healed.

Questions

Questions 1 and 2 relate to the clinical vignette discussed at the beginning of this chapter.

1 In addition to discontinuing ibuprofen, the next step in the management of the patient is which of the following?
   A Upper endoscopy.
   B *H. pylori* test and eradication.
   C Proton pump inhibitor (PPI) for 8 weeks.
   D Computed tomography of the abdomen and pelvis.
   E Prescribe aspirin 81 mg daily

2 The patient returns to your office in 12 weeks stating that she has had minimal improvement after stopping ibuprofen and starting PPI therapy. *H. pylori* serology is negative. The next step in the management of this patient is which of the following?
   A Upper endoscopy.
   B Measure serum gastrin.
   C Increase the dose of the PPI to twice daily.
   D Switch to another PPI.
   E Test the urine for surreptitious NSAID use.

3 A 57-year-old man presents with epigastric pain of 2 months' duration and black tarry stools three times per day over the past 2 days. An upper endoscopy reveals a duodenal ulcer with active bleeding that is treated endoscopically. Gastric biopsies are taken, and a rapid urease test for *H. pylori* is negative. What is the next step in management of this patient?

A No further evaluation.
B Urea breath test.
C *H. pylori* fecal antigen.
D Urea breath test 2 weeks after completion of PPI therapy.
E Repeat upper endoscopy in 2 months.

4 A 40-year-old man who has osteoarthritis of his knee requires long-term use of an NSAID. He smokes a half a pack of cigarettes a day. He is concerned about PUD as a result of NSAID use. What would you advise him?
A Stop smoking.
B Stop the NSAID.
C Test for *Helicobacter pylori* and eradicate if present.
D Use amoxicillin.
E Upper endoscopy.

5 Which of the following statements regarding *H. pylori* is false?
A It is the cause of the majority of duodenal ulcers.
B It causes a decrease in the number of antral G-cells.
C It colonizes surface epithelial cells in the antrum of the stomach.
D The majority of people infected acquire *H. pylori* during childhood.
E Treatment of *H. pylori* infection results in regression or cure of 90% of cases of early-stage MALT lymphoma.

6 A 30-year-old man presents to the emergency department with the sudden onset of severe abdominal pain. He states that he has been training for a marathon and has been taking ibuprofen for myalgias. Physical examination reveals a distended, rigid abdomen, and rebound tenderness. Bowel sounds are absent. You suspect perforation of a gastric or duodenal ulcer. Which of the following tests can confirm a perforation?
A Upright abdominal film.
B Chest X-ray.
C Computed tomography (CT) of the abdomen.
D All of the above.

Answers

1 B
This patient presents with dyspepsia. She has no alarm symptoms and is less than 55 years of age, so rather than proceeding with endoscopy, it would be reasonable to either empirically treat with PPI or to test and treat for *H. pylori* depending on the prevalence of *H. pylori* in her area.

2   A

This patient has had no response to PPI therapy and has had negative *H. pylori* testing, so the next step in evaluation is to proceed with upper endoscopy.

3   D

In the setting of active GI bleeding, the sensitivity of urease-based tests, and even histology, may be reduced. A negative result should be confirmed with another test such as an antibody test or a urea breath test or fecal antigen 2 weeks after completion of PPI therapy. Although a repeat upper endoscopy should be considered to confirm healing of a gastric ulcer and *exclude gastric cancer, it is not necessary for a duodenal ulcer.

4   A

This patient has no risk factors (age >60 years, concomitant use of glucocorticoids, use of multiple or high doses (≥2× normal) of NSAIDs, prior history of PUD, or anticoagulant use) for developing PUD from the use of NSAIDs. *H. pylori* eradication in NSAID users is insufficient to prevent NSAID-related ulcer disease. On the other hand, smoking cessation has been shown to reduce the incidence of NSAID-induced PUD. Amoxicillin has not been shown to prevent NSAID-induced PUD. Upper endoscopy is not indicated in this patient.

5   B

H. pylori does not cause a decrease in the number of antral G-cells. *H. pylori* colonizes surface epithelial cells in the antrum and causes destruction of antral epithelial cells, which results in ulcer formation. *H. pylori* infection reduces the number of antral D-cells, resulting in relative hypofunction of the inhibitory action of D-cells against G-cells, which may explain the increased gastrin secretion seen in *H. pylori* infection.

6   D

Any of the tests listed can detect signs of a perforated ulcer (free air in the abdomen). The most sensitive test is CT of the abdomen (see Chapter 27).

Further Reading

Chan, F.K.L. and Lau, J.Y.W. (2016) Peptic ulcer disease, in *Sleisenger and Fordtran's Gastrointestinal and Liver Disease: Pathophysiology/Diagnosis/Management*, 10th edition, (eds M. Feldman, L.S. Friedman, and L.J. Brandt), Saunders Elsevier, Philadelphia, pp. 884–900.

Chey, W.D. and Wong, B.C.Y. (2007) American College of Gastroenterology guideline on the management of *Helicobacter pylori* infection. *American Journal of Gastroenterology*, **102**, 1808–1825.

Fallone, C.A., Chiba, N., Zanten, S.V.V., et al. (2016) The Toronto consensus for the treatment of *Helicobacter pylori* infection in adults. *Gastroenterology*, **151**, 51–69.

Lanas, A., and Chan, F.K.L. (2017) Peptic ulcer disease. *The Lancet*, **390**, 613–624.

Moayyedi, P.M., Lacy, B.E., Andrews, C.N., et al. (2017) ACG and CAG clinical guideline: Management of dyspepsia. *Am J Gastroenterol*, **112**, 988–1013.

Patel, K.A. and Howden, C.W. (2015) Update on the diagnosis and management of *Helicobacter pylori* infection in adults. *Journal of Clinical Gastroenterology*, **49**, 461–467.

Weblinks

http://www.merckmanuals.com/professional/sec02/ch013/ch013e.html
http:// www.aafp.org/afp/2015/0215/p236.html

4

Common Upper Gastrointestinal Surgeries

Rebecca G. Lopez and Edward Lin

Clinical Vignette

A 64-year-old man with a 40 pack-year smoking history presents with a complaint of severe dysphagia for solids and worsening dysphagia for liquids. He has had a 5 lb (2 kg) weight loss. On esophagogastroduodenoscopy (EGD), a 3-cm ulcerated lesion in the distal third of the esophagus is found, and on histologic examination of biopsy specimens it proves to be a squamous cell carcinoma. Endoscopic ultrasonography (EUS) reveals no regional lymphadenopathy, and computed tomography (CT) shows no evidence of distal metastases.

Esophagectomy

Procedure

- Decisions regarding the surgical resection of esophageal neoplasms are determined by the location of the tumor in the esophagus, the need for lymphadenectomy, and the surgeon's expertise. Approaches include a transhiatal approach, the Ivor Lewis approach, the three-hole, or McKeown, approach, and a minimally invasive approach (Figure 4.1).
- For each approach, the resulting esophageal conduit depends on the greater curvature of the stomach supplied by the right gastroepiploic artery (Figure 4.2). If the stomach cannot serve as a conduit, a more complex colonic or jejunal interposition may be performed instead.

Sitaraman and Friedman's Essentials of Gastroenterology, Second Edition.
Edited by Shanthi Srinivasan and Lawrence S. Friedman.

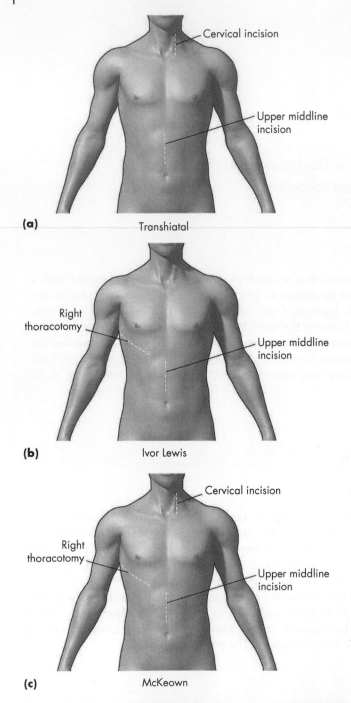

Figure 4.1 Incisions for the (a) Transhiatal, (b) Ivor Lewis, and (c) McKeown esophagectomy approaches.

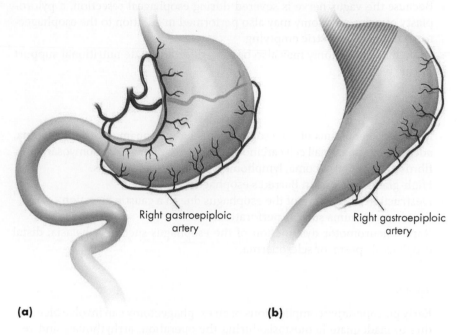

(a)   **(b)**

Figure 4.2 Esophageal conduit supplied by the right gastroepiploic artery following esophagectomy. (a) Normal anatomy. (b) Postsurgical anatomy showing the conduit (shaded).

- The **transhiatal approach** involves an upper midline incision to create a gastric conduit and a left transverse supraclavicular or left neck incision parallel to the sternocleidomastoid to access and dissect the cervical esophagus. The gastric conduit is then delivered into the posterior mediastinum to create the esophagogastric anastomosis in the cervical region.
- The **Ivor Lewis approach** involves an upper midline incision to create a gastric conduit in a manner similar to that for the transhiatal approach, followed by a right thoracotomy to mobilize the intrathoracic esophagus for an intrathoracic anastomosis.
- The **three-hole, or McKeown, approach** is carried out through separate upper midline, thoracic, and cervical incisions. This approach is thought to provide a better exposure to the surrounding structures and to decrease the risk of idiopathic injury; it also allows an extensive lymphadenectomy to be performed.
- Laparoscopic, thoracoscopic, and robot-assisted approaches have also been employed in the hope of decreasing the morbidity of multiple incisions while replicating the results of the open approaches.

- Because the vagus nerve is severed during esophageal resection, a pyloroplasty or pyloromyotomy may also performed in addition to the esophagectomy to improve gastric emptying.
- A feeding jejunostomy may also be placed for adequate nutritional support during recovery.

Indications

- Malignant neoplasms of the esophagus, including squamous cell carcinoma, adenocarcinoma, small cell carcinoma, leiomyosarcoma, rhabdomyosarcoma, fibrosarcoma, liposarcoma, lymphomas, and metastatic lesions.
- High-grade dysplasia in Barrett's esophagus.
- Destruction or stricture of the esophagus due to a caustic ingestion.
- Esophageal trauma such as perforation.
- Rarely, neuromotor dysfunction of the esophagus such as achalasia, distal esophageal spasm, or scleroderma.

Complications

- Early postoperative complications of an esophagectomy can involve bleeding due to inadequate hemostasis during the operation, arrhythmias, and respiratory complications such as atelectasis and pneumonia.
- Ischemia of the conduit typically manifests in the first 2–3 days following surgery, with unexplained tachycardia, cardiac arrhythmias, and poor oxygenation. Endoscopic examination revealing gross ischemia of the conduit requires immediate takedown of the conduit and wide drainage, with plans for a staged reconstruction. Rarely, if only a small portion of the stomach is ischemic, the ischemic portion can be resected with immediate reconstruction.
- Anastomotic leaks manifest in the first few days following surgery:
  - Thoracic anastomotic leaks typically present as sepsis. The chest tube output will often be noted to be abnormally turbid in color. A water-soluble contrast study can help to identify the location and magnitude of the leak. Depending on the size, treatment can range from CT-guided drainage for a small leak to re-exploration and drainage for a large leak.
  - One of the first signs of a leak of a cervical anastomosis is drainage of turbid fluid from the neck wound. Opening of the neck wound and daily dressing changes are usually sufficient management for leaks confined to the neck. For a leak arising from the mediastinum, exploration and drainage are often required.
  - For all leaks, patients should be placed on broad-spectrum antibiotics guided by culture sensitivities, and adequate nutritional support should be administered.

Complete or Partial Fundoplication

Clinical Vignette

A 42-year-old man complains of a persistent burning sensation in the epigastrium, acid taste in his mouth, and intermittent regurgitation. The physical examination is unremarkable except for a body mass index of 26. Initially, diet, lifestyle modifications, and daily proton pump inhibitor (PPI) therapy provided symptomatic relief, but the symptoms have slowly recurred. Despite a maximum dose of antisecretory medication, upper endoscopy shows Los Angeles Class B esophagitis and a small hiatal hernia (see Chapter 1). A 24-hour ambulatory esophageal pH study correlates the symptoms with reflux episodes. Esophageal manometry indicates a decreased lower esophageal sphincter pressure. The patient is concerned about the long-term use of medications and is willing to consider a surgical procedure for his gastroesophageal reflux disease (GERD).

Procedure

- The Nissen fundoplication entails dividing the short gastric vessels that are attached to the spleen, and mobilizing the entire gastric fundus so that it can be delivered behind the gastroesophageal junction to create a 360° wrap around the distal 3–4 cm of the esophagus (Figure 4.3). The fundoplication essentially increases the pressure of the lower esophageal sphincter (LES).

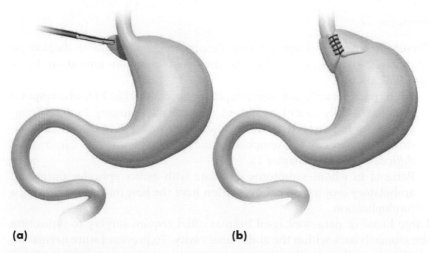

(a)　　　　　　　　　　　　　　**(b)**

Figure 4.3 Nissen fundoplication. (a) Mobilization of fundus; (b) 360° wrap around the distal 3–4 cm of esophagus.

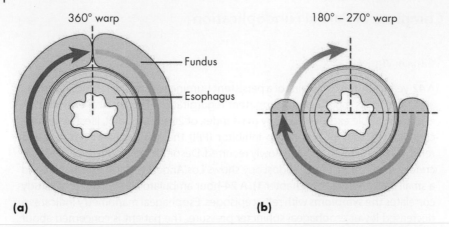

Figure 4.4 Cross-sections of (a) a Nissen fundoplication and (b) a Toupet fundoplication.

- Partial fundoplications, such as the Toupet fundoplication (270° posterior wrap), are employed when there is concern that a complete fundoplication may result in a hypercontinent LES, which may lead to gas-bloat syndrome, dysphagia, and other complications associated with a complete fundoplication (Figure 4.4). Other reasons to pursue a partial fundoplication include:
  - Esophageal dysmotility that limits bolus propagation.
  - Insufficient gastric fundus for a complete fundoplication.
  - Fundoplication used with a Heller cardiomyotomy for achalasia (see Chapter 2 and later).

Indications

- Persistent gastroesophageal reflux despite maximal medical therapy to suppress gastric acid secretion is the most common indication for a fundoplication.
  - Young patients with gastroesophageal reflux disease (GERD) who respond symptomatically to PPI treatment may consider surgery to defer long-term costs and associated concerns about chronic PPI use (such as a possible increased risk of osteoporosis and an increased risk of *Clostridium difficile* colitis; see Chapter 1).
  - Patients in whom symptoms correlate with reflux episodes during an ambulatory esophageal pH evaluation have the best outcome following a fundoplication.
- Large hiatal or paraesophageal hernias often require surgery to reposition the stomach back within the abdominal cavity. To prevent future herniation of the stomach into the thoracic cavity, some surgeons believe that a

fundoplication that serves as a buttress should be performed after repair of the diaphragmatic crura; however, postsurgical dysphagia may occur following a fundoplication.

- A fundoplication may also be considered for nongastrointestinal manifestations of GERD, such as cough, asthma, esophageal stenosis, and aspiration pneumonia.
  - Many lung transplant center protocols offer a fundoplication at the time of lung transplantation to prevent aspiration into the transplanted lung(s).
- Patients with GERD and morbid obesity should consider weight-loss surgery in the form of a Roux-en-Y gastric bypass (see later).

Complications

- Gas-bloat syndrome, the sensation of needing to belch but being unable to, occurs in less than 5% of patients and seems to dissipate as time progresses after surgery.
  - Management is conservative and includes avoidance of caffeine, the use of a straw to drink liquids, and simethicone (an anti-gas agent). In some patients, motility agents or even balloon dilation may be necessary to improve symptoms.
- Dysphagia occurs in approximately 20% of patients in the early postoperative period (first 12 weeks). Dysphagia is managed by modifying the diet to consist mostly of liquids until the symptoms resolve.
  - Persistent dysphagia requiring frequent dilations and even reoperation to convert a 360° complete wrap into a 270° or 180° partial wrap occurs in 5–15% of patients.
  - In some patients, antisecretory medications may be necessary.

Heller Cardiomyotomy

Clinical Vignette

A 28-year-old woman presents with acid reflux and a 15 lb (6.8 kg) weight loss over 4 months. EGD demonstrates a dilated esophagus with retained food debris. A barium swallow demonstrates esophageal dysmotility and a bird's beak appearance of the lower esophageal sphincter. A 12.5-mm barium tablet becomes lodged at the gastroesophageal junction. Esophageal manometry shows aperistalsis, an elevated resting lower esophageal sphincter (LES) pressure, and inability of the LES to relax with a swallow, consistent with achalasia (see Chapter 2).

Procedure

- The initial esophageal mobilization is similar to a fundoplication, as described earlier. Prior to closing the diaphragmatic crura, the muscular layer of the lower esophagus and the seromuscular layer of the gastric cardia are completely divided, leaving the mucosal layer intact. To avoid an incomplete myotomy, it is recommended that the myotomy extend at least 6 cm above the squamocolumnar junction and 2 cm below the squamocolumnar junction (Figure 4.5). The crura are then closed after the myotomy is performed.
- Whenever possible, a partial fundoplication is performed to reduce the amount of acid reflux into the esophagus.

Indication

- Myotomy of the LES is curative for achalasia.
  - Young patients and persons with early achalasia tend to have better outcomes with a Heller cardiomyotomy than older patients or those in whom the disease has progressed to a megaesophagus. Furthermore, young patients generally tolerate complications better than the elderly.

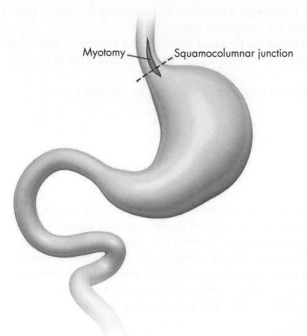

Figure 4.5 Heller cardiomyotomy.

Myotomy — Squamocolumnar junction

Complications

- Immediate postmyotomy complications include gastric or esophageal perforations.
- Persistent dysphagia, even several months after surgery, may be the result of an incomplete myotomy or adhesion formation. Treatment options include endoscopic dilation and repeat myotomy.
- GERD occurs in up to 40% of patients who undergo a myotomy without a concomitant antireflux procedure.
- Barrett's esophagus may occur with longstanding GERD. Postsurgical endoscopic surveillance for Barrett's esophagus should be performed (see Chapter 1).

Roux-en-Y, Billroth I, and Billroth II Gastroenterostomy

Clinical Vignette

A 53-year-old man undergoes an EGD for nausea and abdominal discomfort associated with melena and a 3.6-kg weight loss. On endoscopy, a 1.5-cm mass lesion in the stomach is found to be an adenocarcinoma on histologic examination. EUS reveals neither submucosal invasion nor lymphadenopathy, and CT confirms antral thickening without surrounding lymphadenopathy.

Procedure

- Surgical resection of gastric neoplasms or for complicated peptic ulcer disease involves a partial resection of the stomach and re-establishment of gastrointestinal continuity by reconnecting the gastric pouch to the small intestine. This can be accomplished by a Roux-en-Y gastrojejunostomy, Billroth I gastroduodenostomy, or Billroth II gastroenterostomy (Figure 4.6).
- The Roux-en-Y procedure is a gastrojejunostomy. The gastrojejunal, or 'Roux', limb is anastomosed to the biliopancreatic limb approximately 40–60 cm downstream from the gastrojejunostomy. This is performed to decrease alkaline reflux into the stomach pouch.
- The Billroth I procedure is an end-to-end gastroduodenostomy. The duodenal bulb, gastric pylorus, antrum, and a small portion of the body of the stomach are resected, and an anastomosis between the gastric remnant and proximal portion of the remaining duodenum is made, thereby preserving a physiologic flow of chyme.

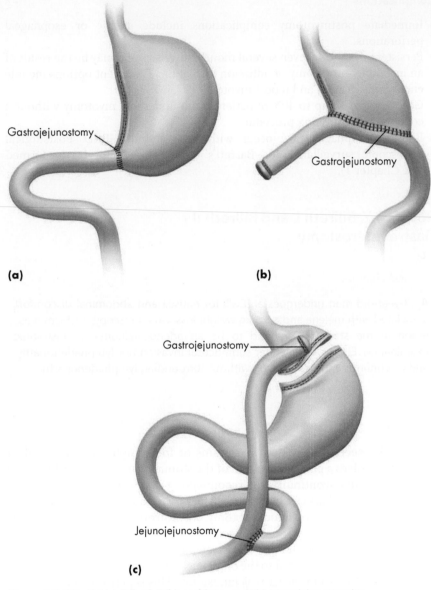

Gastrojejunostomy

Gastrojejunostomy

(a)

(b)

Gastrojejunostomy

Jejunojejunostomy

(c)

Figure 4.6 Billroth I (a), Billroth II (b), and Roux-en-Y (c) gastrojejunostomies.

- The Billroth II gastroenterostomy is an end-to-side gastrojejunostomy with partial gastric and proximal duodenal resection. The remaining duodenum containing the ampulla of Vater drains into the stomach as the afferent limb; the loop of jejunum connected by an end-to-side anastomosis to the stomach forms the efferent limb.

- In the case of a gastrectomy for malignancy, lymphadenectomy is often added and involves removal of the pyloric, portal, celiac, splenic, and cardiac lymph nodes.
- In the case of a gastrectomy for ulcer disease, truncal vagotomy may be performed. Vagotomy is not required when gastrectomy is performed for gastric adenocarcinoma because the patients are often achlorhydric.

Indications

- **Complicated peptic ulcer disease**: this is defined as an ulcer associated with bleeding, perforation, or gastric outlet obstruction or refractory to medical and endoscopic management.
- **Malignant antral adenocarcinoma** (stages I–III – limited local and regional spread on cross sectional imaging [CT, magnetic resonance imaging] and EUS); or other tumors.

Complications

Anastomotic Leak

This is a dreaded postoperative complication that can result in peritonitis and septic shock. Early management is imperative, and occurrence in a patient with a Billroth I gastroenterostomy often requires conversion to a Billroth II gastroenterostomy.

Postgastrectomy Syndromes

- **Postvagotomy diarrhea** likely results from colonic hypersecretion due to excess bile acids and bile salts that are unabsorbed in the small intestine (see Chapter 20). Initial treatment consists of small, frequent, low-fat meals in conjunction with fluid restriction and bulking agents. If conservative management fails, the entire gastrointestinal (GI) tract should be evaluated before surgical treatment aimed at slowing small bowel transit is considered.
- **Alkaline reflux gastritis** results from the reflux of bile into the gastric remnant. Sucralfate, a bile-salt binding agent such as cholestyramine, or a PPI, may be used for symptomatic relief. In patients who do not respond to medical therapy for alkaline reflux gastritis, the gastrojejunostomy can be converted to a Roux-en-Y configuration, which diverts the bile further downstream.
- **Dumping syndrome** is defined as a constellation of symptoms that include lightheadedness, palpitations, hypoglycemia, and diarrhea that occurs after a meal. Dumping syndrome results from the reduced capacity of the stomach and a dysregulated hormonal response to calorie-dense nutrients.
  - 'Early' dumping syndrome typically occurs 15–30 minutes after a meal due to rapid emptying of hyperosmolar chyme into the small intestine, thereby leading to intravascular shifts of fluid into the small intestinal lumen.

- – 'Late' dumping occurs 2–3 hours after a meal due to a hyperinsulinemic response to the large carbohydrate load.
- – Dietary modifications that include avoidance of simple carbohydrates and frequent small meals consisting of complex carbohydrates and high-fiber foods and avoidance of drinking beverages with meals are the mainstays of treatment.
- **Afferent loop syndrome** results from obstruction of the afferent limb that prevents emptying of biliary and pancreatic fluid into the stomach. The obstruction, caused by a stricture, kinking of the bowel, adhesions, or narrowing of the anastomosis (due to recurrent ulcer or malignancy), may lead to bowel ischemia, pancreatitis, or cholangitis.
- **Roux stasis syndrome** occurs after Roux-en-Y reconstruction and manifests as nausea, vomiting, early satiety, and abdominal pain. It can be due to Roux limb stasis, delayed gastric emptying, or both. Prokinetic agents, antiemetics, and limiting use of narcotics may improve symptoms. Mechanical obstruction of the Roux limb should be ruled out; such mechanical obstructions can occur from adhesions, intussusception, or internal hernia.

Weight-Loss Surgery

Clinical Vignette

A 45-year-old man with morbid obesity, diabetes mellitus, hypertension, and dyslipidemia presents for a routine annual health check-up. He complains of arthralgias of his knees that limit his physical activities. He routinely visits a nutritionist but is unable to lose weight despite aggressive dietary modifications.

Procedures (see Table 4.1)

Roux-en-Y Gastric Bypass (RYGB)
- A small, 15–30 ml, gastric pouch is separated from the larger, remnant stomach. The pouch is then connected to a jejunal limb to create a gastrojejunal anastomosis. The gastrojejunostomy (Roux) limb is connected downstream (75–150 cm) to the biliopancreatic limb via a Roux-en-Y configuration (Figure 4.7).
- Weight loss occurs due to the restrictive nature of the gastric pouch as well as intestinal malabsorption. There is no nutrient absorption within the Roux limb, and caloric and nutrient absorption can be further reduced by creating a longer Roux limb.
- A longer Roux limb portends greater malabsorption; thus, patients need life-long micronutrient and vitamin supplementation. The procedure provides sustained, continued weight loss over many years.

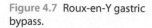

Figure 4.7 Roux-en-Y gastric bypass.

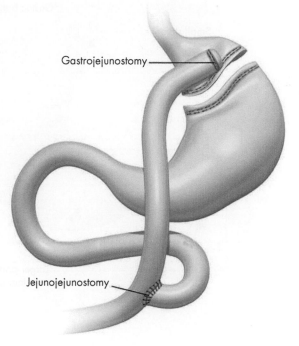

Gastrojejunostomy

Jejunojejunostomy

Laparoscopic Adjustable Gastric Banding (LAGB)

- A restrictive band is placed circumferentially around the cardia of the stomach to create a small reservoir. The band is connected to a reservoir port placed under the abdominal skin pad. The port can be accessed by a needle that contains saline, and the band can be tightened or loosened to constrict or enlarge, respectively, the size of the stoma (Figure 4.8).
- No anastomoses are created.
- Because the procedure has no malabsorptive properties and is solely restrictive, patients who continue on a soft, liquid, high-caloric diet may not lose weight despite a restricted gastric capacity.
- Weight loss is not as profound as it is in a RYGB and is frequently temporary despite repeated tightening of the band.

Sleeve Gastrectomy

- This is a restrictive procedure in which a significant portion of the fundus and greater curve (approximately 65–80% of the stomach) is removed to create a tubular stomach reservoir (Figure 4.9).
- As solely a restrictive procedure, nutrient malabsorption is less severe than after a RYGB.

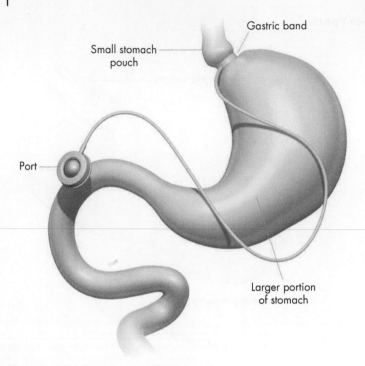

Small stomach
pouch

Gastric band

Port

Larger portion
of stomach

Figure 4.8 Laparoscopic adjustable gastric band.

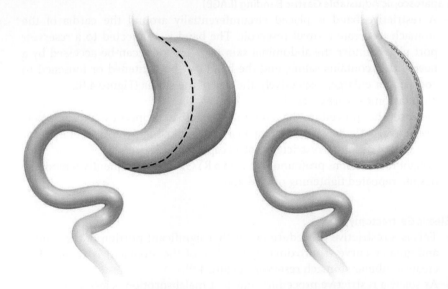

Figure 4.9 Sleeve gastrectomy.

Indications

- Morbidly obese persons (body mass index [BMI]) >40) and moderately obese persons (BMI >35) with significant comorbidities (e.g., diabetes mellitus, hypertension, coronary artery disease) are candidates for a weight-loss procedure.
- Prior to bariatric surgery, patients must have attempted and failed prior weight-loss programs, including strict compliance with a low-calorie diet as well as an aggressive exercise program.
- Mental illness and the inability to cope can be contraindications to a weight-loss procedure.

Complications

- Vitamin and mineral deficiencies are the most significant complications associated with malabsorptive weight-loss procedures, particularly the RYGB.
  - Vitamin B_{12} deficiency occurs when the fundus and body of the stomach are removed. Intrinsic factor, the peptide necessary for intestinal absorption of vitamin B_{12}, is synthesized by the parietal cells of the stomach.
  - Iron deficiency arises from bypass of the proximal duodenum (RYGB) or decreased acid production as a result of parietal cell loss due to resection of the fundus (sleeve gastrectomy).
  - Like iron absorption, calcium absorption occurs in the proximal duodenum, and procedures that bypass the duodenum require that the patient take supplements to try to prevent osteoporosis.
  - Malabsorption of vitamins A and D may occur due to disruption of the enterohepatic circulation (see Chapter 20).
- Others:
  - Because of multiple anastomoses, a RYGB is associated with a slightly increased risk of internal hernias, anastomotic leak, ulceration, and stomal stenosis.
  - The LAGB procedure is associated with the highest rate of failure to lose weight. Occasionally, the stomach pouch proximal to the band can distend because of slippage of the band, thereby causing GERD, dysphagia, and esophageal obstruction. High-calorie nutrient intake also leads to failure to lose weight. Band erosions through the stomach wall can occur with the LABG and can be detected by endoscopy or a skin port-site infection.

A comparison of the weight-loss operations is shown in Table 4.1.

Table 4.1 A comparison of weight-loss surgical procedures.

	Roux-en-Y-gastric bypass (RYGB)	Laparoscopic adjustable gastric band	Sleeve gastrectomy
Mechanism of weight-loss	Restrictive + malabsorption	Restrictive	Restrictive
Weight-loss outcomes	50–70% in 3–8 years; 'gold standard'; weight loss is more sustained and predictable	25–80% in 3–8 years; high failure rate; weight loss is reversible because band may be removed	Data beyond 5 years are not available; weight loss is significant but may not be sustained
Nutrient deficiencies	Minerals absorbed in duodenum or requiring acid; fat-soluble vitamins	None	Vitamin B_{12}, iron, calcium
Complications	Internal hernia, anastomotic leak, ulceration, or stenosis	Weight-loss failure; band erosion or infection	Gastroesophageal reflux, weight gain, conversion to RYGB

Whipple Resection

Clinical Vignette

A 62-year-old woman is evaluated for jaundice, dark urine, and weight loss of 4.5 kg over the previous 2 months. Her past medical history is unremarkable. She takes no prescription or over-the-counter medications. Physical examination shows conjunctival icterus and a painless palpable gallbladder (Courvoisier's sign). Laboratory tests reveal a serum total bilirubin level of 6 mg dl^{-1} (direct 5.2 mg dl^{-1}) and alkaline phosphatase 280 U l^{-1}. The remainder of the routine laboratory tests are normal. Abdominal CT reveals a 3-cm mass in the head of the pancreas and dilated intra- and extra-hepatic bile ducts. An EUS-guided biopsy of the mass confirms adenocarcinoma. The tumor does not involve lymph nodes or invade vascular structures or distant organs.

Procedure

- A Whipple resection is a pancreaticoduodenoctomy (Figure 4.10).
- A conventional Whipple resection involves resection of the head and uncinate process of the pancreas, distal third (antrum and pylorus) of the stomach, duodenum, gallbladder, and distal bile duct.

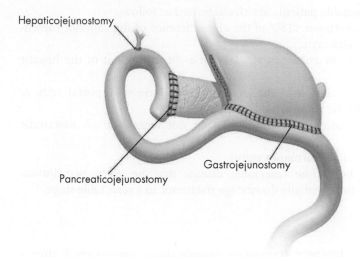

Figure 4.10 **Whipple resection.**

- A pylorus-preserving Whipple resection, which marks the proximal resection line 3–4 cm distal to the pylorus, may be employed for benign disease or for small periampullary tumors, and is thought to improve long-term upper GI function and potentially mitigate dumping syndrome.
- Three anastomoses are created to restore intestinal continuity:
  - End-to-side gastrojejunostomy.
  - End-to-side hepaticojejunostomy.
  - End-to-end or end-to-side pancreaticojejunostomy.

Indications

- A malignant tumor of the head of the pancreas is the most common indication for performing a Whipple resection:
  - Resectability of a malignant lesion is determined by the absence of invasion of surrounding arteries and lack of distant metastatic spread.
  - Unlike arterial invasion, invasion of the portal venous structures is no longer considered an absolute contraindication to resection because harvested vein grafts or prosthetic vascular conduits may be used to re-establish portal blood flow.
- Other reasons for performing a Whipple resection include duodenal tumors, symptomatic benign tumors of the head of the pancreas, chronic pancreatitis, and premalignant or malignant lesions of the ampulla of Vater or distal bile duct.

- Borderline resectable patients are characterized as follows:
- Tumor-artery abutment ≤180° of the circumference of the superior mesenteric artery or celiac axis.
- Tumor abutment or encasement >180° of a short segment of the hepatic artery.
- Short-segment occlusion of the superior mesenteric vein, portal vein, or superior mesenteric vein-portal vein confluence.
- MRI and CT findings suspicious for, but not diagnostic of, metastatic disease.
- Marginal physical performance status.
- Patients with borderline resectable disease may be given neoadjuvant chemotherapy to potentially downstage the tumor to a resectable stage.

Complications

- The two most frequent immediate complications encountered after a Whipple resection are delayed gastric emptying and pancreatic fistula formation.
  - Up to 25% of patients experience delayed gastric emptying after a Whipple resection. Delayed gastric emptying is diagnosed by the requirement for a nasogastric tube for more than 10 postoperative days as well as continued inability to tolerate oral feeding on postoperative day 14. Delayed gastric emptying is managed with a nasojejunal tube, gastrojejunal tube, or total parental nutrition. Gastric emptying is restored in 4–6 weeks in most patients. Persistent delayed gastric emptying beyond this timeframe may require evaluation for mechanical obstruction or the need for surgical feeding access.
  - Pancreatic fistula is defined by leakage of pancreatic secretions into the surgical bed, as confirmed by a fluid collection and an elevated serum amylase level. A fistula is often suspected because of a large output from surgical drains. A fistula is more common in patients having a Whipple resection for causes other than a malignant pancreatic head mass. Patients with a pancreatic fistula are at higher risk of developing a biliary fistula, bile leak, intra-abdominal abscess, and prolonged hospitalization, and they therefore have an increased mortality rate.
- Postoperative gastrointestinal or drain tract bleeding should be evaluated quickly, because these complications could serve as herald signals for a gastroduodenal stump blowout. Interventional radiology can help isolate vascular sources of bleeding, detect pseudoaneurysms, and often embolize the bleeding vessels.

- Long-term complications of a Whipple resection are generally related to reduced exocrine and endocrine function of the remaining pancreas.
  - Patients with diabetes mellitus prior to the procedure often require escalating therapy for glucose control. Those without diabetes mellitus preoperatively typically develop glucose intolerance or diabetes mellitus postoperatively.
  - Intestinal malabsorption of fat (including fat-soluble vitamins A, D, E, and K) can occur due to the lack of exocrine pancreatic enzymes, with resulting steatorrhea and malnutrition. Pancreatic enzyme and vitamin supplements should be provided routinely to patients who have undergone a Whipple resection.
  - All patients who have undergone a Whipple procedure should be prescribed supplementation of iron, calcium, and copper, which are normally absorbed in the duodenum.

Pearls

- When evaluating a patient after any gastrointestinal surgical procedure, it is important to understand the anatomy and the physiologic consequences. For example, a RYGB or Whipple resection leads to absent duodenal nutrient absorption and therefore to micronutrient (e.g., iron, calcium) deficiency.
- Most patients with peptic ulcer disease are now effectively treated with a combination of endoscopic procedures, aggressive acid suppression, avoidance of nonsteroidal anti-inflammatory drugs, and eradication of *Helicobacter pylori*. Persistent ulcer disease not responsive to conservative management or complications of peptic ulcer disease can be treated with either a Billroth I or II procedure.
- The RYGB remains the 'gold standard' for weight-loss surgery because it leads to persistent and predictable weight loss, but the sleeve gastrectomy has surpassed the Roux-en-Y gastric bypass in popularity because of its lower morbidity despite less predictable weight loss. The LAGB is associated with band erosion into the stomach and is now utilized less frequently.
- A Whipple resection, most commonly performed for pancreatic adenocarcinoma, entails an extensive resection that leaves patients with consequences from altered gastrointestinal luminal anatomy as well as pancreatic exocrine and endocrine deficiencies.
- Patient selection is critical for a good outcome from any surgical procedure; understanding the indications while explaining possible complications and side effects of a procedure to the patient will help create reasonable expectations.

Questions

1 A surgeon is consulted on a patient with dysphagia and weight loss despite maximum gastric acid suppressive therapy. Upper endoscopy is unremarkable. The surgeon agrees with the gastroenterologist's concern for achalasia. Which combination of diagnostic tests and therapeutic procedures is indicated?
   A Esophageal manometry and Nissen fundoplication.
   B Esophageal manometry and Heller cardiomyotomy.
   C Bravo pH probe and Heller cardiomyotomy.
   D Barium esophagogram and Heller cardiomyotomy.
   E Barium esophagogram and Nissen fundoplication.

2 A 42-year-old man is diagnosed with gastric adenocarcinoma. Four weeks after curative surgery, he presents with palpitations, headache, and light-headedness that occur approximately 30 minutes after each meal. Which of the following is the most appropriate recommendation for this patient?
   A Referral to a cardiologist.
   B High-caloric, large meals
   C Frequent, small meals with reduced simple carbohydrates.
   D Referral for exploratory laparotomy.
   E Referral to a neurologist.

3 A 19-year-old college football player presents to the emergency department with melena and fatigue. He had been taking ibuprofen 1–2 g every 6 hours following a knee injury. Upper endoscopy reveals a large ulcer in the duodenal bulb without bleeding stigmata but with surrounding edema creating gastric outlet obstruction. Despite intensive gastric acid suppression with a proton pump inhibitor (PPI) for 8 weeks, as well as empiric antibiotic therapy to eradicate *Helicobacter pylori,* he develops refractory nausea and vomiting, followed by recurrent melena and fatigue. Imaging studies are consistent with gastric outlet obstruction. Which of the following surgical procedures should be considered?
   A Billroth I gastroenterostomy.
   B Billroth II gastroenterostomy.
   C Whipple resection.
   D Roux-en-Y bypass.
   E Heller cardiomyotomy.

4 Which of the following interventions in a morbidly obese person results in the most predictable and sustained weight loss?

    A Laparoscopic gastric band.
    B Roux-en-Y bypass surgery.
    C Sleeve gastrectomy.
    D 800-kcal diet and intensive exercise program.

5   A 53-year-old woman is lost to follow-up after gastric bypass surgery until she presents years later with numbness in her fingertips, fatigue, and confusion. Which of the following tests will likely reveal the cause of her symptoms?
    A Serum vitamin B_{12} level.
    B Serum thyroid-stimulating hormone level.
    C Serum protein electrophoresis.
    D Hemoglobin A1c level.
    E Serum folic acid level.

Answers

1   B
    Esophageal manometry, if available, is the 'gold standard' test for diagnosing achalasia. Characteristic manometric findings in achalasia are aperistalsis of the esophagus and a high resting lower esophageal sphincter (LES) pressure. A Heller cardiomyotomy, which divides the LES muscle fibers, is curative. After a myotomy, the fibers of the LES are nonfunctional, and gastroesophageal reflux frequently occurs. Therefore, most surgeons also perform a fundoplication of 180–270°to decrease the frequency of reflux.

2   C
    The patient likely has early dumping syndrome following a Billroth gastrectomy to resect the tumor. Dumping syndrome results from rapid gastric emptying that leads to fluid shifts into the small intestine as a result of high-caloric luminal contents. Smaller meals with reduced simple carbohydrates that result in lower osmolality are recommended to alleviate symptoms. The patient does not need referral to a cardiologist, neurologist, or surgeon at this time. Large meals will worsen his symptoms.

3   B
    A Billroth II gastroenterostomy includes resection of the duodenal bulb and gastric pylorus and antrum, and is appropriate treatment for refractory gastric outlet obstruction. A Billroth I gastroenterostomy involves resection the gastric antrum and pylorus, which may not be sufficient in this patient. The other procedures are not indicated for complicated ulcer disease.

4　B

The Roux-en-Y bypass surgery remains the 'gold standard' weight-loss procedure due to its restrictive and malabsorptive effects. The laparoscopic adjustable gastric banding (LAGB) and sleeve gastrectomy are both restrictive procedures and do not result in malabsorption.

5　A

This patient likely has vitamin B_{12} deficiency as a result of the gastric bypass surgery. Parietal cells synthesize intrinsic factor, which is required for intestinal absorption of vitamin B_{12}. Although other diseases such as hyper- or hypothyroidism, multiple myeloma, and diabetes mellitus may cause the symptoms experienced by this patient, the most likely cause after weight-loss surgery is vitamin B_{12} deficiency. Other micronutrient deficiencies such as copper deficiency should be considered.

Further Reading

Bumm, R. and Siewert, J.R. (2012) Distal gastrectomy with Billroth I or Billroth II reconstruction, in *Fischer's Mastery of Surgery*, 6th edition, (ed. J. Fischer), Lippincott Williams & Wilkins, Philadelphia, pp. 986–1002.

Schwaitzberg, S. (2016) Surgical management of gastroesophageal reflux in adults. https://www.uptodate.com/contents/surgical-management-of-gastroesophageal-reflux-in-adults?source=search_result&search=surgical+gastroesophageal+reflux&selectedTitle=1%7E150

Weblinks

http://www.merckmanuals.com/professional/sec01/ch006/ch006b.html
http://www.win.niddk.nih.gov/publications/gastric.htm
http://www.nlm.nih.gov/medlineplus/ency/article/002925.htm
http://emedicine.medscape.com/article/173594-overview

5

Acute Diarrhea

Jan-Michael A. Klapproth

Clinical Vignette

A 68-year-old recently retired man presents with a 7-day history of acute watery diarrhea and associated intermittent cramping and bloating with abdominal distention. He describes four to six watery, floating, malodorous bowel movements per day and has at least two additional bowel movements at night that awaken him from sleep. In addition, he has malaise. The patient decided to seek medical advice after an episode of incontinence. Three days before the onset of symptoms, he returned from a cruise that took him to Stockholm, Helsinki, and Saint Petersburg. During the trip, he ate at local restaurants with his travel companions, none of whom developed similar symptoms. He denies sick contact, fever, chills, bleeding, or skin symptoms. His past medical history is positive for hypertension, diabetes mellitus controlled by diet, and hyperlipidemia. Current medications include lisinopril, aspirin, and atorvastatin. He drinks a glass of wine with dinner and is a lifetime nonsmoker. The patient's vital signs are normal. The abdomen is distended and tympanic with hyperactive bowel sounds, but nontender to deep palpation. The remainder of his physical examination is unremarkable, including a normal-sized liver and undetectable spleen tip.

Definition

- Diarrhea is defined as the passage of stools of abnormally loose consistency, usually associated with excessive frequency of defecation (three or more stools per day) and with excessive stool output (>0.21 per day).

Sitaraman and Friedman's Essentials of Gastroenterology, Second Edition.
Edited by Shanthi Srinivasan and Lawrence S. Friedman.
© 2018 John Wiley & Sons Ltd. Published 2018 by John Wiley & Sons Ltd.

- Acute diarrhea is defined as diarrhea of ≤14 days' duration, persistent diarrhea as lasting between 14 and 30 days, and chronic diarrhea as lasting longer than one month.

Epidemiology

- In the US, acute diarrhea caused by 31 major pathogens accounts for 9.4 million episodes, 55 961 hospitalizations, and 1351 deaths per year.
- Additional unspecified agents causing acute diarrhea are responsible for approximately 38.4 million episodes of foodborne illnesses in the US, resulting in 71 878 hospitalizations and 1686 deaths.

Etiology

- More than 90% of cases of acute diarrhea are caused by infections of the gastrointestinal tract with bacteria, viruses, protozoa, or parasites.
- Other causes include food allergies and medications.
- In addition, diseases associated with chronic diarrhea such as inflammatory bowel disease (IBD), celiac disease, and intestinal ischemia may present with an acute onset of diarrhea (see Chapter 6).

Pathogenesis

- Pathogens cause diarrhea by one or more of the following mechanisms:
  - Production of enterotoxin, cytotoxin, or preformed toxin:
    - Enterotoxins induce fluid secretion by activation of intracellular signaling pathways (e.g., adenylate cyclase) without causing damage to the mucosa (e.g., *Vibrio cholerae*).
    - Cytotoxins induce fluid secretion and cause damage to the mucosa (e.g., *Clostridium difficile*).
    - Preformed toxins induce rapid fluid secretion (e.g., *Staphylococcus aureus*).
  - Adherence to the mucosa: some bacteria adhere to the mucosa and elicit fluid secretion without elaborating toxins (e.g., enteroadherent *Escherichia coli*, enteropathogenic *E. coli*).
  - Invasion of the mucosa: some organisms invade the epithelial cells and lamina propria, where they elicit an inflammatory response (e.g., *Salmonella* spp., *Shigella* spp.).
- A number of host factors determine the severity of illness once exposure to a pathogen has occurred. These include age, personal hygiene, gastric acidity, intestinal motility, enteric microflora, immune status, and expression of intestinal receptors for enterotoxins.

Classification

Acute diarrhea may be classified as watery or inflammatory.

Watery Diarrhea

- Watery diarrhea implies a defect primarily in water and electrolyte absorption.
- Pathogens that cause watery diarrhea usually infect the small intestine. They adhere to the mucosal surface without invading the epithelium or produce enterotoxins that result in minimal or no mucosal inflammation.
- Patients usually present with large-volume, watery stools without blood, pus, or severe abdominal pain.
- Watery diarrhea has the potential to result in profound dehydration.
- Typically, fever and signs of systemic illness are absent.
- Diarrhea may be accompanied by nausea and vomiting.
- Examples of pathogens that cause watery diarrhea include viruses (rotavirus, norovirus), enterotoxigenic *E. coli, Vibrio cholerae, Staphylococcus aureus, Clostridium perfringens, Giardia lamblia,* and *Cryptosporidium* spp.
- Patients who present with watery diarrhea are treated with rehydration and, in general, do not require extensive evaluation to identify the cause.

Inflammatory Diarrhea

- Inflammatory diarrhea results from direct invasion of the intestinal mucosa by pathogens, and/or from cytotoxins produced by the pathogens and elicit an inflammatory response. The inflammatory response leads to mucosal damage and ulcerations, usually in the colon, resulting in loss of mucus, serum proteins, and blood into the lumen.
- Inflammatory diarrhea is characterized by blood and/or mucus in stool and tenesmus.
- Patients with inflammatory diarrhea usually present with numerous small-volume stools that may be mucoid, grossly bloody, or both.
- Patients usually are febrile and may have signs of systemic illness, such as fever, rash, or joint symptoms.
- Patients are less likely to be dehydrated due to the small stool volumes.
- Examples of microbes that cause inflammatory diarrhea include *Shigella* spp., *Campylobacter* spp., enterohemorrhagic *E. coli, C. difficile, Salmonella* spp., *Yersinia* spp., *and Entamoeba histolytica.*

> Pathogens that cause watery diarrhea typically affect the small bowel, and the diarrhea is caused by altered electrolyte secretion or absorption by an enterotoxin elaborated by the organism. By contrast, inflammatory diarrhea is caused by invasive pathogens that usually infect the colon.

Clinical Features

History

- A thorough history is the cornerstone of the diagnosis of acute diarrhea, and should include the number of daily bowel movements, their consistency and volume, the duration of illness, the presence of blood, mucus, tenesmus, urgency, nocturnal bowel movements, and associated symptoms such as abdominal pain, nausea, vomiting, and fever.
- The history should also include recent travel, previous episodes of acute diarrhea, foods consumed, hospitalizations, exposure to pets and livestock, sick contacts, and possible community outbreaks.
- A number of medications can cause diarrhea, and a thorough history of prescription, over-the-counter, and herbal medication use should be obtained. Examples of medications associated with diarrhea include antibiotics, antacids, colchicine, laxatives, misoprostol, nonsteroidal anti-inflammatory drugs, and olsalazine.
- Comorbid conditions such as vascular disease, collagen vascular diseases, hyperthyroidism, IBD, and human immunodeficiency virus (HIV) infection should be elicited.

Physical Examination

- Physical findings in patients with acute diarrhea are most useful in determining the severity of diarrhea. Patients should be assessed for fever and signs of dehydration such as hypotension, tachycardia, loss of skin turgor, sunken eyes, and dry conjunctivae and mucous membranes.

> Most cases of infectious diarrhea are brief and self-limited, and patients do not seek medical attention. For patients who present to a healthcare provider, a thorough history and physical examination are the cornerstones of diagnosis and of determining the severity and presence of complications and whether diagnostic testing is needed (and, if so, which tests should be used). Diagnostic testing should be kept to a minimum, and treatment should focus on rehydration.

Diagnosis

- Most cases of acute diarrhea are self-limited and do not require further diagnostic testing. Indications for further diagnostic testing are outlined in Table 5.1.
- Complete blood count: leukocytosis usually indicates a bacterial cause of diarrhea, but neutropenia can be caused by *Salmonella typhi* and *Shigella* ssp. Anemia may be associated with an invasive organism.

Table 5.1 Indications for diagnostic testing in patients with acute diarrhea.

- Large-volume diarrhea with dehydration
- Severe abdominal pain
- >3 days of symptoms
- Bloody diarrhea
- Fever >101.5 °F (38.5 °C)
- Recent history of international travel
- Extremes of age (infancy, old age)
- Diabetes mellitus
- Immunodeficiency state (acquired immunodeficiency syndrome, immunosuppressive medications, chemotherapy)
- Malignancy

- Serum electrolytes, blood urea nitrogen, and creatinine are useful for assessing dehydration.
- Stool culture for bacteria should be performed in selected patients (see Table 5.2):
  - A stool culture is positive in only 1.5–3% of cases, and the cost is $427 for every positive test.
- Testing of stool for ova and parasites is indicated in immunocompromised patients, homosexual persons, persons who have been in a daycare center, and those who have been on a camping trip or who have traveled to a developing country.
- A stool test for *C. difficile* toxin A and B by enzyme-linked immunoassay (ELISA) is indicated in persons with the recent use of antibiotics, IBD, diarrhea developing during hospitalization or subsequent to discharge, and immunocompromised persons.
- Fecal leukocytes are helpful in differentiating inflammatory diarrhea from watery diarrhea. Invasive organisms typically produce large quantities of fecal leukocytes.
- Endoscopy: unprepared flexible sigmoidoscopy or colonoscopy and/or upper endoscopy with duodenal biopsy are indicated in patients with persistent symptoms.

Treatment

Fluid Therapy

- Rehydration and replacement of electrolytes remain mainstays of the treatment of acute diarrhea. Oral rehydration solutions are typically used; however, intravenous fluid replacement may be needed in severe cases.

Table 5.2 Specific causes of acute diarrhea.

Causative agent	Characteristics	Setting, risk factors	Clinical features	Diagnosis	Treatment
Viruses					
Rotavirus	Most common cause of diarrhea in children <2 years of age	Daycare centers, hospitals	Large-volume, watery diarrhea	Clinical suspicion	Self-limited disease, supportive management. Rotavirus vaccine recommended for all infants
Norovirus	Any age	Outbreaks on cruise ships, at banquets. Consumption of raw oysters	Large-volume, watery diarrhea	Clinical suspicion	Self-limited disease, supportive management
Bacteria					
Campylobacter jejuni	Most common cause of acute bacterial diarrhea in the US	Consumption of contaminated poultry, meat, raw milk, eggs	Fever, watery or bloody diarrhea, malaise, abdominal cramps. Complications include Guillain–Barré syndrome, reactive arthritis	Stool culture	Mild–moderate disease is self-limited. For severe disease or symptoms >1 week, a macrolide (erythromycin, azithromycin) is the drug of choice.
Clostridium difficile	Most common nosocomial infection. Produces cytotoxins	Increasing age, recent antibiotic use, IBD	Fever, abdominal pain, bloody diarrhea	Stool test for toxins A and B by ELISA	Metronidazole, vancomycin

Organism	Characteristics	Source	Clinical features	Diagnosis	Treatment
Enterotoxigenic *E. coli*, enteropathogenic *E. coli*, enteroaggregative *E. coli*	Mediated by enterotoxin or adherence to brush border epithelial cells. Developing countries. Increased risk in children <2 years of age and immunocompromised hosts	Fecal contamination of food, poor hygiene	Watery diarrhea that occurs within 2 days of ingesting contaminated food and resolves within 3 days	Clinical suspicion	Supportive management. A fluoroquinolone, trimethoprim–sulfamethoxazole, azithromycin, or rifaximin for severe disease
Enteroinvasive *E. coli* and enterohemorrhagic *E. coli* (*E. coli* O157:H7)	Invasive, produces cytotoxin	Consumption of contaminated beef, pesto, alfalfa sprouts	Fever, abdominal cramps, tenesmus, rectal prolapse, bloody diarrhea. Complications include toxic megacolon, sepsis, perforation, thrombotic thrombocytopenic purpura, hemolytic uremic syndrome	Stool culture	Supportive management. Antibiotics and antimotility agents should be avoided
Listeria monocytogenes	Noninvasive or invasive. Resistant to chemical inactivation. Survives even at 4°C. Pregnant women, diabetics, and immunocompromised patients are at increased risk	Consumption of contaminated meat, chocolate milk, unpasteurized cheese	Watery diarrhea, nausea, vomiting, myalgias, arthralgias. Complications include sepsis, meningoencephalitis	Stool culture on selective medium; blood or cerebrospinal fluid cultures	Treatment for severe disease or systemic illness: ampicillin, penicillin G, trimethoprim–sulfamethoxazole.

(Continued)

Table 5.2 (Continued)

Causative agent	Characteristics	Setting, risk factors	Clinical features	Diagnosis	Treatment
Salmonella enteritidis, S. typhimurium, S. Heidelberg, S. Newport, S. typhi	Invasive	Consumption of contaminated poultry, egg yolks, fresh produce, ground beef, milk	Enterocolitis: watery or bloody diarrhea, fever, malaise. Complications include sepsis, meningitis, endovascular lesions. Typhoid fever (caused by *S. typhi*): fever, chills, abdominal pain, rose spots	Blood and stool cultures	Enterocolitis: self-limited illness. Antibiotics indicated for severe disease, systemic symptoms, comorbid conditions: a fluoroquinolone, macrolide, or third-generation cephalosporin. Typhoid fever: a fluoroquinolone
Shigella sonnei, S. flexneri, S. dysenteriae, S. boydii	Invasive, produces enterotoxin. Requires <100 organisms to cause infection	Consumption of undercooked food, contaminated water	Fever, abdominal cramps, tenesmus, rectal prolapse, bloody diarrhea. Complications include toxic megacolon, sepsis, perforation, thrombotic thrombocytopenic purpura, hemolytic uremic syndrome	Stool culture	Antibiotics always recommended: azithromycin, trimethoprim-sulfamethoxazole, a fluoroquinolone, third-generation cephalosporin, rifaximin
Vibrio cholerae	Noninvasive small bowel pathogen that induces cAMP production with subsequent Cl secretion	Consumption of contaminated water	Massive watery diarrhea	Stool culture	Rehydration

Non-cholera vibrios: *Vibrio vulnificus*, *V. parahemolyticus*	Patients with chronic liver disease and iron overload are at highest risk	Consumption of undercooked shellfish	Bloody diarrhea, fever, abdominal cramps	Stool culture	Supportive management
Yersinia enterocolitica, *Y. pseudotuberculosis*	Uncommon in US; common in Northern Europe	Consumption of contaminated milk products, pork (chitterlings)	Bloody diarrhea, right lower quadrant pain (may mimic appendicitis or Crohn's disease), fever. Complications include reactive arthritis, erythema nodosum, myocarditis, osteomyelitis, nephritis	Stool culture	Antibiotics only for severe cases or complications: a fluoroquinolone, trimethoprim–sulfamethoxazole, or doxycycline plus an aminoglycoside
Parasites					
Entameba histolytica	Developing countries	Consumption of contaminated food	Abdominal pain and bloody diarrhea, possibly alternating with constipation. Majority of infected persons are asymptomatic. Complications include liver abscess	Stool examination for trophozoites; serologic testing for antibody in serum by immunofluorescence or hemagglutination	Metronidazole, followed by iodoquinol or paromomycin
Cyclospora cayetanensis	Intracellular pathogen, villous atrophy	Outbreaks due to raspberries from Guatemala, travel to Nepal. Reported in hospital workers in Chicago	Profuse, prolonged diarrhea, nausea, abdominal cramps	Oocysts in stool, blue autofluorescence when examined by ultraviolet epifluorescence microscopy	Trimethoprim–sulfamethoxazole

(Continued)

Table 5.2 (Continued)

Causative agent	Characteristics	Setting, risk factors	Clinical features	Diagnosis	Treatment
Cryptosporidium parvum	Resistant to chemical inactivation	Immunocompromised hosts	Profuse, prolonged diarrhea	Acid-fast stain, immunofluorescence of stool sample, polymerase chain reaction testing	Paromomycin, nitazoxanide, azithromycin
Giardia lamblia	Chronic infection in patients who are immunodeficient. Recurrent disease in 15%	Found in mountain streams. Men who have sex with men are at increased risk	Explosive fatty diarrhea, abdominal distention	Stool ELISA (30% positive), immunofluorescence, duodenal aspiration	Metronidazole, nitazoxanide, quinacrine
Isospora belli	Intracellular pathogen causing villous atrophy	Immunocompromised hosts. May cause self-limited diarrhea in immunocompetent persons	Acute and chronic diarrhea	Stool microscopy, small bowel biopsy	Trimethoprim–sulfamethoxazole, metronidazole and pyrimethamine for persons with a sulfa allergy
Microsporidia	Intracellular pathogen causing villous atrophy	Opportunistic infection	Watery diarrhea, nausea, malabsorption	Modified trichrome stain of stool sample	Albendazole

cAMP, cyclic adenosine monophosphate; *E. coli*, *Escherichia coli*; ELISA, enzyme-linked immunosorbent assay; IBD, inflammatory bowel disease.

Diet

- Soft, easily digestible foods are most acceptable to a patient with acute diarrhea.
- Caffeinated products, chewing gum, and alcohol should be avoided.
- Milk and milk products should also be avoided because secondary lactase deficiency may occur during an episode of acute diarrhea. In some persons secondary lactase deficiency and intolerance to lactose-containing food may persist for up to 1 year.
- Oral rehydration solution (ORS): contains sodium 60–75 mEq l^{-1} and glucose 75–90 mmol l^{-1}; prevents death from acute diarrhea in the elderly, since 80% of deaths in the US caused by acute diarrhea occur in the elderly.

Antibiotics

- Fewer than 10% of patients with an acute diarrheal illness benefit from the use of antibiotics. Antibiotics are not indicated for community-acquired diarrhea, because the vast majority of cases are due to viruses (norovirus, adenovirus, rotavirus).
- Travelers who self-medicate with antibiotics for acute diarrhea due to β-lactamase-producing *Enterobacteria* spp. become colonized with these organisms, thereby promoting the distribution of antibiotic resistance.
- Infections caused by *Shigella* spp., enteroinvasive *E. coli, C. difficile, V. cholerae, E. histolytica*, and *G. lamblia*, and some cases of *Salmonella* infection as well as traveler's diarrhea, benefit from antimicrobial treatment.
- Antibiotics may also benefit patients with prolonged infection caused by *Salmonella, Campylobacter, Aeromonas*, or *Plesiomonas* spp.
- Empiric treatment with a fluoroquinolone (ciprofloxacin, ofloxacin, norfloxacin) is recommended for patients with traveler's diarrhea, patients with fever and bloody diarrhea, immunocompromised patients, those >65 years of age, and those with diarrhea that lasts >3 days and associated with one or more of the following: abdominal pain; fever; vomiting; myalgias; or headache.
- *Campylobacter* is fluoroquinolone-resistant and should be treated with a macrolide (e.g., azithromycin).

Antidiarrheals and Antimotility Agents

- Antidiarrheal or antimotility agents should be used only in patients who have no fever, fecal leukocytes, or increased peripheral white blood cell count.
- Diphenoxylate–atropine, tincture of opium, codeine, and paregoric are commonly used agents (see Chapter 6).
- Bismuth subsalicylate is used for mild to moderate traveler's diarrhea, controlling bowel movement frequency.

- Loperamide in conjunction with antibiotics for traveler's diarrhea decreases duration of diarrhea and promotes clinical improvement.

Probiotics

- Evidence supports the use of probiotics to prevent antibiotic-associated diarrhea with a relative risk reduction of 0.58 and number needed to treat 13, but not diarrhea due to other causes.

Diarrheal Syndromes

Traveler's Diarrhea

- Most frequently caused by enterotoxigenic *E. coli* and to a lesser extent *Shigella* spp., *Campylobacter* spp., *Vibrio* spp., *Salmonella* spp., *Cyclospora cayetanensis*, *G. lamblia*, *Crystosporidium* spp., *E. histolytica*, rotavirus, and norovirus.
- Affects 20–50% of all travelers, predominantly during visits to Latin America, Africa, the Middle East, and Asia.
- Pathogens are usually transmitted through the fecal–oral route. Risk factors include improper disposal of feces, lack of proper hand washing following defecation by food handlers, improper food hygiene, inadequate preservation of food, and consumption of contaminated water.
- Symptoms include the abrupt onset of self-limited watery diarrhea with four to five bowel movements per day within 12–72 hours of ingesting food containing the pathogen.
- Diagnosis is based on history.
- Bismuth subsalicylate may be used for prophylaxis. Bismuth should be used with caution if the patient is allergic to aspirin, pregnant, or taking other medications concomitantly.
- Rehydration is the mainstay of treatment. Empiric treatment with a fluoroquinolone (e.g., ciprofloxacin 500 mg twice daily for 3–5 days) is indicated for patients with three or more loose stools over 8 hours associated with nausea, vomiting, abdominal cramps, fever, or bloody bowel movements.

Food Poisoning

- More than 250 infectious agents have been implicated; the most frequent causes are *E. coli* O157:H7, *Campylobacter jejuni*, *Salmonella* spp., *Shigella* spp., *Listeria monocytogenes*, *S. aureus*, *Bacillus cereus*, scombroid poisoning, and ciguatera fish poisoning.
- Causes 9.4 million illnesses per year in the US.

- Incubation period is 4–6 hours for *S. aureus* and *Bacillus cereus*, 8–12 hours for *Clostridium perfringens*, and 14 hours for invasive pathogens (e.g., *Salmonella* spp.).
- Symptoms include nausea, vomiting, diarrhea within minutes (scombroid) to 72 hours after consumption of the contaminated food.
- Most cases are self-limited. Rehydration is the mainstay of treatment. Ciprofloxacin (500 mg twice daily for 3–5 days) may be used for severe symptoms (nausea, vomiting, abdominal cramps, fever, or bloody bowel movements). Antibiotics should be considered only in patients in whom *E. coli* O157:H7 has been ruled out.
- Ciguatera fish poisoning is the most common nonbacterial food-borne disease:
  - Dinoflagellates such as *Gambierdiscus toxicus* produce ciguatoxin, which enters the food chain through tropical fish that are later eaten.
  - Symptoms include bradycardia, hypotension, perioral tingling, fever, dysesthesias, myalgias, and arthralgias within 30 minutes to 12 hours of consuming contaminated fish; residual symptoms may linger for years.
  - Ciguatera food poisoning is reported to be associated with chronic fatigue syndrome.
  - The diagnosis is made by detecting the toxin in contaminated fish.
- Scombroid poisoning (also called histamine fish poisoning):
  - Acute onset of peppery, metallic taste, oral numbness, headache, and occasional diarrhea that begin within minutes of ingesting contaminated fish. Symptoms resolve within 24 hours.

Nosocomial Diarrhea

- *C. difficile* is the main cause of nosocomial diarrhea in developed countries.
- *C. difficile* is an anaerobic, Gram-positive, spore-forming bacillus.
- The prevalence and mortality related to *C. difficile* colitis have increased substantially due to the emergence of a virulent strain of *C. difficile* designated NAP1/027. This strain harbors mutations that confer antibiotic (fluoroquinolone) resistance, result in increased toxin A and B production, and facilitate sporulation of the bacterium.
- The single most important risk factor for *C. difficile* infection is antimicrobial therapy. Any antimicrobial agent has the potential to cause *C. difficile* infection; antimicrobial agents that are most frequently associated with *C. difficile* infection include amoxicillin or ampicillin, cephalosporins, clindamycin, and fluoroquinolones.
- Other risk factors for *C. difficile* infection include increasing age, hospitalization, chemotherapy, HIV infection, and IBD.
- *C. difficile* colitis is caused by toxin A and toxin B produced by the organism. These toxins bind to, and are internalized by, colonocytes and elicit an inflammatory response. Several host factors, particularly the immune

response to *C. difficile* toxins, determine whether a person remains an asymptomatic carrier or develops colitis.

- The clinical presentation ranges from asymptomatic carriage to life-threatening pseudomembranous colitis. Typical symptoms include fever, abdominal pain, and bloody diarrhea.
- The diagnosis is made by the detection of toxin A and B in a stool sample. Flexible sigmoidoscopy or colonoscopy is usually not required to make the diagnosis but, when performed, may reveal characteristic pseudomembranes (yellow, gray, or white plaques 2–5 mm in diameter). Histologic examination of the colonic mucosa may show focal ulceration associated with the eruption of inflammatory cells and necrotic debris that covers the area of ulceration, a constellation of findings called the 'volcano lesion' (see Chapter 28).
- Treatment:
  - Discontinue the precipitating antibiotic if possible. In 20–25% of cases, C. *difficile* infection may resolve without further intervention.
  - Metronidazole, 250–500 mg orally three to four times a day for 10–14 days, is the drug of choice for mild–moderate colitis.
  - Vancomycin, 125–500 mg orally four times a day for 10–14 days, may be used in patients with severe colitis, those who are unable to tolerate metronidazole, pregnant women, children <10 years of age, or patients in whom diarrhea does not improve with metronidazole.
  - The response rate to metronidazole or vancomycin is 90–97%.
  - *C. difficile* infection may relapse in up to 20% of patients. Relapse is treated with metronidazole or vancomycin in a tapering schedule. Additional options include probiotics (*Saccharomyces boulardii* or *Lactobacillus* spp.) with and following metronidazole or vancomycin, intravenous immunoglobulin, rifampin, cholestyramine in combination with vancomycin, and fidaxomicin.
  - Fecal microbial transplantation is occasionally performed in patients with repeated recurrences of *C. difficile* colitis.

Pearls

- Most cases of acute diarrhea are a result of an infection; however, a specific organism can be identified in only a minority of cases.
- Most episodes of acute diarrhea are self-limited, and investigations should be performed only if the results will influence management and outcome.
- A thorough history and physical examination enable the clinician to classify an acute diarrheal illness, assess its severity, and determine whether further investigations are needed.
- Antibiotic therapy is not required in most patients with an acute diarrheal illness. Therapy should be directed mainly to preventing dehydration.

Questions

Questions 1 and 2 relate to the clinical vignette at the beginning of this chapter.

1 The patient's laboratory test results, including a complete blood cell count and comprehensive metabolic profile, are normal. Stool cultures, including ova and parasites, are pending. Which of the following should be prescribed next?
A Ciprofloxacin.
B *Lactobacillus acidophilus.*
C Amoxicillin.
D Metronidazole.
E No drug therapy is indicated.

2 The patient returns for a follow-up outpatient visit four weeks later. He states that his symptoms improved initially, but he then developed recurrent symptoms. He reports four to six bowel movements each day without blood and at least one to two bowel movements at night. He has rectal urgency and tenesmus and has had a weight loss of 6 lb (2.7 kg). He has cramping abdominal pain but denies nausea, vomiting, or fever. A repeat complete blood count and comprehensive metabolic profile are normal. Stool cultures for enteric pathogens and an ELISA for *Clostridium difficile* toxin are negative, but an ELISA for trophozoites is positive. Which of the following is the most appropriate next step in the management of this patient?
A Serum immunoglobulins.
B Upper endoscopy with small bowel biopsies.
C Culture and sensitivity testing for resistant *Giardia lamblia.*
D A prolonged course of oral metronidazole.
E Ciprofloxacin.

3 A 55-year-old man is brought to the emergency room by his wife for rapidly progressive difficulty standing upright, walking, and raising himself out of a chair. Since the previous night he has noted oropharyngeal dysphagia and double vision. He had an episode of acute diarrhea 6 weeks earlier that lasted for 7 days and was accompanied by a fever of 39 °C. On physical examination, the patient is tachypneic, tachycardic, and has an oxygen saturation of 89% on room air. Which of the following infectious agents is in the differential diagnoses?
A *Escherichia coli* O157H:7.
B *Clostridium difficile.*
C *Shigella* spp.
D *Campylobacter jejuni.*
E *Entamoeba histolytica.*

4 A 65-year-old man presents with fever, chills, and bloody diarrhea of 3 days' duration. He recently completed a course of ampicillin for otitis media. Laboratory tests show a white blood cell count of 18 000 mm^{-3}. Which of the following is the most likely cause of this patient's diarrhea?

A *Escherichia coli* O157H:7.
B *Clostridium difficile.*
C *Shigella* spp.
D *Salmonella* spp.
E *Entamoeba histolytica.*

Answers

1 D

The patient's symptoms suggest that the diarrhea is due to *Giardia lamblia*. The three most common symptoms caused by *G. lamblia* include diarrhea, malaise, and floating, malodorous stool due to intestinal malabsorption. The patient's history of visiting Saint Petersburg is an additional clue to the correct diagnosis, because the drinking water supply of that city, Lake Ladoga, is known to be contaminated with *G. lamblia*.

2 A

Infection with *G. lamblia* leads to production of serum immunoglobin (IgG) and secretory IgA antibodies against the parasite by the host. The IgA antibodies prevent *G. lamblia* from adhering to epithelial cells in the intestine. Patients with selective IgA deficiency cannot mount an IgA-mediated immune response, leading to persistence of trophozoites and re-infection that is difficult to clear with antibiotics. Therefore, serum immunoglobulin levels should be assessed in patients with refractory *G. lamblia* infection.

3 D

The history of diarrhea and fever 6 weeks earlier raises suspicion for an invasive pathogen that may lead to ascending paralysis, eye muscle weakness, and respiratory failure, all findings consistent with Guillain–Barré syndrome. The likely cause is *Campylobacter jejuni*, which induces an immune response that targets bacterial lipo-oligosaccharides and cross-reacting human peripheral nerve gangliosides GM1 and GD1a.

4 B

Although any of the listed pathogens can cause bloody diarrhea, given the history of recent ampicillin use, *Clostridium difficile* is the most likely cause of the patient's symptoms.

Further Reading

Navaneethan, U. and Giannella, R.A. (2008) Mechanisms of infectious diarrhea. *Nature Clinical Practice. Gastroenterology and Hepatology*, **5**, 637–647.

Newton, J.M. and Surawicz, C.M. (2011) Infectious gastroenteritis and colitis, in Diarrhea, 1st edition, (eds S. Guandalini and H. Vaziri), Springer Science + Business Media, New York, pp. 33–59.

Pawlowski, S.W., Warren, C.A., and Guerrant, R. (2009) Diagnosis and treatment of acute or persistent diarrhea. *Gastroenterology*, **136**, 1874–1886.

Riddle, M.S. and DuPont, H.L. (2016) ACG Clinical Guideline: Diagnosis, treatment, and prevention of acute diarrheal infections in adults. *American Journal of Gastroenterology*, **126**, 1–15.

Weblinks

http://www.bt.cdc.gov/disasters/disease/diarrheaguidelines.asp
  http://www.clevelandclinicmeded.com/medicalpubs/diseasemanagement/gastroenterology/acute-diarrhea/
  http://www.fpnotebook.com/gi/diarrhea/actdrh.htm

6

Chronic Diarrhea

Sonali S. Sakaria and Robin E. Rutherford

Clinical Vignette

A 38-year-old white woman presents with an 8-month history of gradually worsening diarrhea, weight loss, and abdominal discomfort. She describes loose stools three to four times a day. She denies blood in the stool, urgency, tenesmus, or nocturnal bowel movements. There is no history of travel or recent use of antibiotics. Her past medical history is remarkable for osteoporosis, for which she takes alendronate. Her parents are alive and healthy; her mother has had 'intestinal problems.' One of her three siblings also has similar complaints but has never seen a physician. She is married, has no children, and is a homemaker. Review of systems is remarkable for infertility, depression, and easy bruisability. Physical examination reveals a blood pressure of 109/70 mmHg, pulse rate 67/minute, and body mass index 18. She is afebrile. The remainder of the examination is unremarkable. Rectal examination reveals brown stool that is negative for occult blood. Routine laboratory tests show a normal white blood cell count, hemoglobin level of $11.1 \, g \, dl^{-1}$, mean corpuscular volume 75 fl, and normal platelet count. A comprehensive metabolic panel is notable for slightly elevated alanine aminotransferase and aspartate aminotransferase levels and a normal serum albumin level. Iron saturation is 6%. Stool culture for enteric pathogens and stool examination for ova and parasites are negative.

General

- Diarrhea is defined as the passage of stools of abnormally loose consistency, usually associated with excessive frequency of defecation (three or more stools per day) and with excessive stool output (>0.2 l per day) (see Chapter 5).

Sitaraman and Friedman's Essentials of Gastroenterology, Second Edition.
Edited by Shanthi Srinivasan and Lawrence S. Friedman.
© 2018 John Wiley & Sons Ltd. Published 2018 by John Wiley & Sons Ltd.

- Chronic diarrhea is defined as diarrhea that lasts more than 4 weeks.
- The prevalence of chronic diarrhea in the US is 5%.
- With the exception of a few infections (e.g., *Aeromonas* spp., *Yersinia* spp.), chronic diarrhea is usually not caused by an infectious agent in immuno-competent persons.

Classification and Pathophysiology

- The small intestine and colon absorb 99% of the combination of oral fluid intake and endogenous secretions from the salivary glands, stomach, liver, and pancreas, totaling 9–10 l day^{-1} (Table 6.1). Diarrhea ensues when the normal physiologic secretion or absorption process is deranged.
- Normal stool is comprised of 75% water and 25% solid, and stool output is 100–150 g day^{-1}.
- Chronic diarrhea may be classified based on stool volume (small or large volume), stool characteristics (watery, fatty, or inflammatory), or pathophysiology (osmotic or secretory). In this chapter, the classification based on stool characteristics will be used because this classification is clinically useful in that it takes into account the patient's history and simple laboratory tests and thereby focuses the differential diagnosis (Table 6.2) and allows efficient diagnosis.
  - **Inflammatory diarrhea** implies damage to gastrointestinal mucosa due to infection or inflammation, which leads to a passive loss of protein-rich fluids and a decreased ability to absorb fluids and electrolytes. Stools typically contain frank or occult blood and leukocytes. Features of osmotic, secretory, and fatty diarrhea may also be present.

Table 6.1 Daily fluid intake, secretion, and absorption along the gastrointestinal tract (in liters).

Source	Intake or secretion	Absorption
Oral intake	1–2	–
Salivary glands	0.5	–
Stomach	1–2	–
Pancreas/bile	2	–
Jejunum	–	6
Ileum	2–3	2.5
Colon	–	1.4

Table 6.2 Causes of diarrhea according to clinical presentation.

Type of diarrhea	Causes
Inflammatory diarrhea	Inflammatory bowel disease (Crohn's disease, ulcerative colitis)
	Infectious diseases (*Giardia lamblia, Aeromonas* spp., *Pleisomonas* spp.)
	Ischemic colitis
	Microscopic colitis (lymphocytic and collagenous colitis)
	Radiation enteritis
Watery diarrhea	***Osmotic***
	Carbohydrate malabsorption (lactase deficiency, pancreatic insufficiency)
	Ingestion of poorly absorbed sugars (sorbitol, lactulose)
	Ingestion of laxatives that contain magnesium, phosphate, sulfate, or lactulose
	Secretory
	Bile acid malabsorption (following surgical resection of the terminal ileum or after cholecystectomy)
	Endocrine causes:
	Hyperthyroidism
	Addison's disease
	Medications (antacids, antibiotics, antiretroviral medications, chemotherapeutic agents, mineral supplements, nonsteroidal anti-inflammatory drugs, proton pump inhibitors, quinidine, vitamins)
	Neoplasms:
	Carcinoid syndrome
	Colon cancer
	Gastrinoma
	Lymphoma
	Pheochromocytoma
	Somatostatinoma
	Vasoactive intestinal peptide (VIP)oma
	Dysmotility
	Diabetic autonomic neuropathy
	Irritable bowel syndrome
	Postsympathectomy
	Postvagotomy

(*Continued*)

Table 6.2 (Continued)

Type of diarrhea	Causes
Fatty diarrhea	*Maldigestion* Atrophic gastritis Chronic pancreatitis Bile acid deficiency (surgical resection of the terminal ileum, cirrhosis, primary sclerosing cholangitis, primary biliary cholangitis) *Malabsorption* Amyloidosis Celiac disease Chronic mesenteric ischemia Heart failure Constrictive pericarditis *Giardia* infection Lymphangectasia Mastocytosis Short bowel syndrome Small intestinal bacterial overgrowth Whipple disease

- **Watery diarrhea** implies that there is no structural damage to the intestinal mucosa. Watery diarrhea may be:
  - **Osmotic**: results from ingestion of a poorly absorbed substance. Diarrhea stops when the offending agent is stopped.
  - **Secretory**: results from a defect primarily in water absorption as a result of increased secretion or reduced absorption of electrolytes. Diarrhea continues even if there is no oral intake, and the stools are isotonic with plasma (see later).
  - **Dysmotility-related**: diarrhea is typically intermittent and may alternate with periods of constipation. The most common cause of dysmotility-related diarrhea is irritable bowel syndrome (see Chapter 7).
- **Fatty diarrhea** (also called steatorrhea) implies the presence of excess fat in stools. Fatty diarrhea results from malaborption or maldigestion of fat and other nutrients. Stools may float in the toilet bowl due to the presence of excess lipid, may appear oily, and are especially foul-smelling. The most common cause of fatty diarrhea is celiac disease.

Clinical Features

History

- The clinical history helps distinguish inflammatory, watery, and fatty diarrhea, and is one of the most important aspects in the evaluation of a patient with chronic diarrhea.
- The history should include a description of the onset (abrupt, gradual, lifelong), pattern (intermittent, continuous), and duration of symptoms.
- Epidemiologic factors such as travel, exposures to foods, source of water, and sick contacts should be identified.
- Patients should be questioned regarding symptoms of fecal incontinence (patients may mistake incontinence for diarrhea), fecal urgency, presence of nocturnal diarrhea, and persistent diarrhea despite fasting.
- Associated symptoms such as blood in the stool, abdominal pain, fever, weight loss, muscle weakness, arthralgias, and visual disturbances should be elicited.
- Aggravating factors such as diet, medication, and stress should be elicited.
- A thorough medication history including prescription, over-the-counter, and herbal medications should be obtained including the use of laxatives.
- The past medical history including surgical history or prior radiation therapy should be obtained.
- The family history should include lactose intolerance, celiac disease, inflammatory bowel disease (IBD), and cystic fibrosis.
- A history of alcohol and tobacco use should be obtained.
- Previous evaluations and therapeutic trials should be reviewed.

> A thorough history is required to: (1) differentiate 'organic' from 'functional' causes (see Chapter 7); (2) establish the type of diarrhea – inflammatory, watery, or fatty; and (3) narrow the differential diagnosis. Symptoms suggestive of an organic disease include a history of diarrhea of less than 3 months' duration, nocturnal symptoms, daily symptoms, and significant weight loss.

Physical Examination

- The physical examination is normal in the majority of patients.
- Certain signs may give a clue to the cause of diarrhea:
  - dermatitis herpetiformis: celiac disease;
  - angular cheilitis: malabsorption, IBD;
  - erythema nodosum or pyoderma gangrenosum: IBD;
  - edema: protein-losing enteropathy;

- oral ulcerations: IBD;
- hyperpigmentation: Whipple disease, Addison's disease;
- wheezing: cystic fibrosis, carcinoid syndrome;
- arthritis and arthralgias: *Campylobacter jejuni* infection, common variable immunodeficiency, Whipple disease, IBD;
- fistulas or perianal abscess: Crohn's disease;
- decreased rectal sphincter tone: fecal incontinence;
- exophthalmos and lid retraction: hyperthyroidism.

Differential Diagnosis

The differential diagnosis should be narrowed based on the history and physical examination. Laboratory tests, endoscopy, and radiographic studies should be chosen selectively to confirm the suspected diagnosis (Table 6.3).

Diagnosis

Stool Tests

- Fecal occult blood testing: a positive result is suggestive of an inflammatory or invasive infectious etiology.
- Fecal leukocytes: suggestive of intestinal inflammation, ischemia, infection.
  - Techniques: Wright stain and microscopic examination, lactoferrin agglutination test.
- Fecal fat testing: performed when maldigestion or malabsorption is suspected.
  - Qualitative: a random stool sample is examined under the microscope to visualize fat globules after staining with Sudan III. Visible fat globules indicate maldigestion or malabsorption.
  - Quantitative: patients are asked to consume a diet containing 100 g of fat per day, and stool is collected for 72 hours. A stool fat concentration >8% of measured fat intake over the 3-day period or >7 g per 24 hours is consistent with malabsorption or maldigestion. A stool fat of 7–10 g per 24 hours generally indicates malabsorption due to mucosal disease, whereas a stool fat >14 g per 24 hours indicates maldigestion due to pancreatic insufficiency or bile salt deficiency.
- Fecal osmotic gap: this test is used to differentiate osmotic from secretory diarrhea. Stool sodium and potassium concentrations and osmolality are measured. Stool is isotonic with plasma; a low osmolality is suggestive of factitious diarrhea (stool mixed with water or dilute urine). Fecal osmotic gap = $290 - 2([Na^+] + [K^+])$ mOsm kg^{-1}:
  - osmotic diarrhea: osmotic gap >100 mOsm kg^{-1};
  - secretory diarrhea: osmotic gap <50 mOsm kg^{-1}.

Table 6.3 Clinical features and diagnostic work-up of chronic diarrhea.

Type of diarrhea	Clinical history	Laboratory tests	Imaging tests	Endoscopy
Inflammatory	Small volume, frank or occult blood in stool, rectal urgency, tenesmus, abdominal pain, travel, exposure to potentially unclean water	Complete blood count (anemia, leukocytosis); stool occult blood and leukocytes; stool culture, examination for ova and parasites, *Giardia* antigen	Not indicated	Flexible sigmoidoscopy or colonoscopy
Osmotic	Postprandial diarrhea, laxative use, ingestion of sugar-free food (e.g., sorbitol), secondary gain from illness, weight loss	Serum electrolytes (hypokalemia, hyponatremia), stool osmotic gap ($>100\,mOsm\,kg^{-1}$)	Lactose – hydrogen breath test may be considered	Not indicated
Secretory	Typically large-volume watery diarrhea, nocturnal diarrhea, no improvement with fasting, history of recent surgery (e.g., terminal ileal resection, cholecystectomy), use of certain medications	Comprehensive metabolic panel (hypokalemia, hyponatremia); stool osmotic gap ($<50\,mOsm\,kg^{-1}$)	Computed tomography of the abdomen (neoplasms)	Not indicated
Dysmotility	Intermittent small-volume watery diarrhea, no weight loss	Complete blood count (normal), comprehensive metabolic panel (normal)	Not indicated	Not indicated unless patient is at least 45 years of age
Fatty	Foul-smelling, sticky stool with oil droplets or food particles, weight loss, abdominal pain, history of alcohol and/or tobacco use, diabetes mellitus, prior surgical resection of bowel	Complete blood count (anemia, comprehensive metabolic panel (hypoalbuminemia), vitamin B_{12} (low) and folate (high) levels (small-intestinal bacterial overgrowth), tissue transglutaminase and endomysial antibodies (celiac disease), stool fat determination	Computed tomography of the abdomen (chronic pancreatitis, neoplasm), magnetic resonance imaging or angiography, mesenteric angiography (mesenteric ischemia)	Upper endoscopy, small-bowel biopsy and aspirate

- Stool pH:
  - pH <5.3: suggestive of carbohydrate malabsorption;
  - pH 6.0–7.5: seen in generalized malabsorptive states.
- *Clostridium difficile* toxin A and B.
- Culture: chronic diarrhea due to bacteria in immunocompetent adults is rare; bacteria such as *Aeromonas* spp. or *Pleisiomonas* spp. have been associated with chronic diarrhea in this population. A stool culture should be performed in all immunocompromised persons with chronic diarrhea (see Chapter 5).
- Ova and parasites: a fresh stool specimen should be examined for ova and parasites when indicated (e.g., history of camping, swimming in mountain streams, travel to developing countries, immunocompromise). An enzyme-linked immunosorbent assay for *Giardia lamblia* has a higher sensitivity than microscopic examination of a stool specimen.
- Fecal elastase: levels <200 μg g^{-1} are indicative of pancreatic insufficiency, although levels may be falsely low in large-volume diarrhea.
- Fecal calprotectin: levels are increased in intestinal inflammation and can be useful in distinguishing inflammatory from noninflammatory causes of diarrhea.
- Fecal alpha-1 antitrypsin level or clearance: indicated when protein-losing enteropathy is suspected; an increased level or clearance is indicative of protein-losing enteropathy.

> The most common causes of osmotic diarrhea include ingestion of exogenous magnesium, consumption of poorly absorbable carbohydrates (e.g., sorbitol, lactulose), and carbohydrate malabsorption (e.g., lactose intolerance).

Blood Tests

- Complete blood count:
  - Microcytic anemia may indicate gastrointestinal blood loss due to inflammation or celiac disease.
  - Leukocytosis suggests infection or ischemia.
- White blood count and differential cell count:
  - Eosinophilia suggests diarrhea due to a parasite or medication.
  - Lymphocytosis and eosinophilia may be seen in adrenal insufficiency.
- Comprehensive metabolic panel:
  - Electrolyte abnormalities: chronic diarrhea may cause hypokalemia, hypomagnesemia, or hyponatremia.
- Erythrocyte sedimentation rate (ESR) and C-reactive protein (CRP):
  - ESR or CRP are nonspecific markers of inflammation and may be useful as surrogate tests for inflammatory diarrhea such as IBD (see Chapter 8).

- Thyroid function tests may be obtained if hyperthyroidism is suspected.
- Immunoglobulin (Ig) A and IgG tissue transglutaminase antibodies and endomysial antibodies are highly sensitive and specific for celiac disease.

Endocrine tumors of the pancreas are rare causes of chronic diarrhea. The prevalence of functional tumors of the pancreas is approximately 10 per million. Chronic diarrhea occurs as part of a symptom complex, and its frequency varies depending on the tumor type: 100% in patients with a vasoactive intestinal peptide (VIP)oma, 60–65% in those with a gastrinoma, and 15% in those with a glucagonoma. The diagnosis is made by measuring hormone levels in the serum. Therefore, an extensive work-up for endocrine tumors should only be performed after common diagnoses are ruled out.

Screening blood tests in a person with chronic diarrhea should include a complete blood count, comprehensive metabolic panel, ESR, CRP, vitamin B_{12} and folate levels, and thyroid function tests. These blood tests have high specificity but low sensitivity for the presence of organic disease.

Urine Tests

- 5-Hydroxyindole acetic acid (5-H1AA), histamine, or vanillylmandelic acid levels are indicated if carcinoid syndrome or pheochromocytoma is suspected.

Endoscopy

Endoscopic examination of the colon by flexible sigmoidoscopy or colonoscopy is indicated in persons who present with inflammatory diarrhea, or if a neoplasm is suspected. Although flexible sigmoidoscopy may be sufficient to make a diagnosis, some conditions require colonoscopy for examination of the proximal colon and terminal ileum (see later). Random mucosal biopsies should be obtained even if the visualized mucosa is normal, because some diagnoses can only be made by histologic examination.

- Diagnoses made by mucosal biopsy of the colon:
  - Lymphocytic colitis, collagenous colitis, amyloidosis, granulomatous infections, schistosomiasis.
- Diagnoses suggested by endoscopic examination of the proximal colon:
  - Infections: *Campylobacter* spp., cytomegalovirus.
  - Inflammation: Crohn's disease.
  - Neoplasms.

Esophagogastroduodenoscopy (EGD, upper endoscopy) is indicated when intestinal malabsorption is suspected.

- Upper endoscopy with small bowel biopsy:
  - Inflammation: Crohn's disease, celiac disease, eosinophilic gastroenteritis, abetalipoproteinemia, amyloidosis, mastocytosis.
  - Infection: Whipple disease, mycobacteria, *Giardia lamblia*.
  - Neoplasm: intestinal lymphoma.
- Small bowel aspirate:
  - Quantitative bacterial culture of a small bowel aspirate is the 'gold standard' for the diagnosis of small intestinal bacterial overgrowth ($>10^5$ bacteria ml^{-1}) but this is infrequently done in practice.

Imaging

Imaging evaluation is of limited utility in the work-up of chronic diarrhea.

- Small bowel follow-through is indicated when the following conditions are suspected:
  - Small intestinal diverticulosis (with bacterial overgrowth).
  - Ileal stricture (Crohn's disease).
  - Extensive bowel surgery (to define postsurgical anatomy).
  - Entero-enteric or enterocolonic fistula (Crohn's disease).
- Mesenteric angiography or magnetic resonance angiography is indicated when mesenteric ischemia is suspected.
- Computed tomography or magnetic resonance imaging is indicated to evaluate for chronic pancreatitis and neoplasms.

Lactose Hydrogen Breath Test

- Lactose hydrogen breath testing is used to diagnose lactose intolerance and small intestinal bacterial overgrowth.
- The patient ingests 20–25 g of lactose, and blood is collected at 15, 30, 60, 120, and 180 minutes. A rise in breath hydrogen by 20 ppm at 120 or 180 minutes over the previous value indicates lactose malabsorption.
- An early rise in breath hydrogen of 20 ppm over the previous value at 30 or 60 minutes is suggestive of small intestinal bacterial overgrowth.

In persons less than 45 years of age with symptoms typical of functional bowel disease (see Chapter 7), a normal physical examination, and normal screening blood test results, no further investigation is necessary. In persons 45 years of age or older, colonoscopy may yield a diagnosis in up to 30% of cases.

Treatment

- The treatment of chronic diarrhea depends on the cause. A few examples are given below:
  - Celiac disease: gluten-free diet.
  - Lactose intolerance: avoidance of lactose-containing food (e.g., milk products, ice cream) and use of lactase supplements.
  - Mesenteric ischemia: definitive treatment with open surgical repair (transaortic endarterectomy, direct reimplantation of the aorta, or antegrade or retrograde bypass grafting) or endovascular repair (angioplasty and/or stent placement of atherosclerotic lesions within the mesenteric vasculature). Medical treatment is usually reserved for patients who are not healthy enough to be treated surgically or by endovascular techniques. Medical management includes anticoagulation therapy.
  - IBD: topical and systemic anti-inflammatory medications (see Chapter 8).
  - Eosinophilic gastroenteritis: dietary elimination and glucocorticoids.
  - Pancreatic insufficiency: pancreatic enzyme supplements and gastric acid suppression.
  - Small intestinal bacterial overgrowth: antibiotics.
- General antidiarrheal agents:
  - Nonspecific antidiarrheal agents (Table 6.4) are frequently used to reduce the frequency and volume of bowel movements and abdominal cramps.

Table 6.4 Antidiarrheal agents.

Medication class	Agent	Representative dose*
Luminally acting		
Fiber supplements	Psyllium (Metamucil, Fiberall)	10–20 g daily
Bile acid-binding agents	Cholestyramine, Colestipol	1–4 g four times daily
Systemically acting		
α-Adrenergic agonists	Clonidine	0.1–0.3 g three times daily
Somatostatin analogs	Octreotide	25–250 mg subcutaneously three times daily
Opiates and other antimotility agents	Loperamide (Imodium)	2–4 mg four times daily
	Diphenoxylate with atropine (Lomotil)	2.5–5 mg four times daily
		15–30 mg four times daily
	Codeine	2–20 drops four times daily
	Tincture of opium	

* Taken orally unless otherwise indicated.

Pearls
• Stools may look normal in the presence of excess fat.
• Patients with carbohydrate malabsorption (e.g., lactose intolerance) often present with watery diarrhea, flatulence, and bloating, typically occurring within 90 minutes after a meal.
• Abdominal pain is uncommon in patients with chronic diarrhea, except in those with irritable bowel syndrome, chronic pancreatitis, Crohn's disease, or mesenteric ischemia.
• The most common cause of fatty diarrhea is celiac disease. Tissue transglumi-nase and endomysial antibodies should be obtained in patients who present with fatty diarrhea. The clinical presentation of celiac disease can be subtle, and a history of childhood illness, celiac disease in the family, iron-deficiency anemia, growth retardation, diabetes mellitus, osteopenia, and mild liver biochemical test abnormalities should be elicited.
• Symptomatic treatment with an antidiarrheal agent is often necessary in a patient with chronic diarrhea because specific treatment may not be available.

Questions

Question 1 relates to the clinical vignette at the beginning of this chapter.

1   What is the next step in the management of this patient?
   A Colonoscopy.
   B Computed tomography (CT) of the abdomen.
   C Tissue transglutaminase antibodies.
   D Serum immunoglobulins.
   E Stool test for fecal fat.

2   A 28-year-old Asian woman presents with a 6-month history of intermittent bloating, diarrhea, and flatulence. She denies blood in the stool, nocturnal bowel movements, or weight loss. Her past medical history is unremarkable. She takes no prescription, herbal, or over-the-counter medications. She recently moved to the US. Physical examination is unremarkable. Laboratory tests including a complete blood count, comprehensive metabolic panel, and stool cultures, examination for ova and parasites, *Clostridium difficile* toxin, occult blood test, and Sudan stain are normal. Which of the following would be most helpful in determining the cause of her diarrhea?
   A Colonoscopy.
   B Sigmoidoscopy.
   C CT of the abdomen.
   D Trial of abstinence from milk products.
   E Tissue transglutaminase antibodies.

Questions 3 and 4 relate to the case presented below.

A 63-year-old man complains of a 6-month history of progressively worsening diarrhea and abdominal pain. His symptoms usually occur after a meal. His stools are foul-smelling, sticky, and hard to flush due to the presence of oil droplets on the stool. The abdominal pain is mild, diffuse, and cramping in nature. He reports a 15 lb (7 kg) weight loss but denies nausea, vomiting, reflux symptoms, fever, or chills. His past medical history is notable for hypertension, type 2 diabetes mellitus, retinopathy, and mild chronic kidney disease. He smokes one pack of cigarettes and drinks a six-pack of beer daily. Physical examination is notable for mild muscle wasting. The remainder of the examination is normal. Laboratory tests show a normal complete blood count and comprehensive metabolic panel except for a serum creatinine level of $2 \, mg \, dl^{-1}$ (unchanged from previous values). A fecal occult blood test is negative. A Sudan stain of the stool is highly positive. A stool lactoferrin test is negative.

3   Which of the following is/are possible cause(s) of the patient's diarrhea?
    A Chronic pancreatitis.
    B Chronic mesenteric ischemia.
    C Small intestinal bacterial overgrowth.
    D A or B.
    E A, B, or C.

4   Which of the following is the next appropriate diagnostic step?
    A CT of the abdomen.
    B Colonoscopy.
    C Small-bowel follow-through.
    D 72-hour stool collection for fat.
    E Stool sodium potassium concentrations and osmolality.

5   A 66-year-old woman presents with a 2-year history of progressively worsening watery diarrhea. She describes six to eight small-volume watery bowel movements a day. She denies blood in the stool, mucus, rectal urgency, tenesmus, nocturnal bowel movements, abdominal pain, or weight loss. She is afraid to leave the house because of her symptoms. She denies recent travel or antibiotic use. Her past medical history is remarkable for osteoarthritis, for which she takes ibuprofen. She does not drink alcohol or smoke cigarettes. Physical examination is unremarkable. Laboratory tests including a complete blood count, comprehensive metabolic panel, tissue transglutaminase antibodies, and thyroid-stimulating hormone level are normal. Stool studies including culture, examination for

ova and parasites, *Clostridium difficile* toxin, Sudan stain for fat, and occult blood test are negative. Which of the following diagnostic tests is indicated?

A Colonoscopy with biopsy.

B Barium enema.

C CT of the abdomen.

D Upper endoscopy with small-bowel biopsy.

E Small-bowel follow-through.

Answers

1 **C**

The patient presents with chronic diarrhea associated with weight loss, osteoporosis, anemia, infertility, and easy bruisability suggestive of intestinal malabsorption. Because she is a white woman, suspicion for celiac disease is high in the differential diagnosis of malabsorption. Celiac disease is the most common cause of malabsorption in adults, with a prevalence of 0.5–1 per 100 in the US. There is a female predominance, and the disease is associated with human leukocyte antigen (HLA)-DQ2 or HLA-DQ8. Iron-deficiency anemia is a common presenting symptom in adults with celiac disease. Detection of tissue transglutaminase (or endomysial) antibodies is diagnostic of celiac disease, with a sensitivity and specificity of 98% and 100%, respectively. A stool test for fecal fat will confirm malabsorption but will not indicate a specific diagnosis. CT should be considered if celiac disease is ruled out to evaluate the patient for other causes of steatorrhea, such as chronic pancreatitis. Some patients with celiac disease may have IgA deficiency and falsely negative IgA transglutaminase antibodies; serum immunoglobulins may be obtained to look for IgA deficiency.

2 **D**

Lactose intolerance is seen most commonly in Asians and African Americans; >90% of Asians and African Americans have decreased activity of intestinal lactase. The patient's symptoms, which include diarrhea associated with bloating and flatulence in the absence of nocturnal symptoms, blood in the stool and weight loss, are consistent with the diagnosis of lactose intolerance. The diagnosis can be established with a hydrogen breath test that measures exhaled hydrogen gas following the ingestion of a standard dose of lactose. However, improvement in symptoms with avoidance of lactose-containing foods or use of lactase supplements with dairy products is generally sufficient to make a diagnosis of lactose intolerance. Because the patient has no evidence of inflammatory diarrhea, colonoscopy or sigmoidoscopy is not indicated. Computed tomography is not indicated in this patient. Celiac disease is uncommon in Asians, and testing for tissue transglutaminase antibodies should not be necessary if the patient responds to a therapeutic trial of a lactose-free diet.

3 E

The presence of fat droplets in the stool implies steatorrhea, as confirmed by a Sudan stain. Weight loss along with steatorrhea is suggestive of maldigestion (as may occur with chronic pancreatitis or small-bowel bacterial overgrowth) or malabsorption (as may occur with chronic mesenteric ischemia). The history of alcohol use is a risk factor for chronic pancreatitis. Type 2 diabetes mellitus with end-organ complications, hypertension, and smoking are risk factors for vascular disease, and mesenteric ischemia is a consideration. Diabetes mellitus is also associated with intestinal dysmotility and small-intestinal bacterial overgrowth.

4 A

CT of the abdomen may detect chronic pancreatitis, mesenteric ischemia, or a neoplasm. If the test is unrevealing, a trial of antibiotics for small-intestinal bacterial overgrowth may be considered. Alternatively, an upper endoscopy with small-bowel aspirate for bacterial culture and mucosal biopsy or mesenteric angiography may be considered. Colonoscopy and small-bowel follow-through have a low yield as diagnostic tests in a patient with steatorrhea. Stool determination of sodium and potassium concentrations and osmolality may help differentiate secretory from osmotic diarrhea, and is not indicated in this patient, who has steatorrhea. A Sudan stain for fecal fat is positive, and a quantitative stool fat determination is not needed.

5 A

Microscopic colitis should be considered in a middle-aged woman who presents with watery diarrhea in the face of normal laboratory test and stool study results. The female:male ratio of collagenous colitis is 9:1, and the disorder typically occurs in women over 50 years of age. The mucosa usually appears normal on colonoscopy. The diagnosis is made by histologic examination of colonic mucosal biopsies, which reveal collagen deposition in the lamina propria.

Further Reading

Schiller, L.R. and Sellin, J.H. (2016) Diarrhea, in Sleisenger and Fordtran's Gastrointestinal and Liver Disease: Pathophysiology/Diagnosis/Management, 10th edition, (eds M. Feldman, L.S. Friedman, and L.J. Brandt), Saunders Elsevier, Philadelphia, pp. 221–241.

Sweetser, S. (2012) Evaluating the patient with diarrhea: a case-based approach. *Mayo Clinic Proceedings*, **87**, 596–602.

Weblinks

http://www.fpnotebook.com/gi/diarrhea/ChrncDrh.htm
http://www.acg.gi.org/patients/gihealth/diarrheal.asp

7

Irritable Bowel Syndrome

Kavya M. Sebastian

> ## Clinical Vignette
>
> A 28-year-old woman is seen in the office for intermittent abdominal pain for the past several years. The pain occurs three to four times a week, and is diffuse and cramping in nature. The pain is relieved by a bowel movement. She has alternating episodes of mild diarrhea and mild constipation. Her diarrheal episodes are characterized by watery stool, and they never occur at night. The episodes of constipation are notable for hard, pellet-like stools and a sense of incomplete evacuation. She may vary from diarrhea to constipation every two to three days. She has noted some mucus in the stool and mild bloating, but has not noted any blood in the stools. She denies nausea, vomiting, or weight loss. Her past medical and surgical history is unremarkable. She does not take any prescription or over-the-counter medications. Her family history is unremarkable. She is a single mother solely supporting her three children, and reports working long hours as a law partner. She drinks one or two glasses of wine on weekends, and she has never used tobacco. She has no history of illicit drug use. Physical examination reveals a blood pressure of 121/73 mmHg, pulse rate 70 per minute, temperature 98.6 °F (37 °C), and body mass index 22. The remainder of the examination including an abdominal examination is unremarkable. Routine laboratory tests show a normal complete blood count, blood glucose, and comprehensive metabolic panel.

General

- Irritable bowel syndrome (IBS) is a functional gastrointestinal disorder characterized by abdominal pain and altered bowel habits that occur in the absence of biochemical or structural abnormalities. Alarm symptoms and

Sitaraman and Friedman's Essentials of Gastroenterology, Second Edition.
Edited by Shanthi Srinivasan and Lawrence S. Friedman.
© 2018 John Wiley & Sons Ltd. Published 2018 by John Wiley & Sons Ltd.

signs (weight loss, iron-deficiency anemia, malnutrition, melena or blood in the stools) are absent.

- Based on the predominant symptom, IBS is classified as diarrhea-predominant (IBS-D), constipation-predominant (IBS-C), and mixed (IBS-M).
- Lifetime prevalence of IBS is 10–15% in North America. It accounts for up to 25–50% of referrals to a gastroenterologist, and is the second most common reason for work absenteeism after the common cold. IBS has a 2:1 female predominance in North America. It is more common in persons younger than 50 years of age. Persons who seek care for symptoms are typically found to have less social support than those who do not.

Pathophysiology

- IBS is associated with multiple comorbidities such as somatic pain syndromes (fibromyalgia, chronic fatigue syndrome, chronic pelvic pain) and psychiatric disorders (major depression, anxiety).
- The pathophysiology of IBS is poorly understood. Altered gastrointestinal motility, visceral hypersensitivity, psychosocial distress, genetic predisposition, environmental agents, and alteration of the intestinal and colonic microbiota have been implicated as contributing factors to the development of IBS.
- Increased prevalence of IBS symptoms is seen in persons with chronic inflammatory conditions (inflammatory bowel disease, celiac disease) or after an episode of acute gastroenteritis (post-infection IBS), suggesting a role for altered intestinal immune activation and permeability.
- The presence of true food allergies in IBS is uncommon; however, food intolerances are often present in persons with IBS. Some persons may have poor intestinal absorption of carbohydrates resulting in osmotic diarrhea or increased fermentation, thereby leading to bloating and pain.
- Heightened visceral pain sensitivity is a characteristic feature of patients with IBS. Patients typically perceive the sensation of a balloon distended in the rectum or small bowel at significantly lower volumes than do control subjects. During distention, they are seen to have increased activation of regions of the brain associated with emotional arousal and pain modulation.
- 5-Hydroxytryptamine (5-HT, or serotonin) receptors have been shown to play an important role in diarrhea as well as pain perception. This finding has led to the development of $5-HT_3$ antagonists as a therapy for diarrhea-predominant IBS (see later).
- Women with IBS are more likely to have experienced verbal, sexual, or physical abuse. Early parental response to an individual's pain in childhood or adolescence may lead to permanent alterations of the brain–gut axis with the development of associated poor coping behavioral responses as an adult.

- Patients with IBS are noted to display 'catastrophization,' with heightened emphasis placed on their symptoms, thereby leading to poor coping mechanisms and lower participation in their professional or social lives.

Clinical Evaluation

- The Rome IV criteria for the diagnosis of IBS (Table 7.1) specify that patients have recurrent abdominal pain, on average, at least one day per week during the previous 3 months that is associated with two or more of the following criteria:
  - Related to defecation.
  - Associated with a change in stool frequency.
  - Associated with a change in stool form or appearance.
- Other symptoms that support a diagnosis of IBS include altered stool frequency, altered stool form, altered stool passage (straining and/or urgency), mucus in the stool, and abdominal bloating. The criteria for subtypes of IBS are shown in Table 7.2.
- A thorough history and physical examination, including a rectal examination, should be performed.

Table 7.1 Rome IV criteria for the diagnosis of IBS.*

At least 1 day per week of recurrent abdominal pain or discomfort associated with two or more of the following criteria*:
Related to defecation
Associated with a change in frequency of stool
Associated with a change in form (appearance) of stool

*Criteria should be met for the previous 3 months.

Table 7.2 IBS subtypes.*

IBS-C	Abnormal bowel movements, usually constipation (type 1 and 2 in the BSFS)
IBS-D	Abnormal bowel movements, usually diarrhea (type 6 and 7 in the BSFS)
IBS-M	Abnormal bowel movements, both constipation and diarrhea (>25% are constipation and >25% are diarrhea)
Unclassified IBS	Meets diagnostic criteria for IBS but cannot be accurately categorized into one of the previous three subtypes

BSFS, Bristol Stool Form Scale; C, constipation; D, diarrhea; M, mixed.
* As assessed by the Bristol Stool Form Scale (see Chapter 9).

- Routine laboratory testing should include a complete blood count, comprehensive metabolic panel, thyroid-stimulating hormone, and stool studies for infectious etiologies. Testing for serum tissue transglutaminase antibodies to exclude celiac disease is recommended in persons suspected of having IBS, especially those with possible IBS-D or IBS-M. Hydrogen breath testing may be considered to rule out small-intestinal bacterial overgrowth (SIBO) in persons with IBS-D or IBS-M.
- Upper endoscopy, colonoscopy, or imaging to evaluate for colon cancer, stricture, ischemia, inflammatory bowel disease, or other structural causes is recommended for persons over 50 years of age, and for younger persons with 'alarm' symptoms, such as anemia or substantial weight loss. For patients with IBS-D or IBS-M, colonic mucosal biopsies should be obtained at colonoscopy to exclude microscopic colitis.

Treatment

- The mainstays of therapy are a good doctor–patient relationship, patient reassurance and education, and continuity of care. Initially, the patient should be seen every 6–8 weeks. Goals should be set for long-term control of symptoms rather than expectation of a cure.
- A global approach to management should be undertaken. A guide to the treatment of IBS is provided in Table 7.3. Dietary changes may be beneficial, given the common association of IBS symptoms with food intake. Evidence has emerged to support a diet that is low in fermentable oligosaccharides, disaccharides, monosaccharides, and polyols (FODMAPs). Those who respond to a so-called 'low-FODMAP' diet should gradually and sequentially reintroduce FODMAP-containing foods to attempt to reduce the need for long-term dietary restriction.
- Structured exercise has been demonstrated to lead to improvement in overall IBS symptoms, and patients should be encouraged to pursue daily physical activity.
- Pharmacotherapy is directed at the presumed pathophysiology of altered gastrointestinal motility. Use of low-dose antidepressants such as tricyclic antidepressants and selective serotonin reuptake inhibitors may decrease visceral hypersensitivity. Rifaximin is recommended for IBS-D when SIBO is suspected or confirmed (see Chapter 6), and may reduce bloating, flatulence, and diarrhea. Some patients may benefit from behavioral therapy such as counseling and cognitive psychotherapy by a psychologist or psychiatrist or another alternative therapy such as hypnosis, yoga, acupuncture, or acupressure.

> The primary goal of treatment for IBS is relief of symptoms. Therefore, treatment should be individualized based on the predominant symptom (pain, constipation, diarrhea).

Table 7.3 Treatment options for IBS.*

Category	Agent	Suggested dose
Dietary modification	Increased soluble fiber intake	20 g daily
	Low-FODMAP diet	–
	Avoidance of caffeine or alcohol	–
Antispasmodic agents	Dicyclomine	20 mg four times daily as needed
	Hyoscamine	0.125–0.25 mg every 4 hours as needed
Antiflatulence agent	Simethicone	250–500 mg as needed
Motility agents		
Diarrhea-predominant	Imodium	2 mg two to four times daily as needed
Constipation-predominant	Polyethylene glycol	17–26 g daily
	Magnesium hydroxide	5–15 ml one to four times daily as needed
	Lubiprostone	8 µg twice daily
Antibiotic	Rifaximin	550 mg three times daily × 14 days
Tricyclic antidepressants	Amitriptyline	12.5–150 mg daily
	Desipramine	25–100 mg daily
	Doxepin	25–150 mg daily
	Imipramine	10–50 mg daily
	Nortriptyline	10–75 mg daily
	Trimipramine	25–150 mg daily
Selective serotonin reuptake inhibitors	Fluoxetine (Prozac)	20–40 mg daily
	Citalopram (Celexa)	20–60 mg daily
Psychotherapy	Cognitive behavioral therapy by a psychologist or psychiatrist	
Alternative therapies	Probiotics[†]	–
	Peppermint oil	0.2–0.4 ml in enteric-coated capsules
	Hypnosis	–
	Yoga	–
	Acupuncture or acupressure	–

FODMAP, fermentable oligosaccharides, disaccharides, monosaccharides, and polyols.

* All medications are administered orally.

[†] e.g., *Lactobacillus plantarum, Bifidobacteria infantis.*

Pearls

- The pathophysiology of IBS is complex and involves altered central and intrinsic neuronal sensitivity to pain perception.
- A thorough history, physical examination, and simple laboratory testing are of utmost importance in diagnosing IBS.
- The primary goal of treatment is relief of symptoms; therefore, treatment should be individualized, based on the predominant symptom of abdominal pain, constipation, or diarrhea.
- The mainstays of therapy are a good doctor–patient relationship, patient reassurance and education, and continuity of care.
- Patients with a shorter duration of symptoms, no previous surgeries, or postinfection IBS respond the best to treatment.

Questions

Questions 1 and 2 relate to the clinical vignette at the beginning of this chapter.

1 The most likely diagnosis in this patient is:
   A Colon cancer.
   B Irritable bowel syndrome.
   C Inflammatory bowel disease.
   D Intestinal obstruction.

2 The initial approach to treatment of this patient's condition is:
   A Increased dietary fiber and fluid intake.
   B Osmotic laxative.
   C Stimulant laxative.
   D Rectal enemas.

3 The Rome IV criteria for the diagnosis of IBS include recurrent abdominal pain or discomfort for at least 1 day per week in the past 3 months. An additional principal criterion is which of the following?
   A Abdominal distension, incomplete evacuation, or passage of mucus.
   B Change in the frequency of stool, change in the form of stool, or abdominal pain relieved by defecation.
   C Abdominal pain relieved by defecation, presence of bloating, or a major psychiatric illness.
   D Weight loss, blood in stool, or nocturnal bowel movements.

4 The risk factor most strongly associated with IBS is which of the following?
   A Depression.
   B Food intolerance.

C Bacterial gastroenteritis.

D Hypochondria.

E Oral glucocorticoid use.

5 Which of the following best describes irritable bowel syndrome?

A A functional gastrointestinal disorder most commonly seen in women less than 50 years of age.

B A functional gastrointestinal disorder associated with abdominal pain that is continuous and not relieved with defecation.

C A functional gastrointestinal disorder that exclusively affects the gastrointestinal tract.

D A functional gastrointestinal disorder that is rarely associated with altered pain perception.

E A degenerative disorder of the enteric nervous system.

Answers

1 B

The patient meets the Rome IV diagnostic criteria for irritable bowel syndrome. She has chronic abdominal pain that is worse when she eats and is relieved by a bowel movement. She has no alarm symptoms such as weight loss or anemia. Her physical examination, laboratory tests, and colonoscopy results are normal. Hence, the diagnoses of colon cancer, inflammatory bowel disease, and intestinal obstruction are unlikely.

2 A

In a stepwise approach to treat IBS, the patient should be educated regarding her condition, and dietary fiber and fluid intake should be increased. If symptoms persist despite dietary and lifestyle modifications, pharmacotherapy can be used to treat the predominant symptom of constipation, diarrhea, or pain. Symptoms may be triggered by stress; therefore, psychologic therapy or stress management may be considered if symptoms do not improve with dietary and lifestyle modifications.

3 B

4 C

Studies have shown the correlation between bacterial gastroenteritis and the subsequent occurrence of IBS to be strongest. Depression is prevalent among IBS patients, but a causal association has not been demonstrated.

5 A

Further Reading

Camilleri, M. (2012) Peripheral mechanisms in irritable bowel syndrome. *The New England Journal of Medicine*, **367**, 1626–1635.

Chey, W.D., Kurlander, J., and Eswaran, S. (2015) Irritable bowel syndrome: a clinical review. *Journal of the American Medical Association*, **313**, 949–958.

Ford, A.C. and Talley, N.J. (2016) Irritable bowel syndrome, in Sleisenger and Fordtran's Gastrointestinal and Liver Disease: Pathophysiology/Diagnosis/ Management, 10th edition (eds M. Feldman, L.S. Friedman, and L.J. Brandt), Saunders Elsevier, Philadelphia, pp. 2139–2153.

Weblinks

http://www.gastrojournal.org/article/S0016-5085%2814%2901089-0/abstract
http://www.niddk.nih.gov/health-information/health-topics/digestive-diseases/
  irritable-bowel-syndrome/Pages/overview.aspx

8

Inflammatory Bowel Disease

Jan-Michael A. Klapproth

Clinical Vignette

A 22-year-old female college student on the track team is questioned by her coach regarding a lack of performance during a recent track meet. She admits to a 6 lb (2.7 kg) weight loss over the previous 6 months, accompanied by a lack of appetite and amenorrhea. She also reports persistent, nonradiating, right lower quadrant pain that she describes as cramping and dull in nature. She has one to two bowel movements per day. The stools are watery in consistency, but she reports no rectal bleeding. The concerned coach sends her to the Student Health Service, and laboratory tests are remarkable for a hematocrit value of 21% and mean corpuscular volume 75 fl.

General

- Inflammatory bowel disease (IBD) is comprised of two major chronic intestinal diseases – Crohn's disease (CD) and ulcerative colitis (UC). The distinguishing features of CD and UC are outlined in Table 8.1.
- Approximately 1.4 million persons are affected with IBD in the US.

Epidemiology

- Age of onset: IBD can occur at any age, but the mean age of onset appears to be increasing. IBD has bimodal age distribution; the first peak is at 15–30 years, and the second peak is after age 60 years; 10–15% of patients are diagnosed before age 18.

Sitaraman and Friedman's Essentials of Gastroenterology, Second Edition.
Edited by Shanthi Srinivasan and Lawrence S. Friedman.
© 2018 John Wiley & Sons Ltd. Published 2018 by John Wiley & Sons Ltd.

Table 8.1 Distinguishing features of ulcerative colitis and Crohn's disease.

Feature	Ulcerative colitis	Crohn's disease
Age of onset (years)	15–30	15–30
Male:female ratio	1:1	1:1
Disease location	Colon only Pancolitis: 45–50%; Proctosigmoiditis: 15–35%; Left-sided colonic disease: 35–40%	Any portion of the GI tract Ileocolonic: 40%; Small bowel alone: 30%; Colon alone: 30%; 90% of patients <20 years of age have small-bowel involvement compared with 60% of those >40 years of age
Distribution	Continuous inflammation that extends proximally from the anorectal junction; the rectum is almost invariably involved	Skip lesions Rectal sparing
Depth of inflammation	Mucosa/submucosa	Transmural
Ulcerations	Small, superficial	Deep, serpiginous
Terminal ileal involvement	Typically not involved; backwash ileitis may be present in 15–20% of patients with pancolitis	Commonly involved; ulcerations, strictures, or fistulas
Extraintestinal disease	Yes	Yes
Strictures or fistulas	No	May be present
Postoperative* recurrence	No	Frequent
Serology	pANCA: 60–65% ASCA: 5%	pANCA: 20–25% ASCA: 40–76%

ASCA, anti-*Saccharomyces cerevisiae* antibodies; pANCA, perinuclear antineutrophil cytoplasmic antibodies; GI gastrointestinal. *Colectomy for ulcerative colitis, resection for Crohn's disease.

- Geographical distribution: there is a North–South gradient, with the highest incidence rates in the US and United Kingdom, and the lowest in Croatia and Africa.
- Race: the incidence of IBD is highest in Caucasians and Ashkenazi Jews and lowest in Hispanics, African Americans, and Asian Americans.

Etiology and Pathogenesis

> The etiology of IBD is largely unknown. IBD is thought to result from an inappropriate or aberrant inflammatory response to intestinal microbes in a genetically susceptible host.

Genetic Factors

- First-degree relatives of affected persons have a four- to 20-fold increased risk of developing IBD.
- A family history of IBD is present in 25% of patients with CD, and in 20% of patients with UC.
- Mutations in multiple genes involved in bacterial antigen presentation and the innate immune response have been associated with IBD. A few important genes are as follows:
  - Autophagy-related 16-like 1 (*ATG16L1*): protective of or increased risk for CD, depending on a single nucleotide polymorphism.
  - Nucleotide-binding oligomerization domain containing 2 (*NOD2*, also called caspase recruitment domain family, member 15 [*CARD15*]): three mutations in leucine-rich repeats increase the risk for CD.
  - Immunity-related GTPase (*IRGM*): increased risk for CD.
  - Interleukin-23 receptor (*IL-23R*): increased risk for CD.

Environmental Factors

- Social status:
  - Upper middle class is associated with a higher risk of developing IBD.
  - Male bricklayers, unskilled laborers, security personnel, and women working in the cleaning and maintenance business have lower risks of developing IBD.
- Smoking: protective for UC but increased risk for CD; patients with CD who smoke have more severe disease, require more medications to control the disease, and have an increased rate of recurrent disease activity.
- Appendectomy reduces the risk of developing UC; unclear role in CD.
- Breastfeeding appears to be protective for IBD.
- Nonsteroidal anti-inflammatory drugs (NSAIDs) have been implicated in exacerbations and as potential precipitants of new cases of IBD.

Immune Factors and Microbes

- The intestinal epithelium acts as a barrier between the luminal contents and the mucosal immune system. Loss of intestinal barrier function is thought to precede the development of inflammation in patients with IBD. A defective intestinal barrier has been reported in first-degree relatives of patients with CD.
- Intestinal microbes are documented to play an important role in the inflammatory response. Although no single bacterial strain has been identified conclusively as playing a causal role in IBD, depletion and reduced diversity of members of the mucosa-associated phyla Firmicutes and Bacteroidetes have been documented in patients with IBD compared with control subjects, termed **dysbiosis**. In addition, bacteria that can adhere to and invade the intestinal mucosa, such as *Escherichia coli*, have been implicated.
- The histological hallmark of active IBD is a prominent infiltration of innate immune cells (polymorphonuclear neutrophils, macrophages, dendritic cells, and natural killer T cells) and adaptive immune cells (B cells and T cells) into the lamina propria. Immune activation in the mucosa leads to elevated levels of several cytokines and chemokines, such as tumor necrosis factor alpha (TNF-α), interleukin-1β, interferon-γ, and the interleukin-23–Th17 pathway. Although the precise molecular pathway is unknown, a defective innate and adaptive immune response has been implicated in the pathogenesis of IBD.

Clinical Features

- Characteristic symptoms of IBD include chronic diarrhea and abdominal pain.
- Constitutional symptoms such as fatigue, fever, and weight loss are frequently present.
- The onset of symptoms is usually insidious.
- Typical symptoms of UC include left lower quadrant pain, rectal urgency, tenesmus, mucoid discharge, and bloody diarrhea.
- Depending on the segment of bowel involved, patients with CD may present with right lower quadrant pain associated with diarrhea, obstructive symptoms (nausea, vomiting, abdominal pain and distention), fever, and weight loss.
- A thorough history should be obtained to exclude other causes of diarrhea (see Chapters 5 and 6).
- Physical examination helps to assess the clinical status of a patient with IBD (for signs of dehydration, anemia, and muscle wasting). In patients with CD, an abdominal mass, abdominal tenderness, or perianal fissures, fistulas and abscesses may be present. In addition, a dermatologic examination may reveal erythema nodosum, pyoderma gangrenosum, or aphthous ulcers (see Chapter 26).

Extraintestinal Manifestations

- Extraintestinal manifestations of IBD may be related to bowel activity, have an independent course or, in the case of CD, be related to intestinal malabsorption.
- Related to bowel activity: peripheral arthritis, erythema nodosum, episcleritis, aphthous stomatitis, pyoderma gangrenosum (see Chapter 26).
- Independent course: ankylosing spondylitis, sacroileitis, uveitis, primary sclerosing cholangitis.
- Related to malabsorption: anemia, cholelithiasis, nephrolithiasis, metabolic bone disease.

Diagnosis

> The diagnosis of UC or CD is based on the combination of the clinical presentation and results of laboratory, imaging, and endoscopic studies. No single test is considered diagnostic of CD or UC.

Laboratory Features

- Laboratory tests are useful in assessing the severity of disease.
- A complete blood count may reveal leukocytosis, anemia, or thrombocytosis.
- A comprehensive metabolic profile may reveal electrolyte abnormalities related to fluid loss, and hypoalbuminemia related to intestinal malabsorption.
- Markers of inflammation:
  - Serum C-reactive protein and erythrocyte sedimentation rate levels.
    - These markers are neither sensitive nor specific for IBD, but may be useful to assess disease activity in individual patients.
    - Levels correlate positively with clinical, endoscopic, and radiologic measures of disease activity.
    - Elevations predict relapsing disease.
    - Elevations may identify patients likely to progress to colectomy for severe UC.
  - Fecal calprotectin levels.
    - >250 µg g^{-1}: correlates with the presence of large ulcerations in CD (sensitivity 60%, specificity 80%).
    - ≤ 250 µg g^{-1}: correlates with mucosal healing in CD (sensitivity 94%, specificity 62%).
    - >203 µg g^{-1}: predicts postoperative recurrence of CD.
    - >1900 µg g^{-1}: predicts 87% colectomy rate at one year in UC.
- Stool culture for bacterial pathogens and stool examination for ova and parasites should be performed in patients during their initial presentation.

- The incidence of *Clostridium difficile* colitis is increased in patients with IBD. Stool samples for *C. difficile* toxin should be obtained during acute flares of IBD, whether or not there is history of antibiotic use or recent hospitalization.
- Serologic markers:
  - A serology panel including perinuclear antineutrophil cytoplasmic antibodies (pANCA), anti-*Saccharomyces cerevisiae* antibodies (ASCA), anti-CBir1, anti-I2, and anti-outer membrane porin from *E. coli* (OmpC) antibodies is available to help diagnose IBD.
  - 'Atypical' ANCA yielding a perinuclear staining pattern (pANCA) with alcohol-fixed neutrophils are found in 60–65% of patients with UC; pANCA are also detectable in 20–25% of patients with CD.
  - ASCA, anti-Bir, and anti-OmpC are detected primarily in patients with CD; ASCA are detectable in 46–70% of patients with CD, and in 5% of those with UC.
  - Anti-CBir1 expression is associated independently with small-bowel, penetrating, and fibrostenosing CD.

> Serologic tests lack sensitivity to diagnose IBD and are not recommended for routine use. There does not seem to be any correlation between pANCA or ASCA titers and disease activity, duration of illness, extent of disease, extraintestinal manifestations, or need for surgical or medical treatment in patients with IBD.

Imaging (see Chapter 27)

- Small-bowel follow-through and enteroclysis:
  - These tests are no longer used as first-line diagnostic tests.
  - Small-bowel imaging may be helpful for the detection of small-bowel strictures ('string sign' indicates a long-segment stricture) and fistula.
  - Mucosal edema alternating with ulcerations is described on imaging tests as 'cobblestone' pattern.
- Computed tomography (CT):
  - Useful in the detection of extraluminal disease and complications of CD such as perforation and abscess.
  - The sensitivity is 80–88% for the diagnosis of suspected CD.
- Magnetic resonance imaging (MRI) and MR enterography:
  - MRI and MR enterography are used to assess inflammatory processes in the bowel wall, submucosal inflammation and fibrosis, as well as complications such as abscess and fistula.
  - MR enterography is highly sensitive and specific for the diagnosis of small-bowel ulceration, strictures, and fistulas with a specificity approaching 100% and sensitivity of 80–100%.

- Consider MR enterography for women of childbearing age instead of CT enterography, small-bowel follow-through, or small-bowel enteroclysis (slow-infusion small-bowel follow-through).

Endoscopy

- Indications:
  - Establishing a diagnosis of IBD: endoscopic examination with biopsies for microscopic examination is considered an integral part of the initial evaluation in order to diagnose IBD, assess the severity, and institute appropriate medical therapy (Figure 8.1).
    - ○ Colonoscopy with intubation of the terminal ileum is recommended.
    - ○ Depending on the symptoms, upper endoscopy (esophagogastroduodenoscopy, EGD) may be considered. Endoscopic features that distinguish CD from UC are outlined in Table 8.2.
    - ○ Microscopic examination of the mucosa (see Chapter 28) typically show crypt abscess, crypt distortion, and increased cellularity in the lamina propria. These finding do not distinguish IBD from infectious diseases of the colon.
  - Colon cancer and dysplasia (precancer) surveillance with colonoscopy is indicated in patients with pancolonic CD or UC of at least 8 years' duration. Four-quadrant mucosal biopsies should be obtained every 10 cm, starting in the terminal ileum as the colonoscope is withdrawn for a minimum 33 biopsies; in addition, all suspicious lesions should be biopsied. The yield of surveillance can be increased by using techniques such as chromoendoscopy and narrow band imaging to identify areas of dysplasia.
- Wireless capsule endoscopy (WCE)
  - 30% of patients with CD have small-bowel disease alone, and WCE has a higher diagnostic yield for small-bowel CD compared with radiologic studies. In some cases, intestinal obstruction can be excluded by enteroclysis, small-bowel follow-through, or with a self-dissolving, radiopaque patency capsule prior to WCE delivery to avoid acute obstruction.

> The presence of noncaseating granulomas on histologic examination, present in 20–40% of patients with suspected CD, is specific for the diagnosis of CD.

Differential Diagnosis

- Acute infectious colitis (e.g., *Salmonella* spp., *Shigella* spp., *C. difficile* infection, *Campylobacter jejuni*, cytomegalovirus, amebiasis, intestinal tuberculosis).
- Behçet's disease.

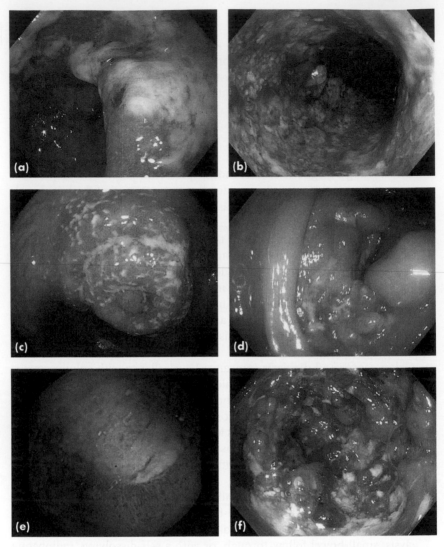

Figure 8.1 Endoscopic views of IBD. (a) Moderately and (b) severely active UC with loss of haustrations, friability, exudate, and pseudopolyps; (c) A cecal patch characterized by inflammation of the appendiceal orifice; (d) Moderately inflamed ileocecal valve; (e) Small-bowel ulceration in CD; (f) Severely inflamed ascending colon in UC.

Table 8.2 Microscopic features of ulcerative colitis and Crohn's disease.

Feature	UC (%)	CD (%)
Crypt distortion	57–100	21–71
Lamina propria cellularity	76–92	72–81
Crypt abscess	41	19
Granuloma	0	21–37
Irregular mucosal surface	17–30	12

- Diverticulitis.
- Drugs and toxins (e.g., chemotherapy, gold, penicillamine).
- Ischemic colitis.
- Microscopic colitis (collagenous colitis and lymphocytic colitis).
- Neutropenic colitis.
- NSAIDs.
- Radiation colitis.

Treatment

- The goals of treatment are to induce and maintain remission and to improve the patient's quality of life.
- The choice of medical therapy depends on the extent, location, and severity of the disease and the presence or absence of fistulas.
- Several scoring systems are available to assess disease activity in CD and UC. These systems (e.g., the Crohn's Disease Activity Index) are typically used for clinical studies. In daily practice, the severity of IBD is assessed on the basis of the patient's symptoms, signs, and laboratory test results.
- Medical therapy varies between UC and CD, with significant overlap between the two (see Table 8.3).
- Certain drugs are used for the induction of remission (IOR), and others for the maintenance of remission (MOR). Some agents may be used for both IOR and MOR.

> Surgery is generally reserved for patients who are refractory to medical therapy or who have fulminant disease (such as toxic megacolon), a complication (such as perforation), dysplasia, or malignancy.

5-Aminosalicylic acid (5-ASA)

- Sulfasalazine (sulfapyridine bound to 5-ASA) and mesalamine (5-ASA), collectively referred to as aminosalicylates, are considered first-line agents for mild-to-moderate UC.
- The therapeutic effect of aminosalicylates depends on the local concentration at the inflamed mucosa.
- Various 5-ASA preparations have been developed to increase local concentration: Balsalaside (5-ASA conjugated to an inactive compound; Colazol®); olsalazine (5-ASA dimer; Dipentum®); Asacol® and Lialda® (mesalamine with delayed-release coating); Pentasa® (5-ASA encapsulated in ethylcellulose microgranules that release 35% of the drug in the small bowel); 5-ASA enema (Rowasa®); and suppositories (Canasa®).

Table 8.3 Commonly used medications for the treatment of UC and CD.

Class of drug	Medication	Dose	Indication	IOR/MOR
5-ASA				
	Mesalamine: oral 5-ASA (various formulations)	2–4 g daily	Mild-to-severe UC	IOR and MOR
	Sulfasalazine (5-ASA bound to sulfapyridine)	1–4 g daily	Mild-to-severe UC	IOR and MOR
	Topical (enema or suppository)	1–4 g daily	Mild-to-moderate left-sided UC	IOR and MOR
Glucocorticoids				
	Oral	Varies with the formulation. Typically, starting dose is prednisone 40 mg daily for mild disease and 60 mg daily for moderate disease, tapered over at least one month	Moderate-to-severe UC, moderate-to-severe small-bowel or colonic CD	IOR
	Oral (high first-pass metabolism)	Budesonide 9 mg daily	Mild-to-moderate small-bowel and colonic CD, mild-to-moderate UC	IOR and MOR
	Intravenous	Typically, solumedrol 40 mg daily	Moderate-to-severe UC and CD, hospitalized patient	IOR
	Enema	Hydrocortisone 100 mg daily	Moderate-to-severe left-sided UC	IOR and MOR
Immunomodulators				
	Azathioprine	2–4 mg daily orally	UC and CD	MOR
	6-Mercaptopurine	1.5–2.5 mg daily orally	UC and CD	MOR
	Methotrexate	15–25 mg weekly intramuscularly, subcutaneously, or orally	Small bowel CD	IOR and MOR

Drug	Dosage	Indication	
Cyclosporine	4 mg kg^{-1}day^{-1} titrated to therapeutic blood levels	Severe UC	IOR and MOR; transition to azathioprine or 6-mercapto-purine
Biologics			
Anti-TNF-α agents			
Infliximab	5 mg kg^{-1} intravenously 0, 2, and 6, and then every 8 weeks	CD, small bowel and colon, fistula; Severe UC	IOR and MOR
Adalimumab	Variable dose and schedule, 40–160 mg subcutaneously	Moderate-to-severe CD or UC	IOR and MOR
Certolizumab pegol	400 mg 0, 2, and 4 weeks and then 200 mg every 4 weeks subcutaneously	Moderate-to-severe CD	IOR and MOR
Golimumab	200 mg at week 0, 100 mg at week 2, then 100 mg every 4 weeks	Moderate-to-severe UC	IOR and MOR
α$_4$/β$_7$ integrin antibody			
Vedolizumab	300 mg intravenously every 4 weeks	Moderate-to-severe UC or CD refractory to anti-TNF agents	IOR and MOR IOR and MOR
Interleukin-12 and -23 antibody			
Ustekinumab	260–520 mg intravenously, then 90 mg subcutaneously every 8 weeks	Moderate-to-severe CD refractory to immunosuppressants or anti-TNF agents	IOR and MOR
Antibiotics			
Metronidazole	10–20 mg kg^{-1} daily orally	Perianal CD	IOR
Ciprofloxacin	500 mg twice daily orally	Used in conjunction with metronidazole for perianal CD	IOR

ASA, aminosalicylic acid; CD, Crohn's disease; IOR, induction of remission; MOR, maintenance of remission; TNF, tumor necrosis factor; UC, ulcerative colitis.

- Side effects of sulfasalazine (attributed to the sulfa moiety) include nausea, dyspepsia, headache, interference with folic acid absorption, and occasionally hemolytic anemia, agranulocytosis, hepatitis, or pneumonitis. Patients taking sulfasalazine should be given folate 1 mg daily.
- Side effects of 5-ASA include hair loss, headache, and abdominal pain. Rarely, 5-ASA may be associated with interstitial nephritis.
- Olsalazine can be associated with diarrhea.

Glucocorticoids

- Glucocorticoids are used to induce remission in mild-to-severe UC and CD.
- They are available in oral (prednisone, prednisolone, budesonide), intravenous (hydrocortisone, methylprednisolone), and enema (hydrocortisone) formulations.
- Budesonide is a glucocorticoid with high (>90%) first-pass liver metabolism; as a result, budesonide has considerably fewer side effects than conventional glucocorticoids; it has a slow onset of action.
- Budesonide is available in two formulations: controlled-ileal-release budesonide is used to treat mild-to-moderate terminal ileal and ileocolonic CD; multimatrix (MMX) budesonide is used to treat mild-to-moderate UC.
- Side effects of glucocorticoids include acne, hypertension, hirsutism, cataracts, striae, hyperglycemia, hyperlipidemia, insomnia, hyperactivity, acute psychotic episodes, adrenal suppression, and weight gain.

Immunomodulators

- Methotrexate:
  - This agent is used primarily for the treatment of patients with glucocorticoid-refractory or glucocorticoid-dependent CD. It is not effective for UC.
  - Side effects include stomatitis, nausea, diarrhea, hair loss, leukopenia, hypersensitivity pneumonitis, and hepatotoxicity.
  - Folic acid 1–2 mg per day orally should be administered with methotrexate to prevent folic acid deficiency.
  - Methotrexate is contraindicated in women who are pregnant or considering pregnancy.
- Azathioprine and 6-mercaptopurine (6-MP):
  - Azathioprine is a prodrug that is converted to 6-MP through a nonenzymatic reaction.
  - These drugs are used to maintain remission in UC and CD.
  - They have a slow onset of action.
  - Side effects
    - Dose-dependent: hepatitis, bone marrow suppression.
    - Idiosyncratic (dose-independent): acute pancreatitis, nausea, vomiting, diarrhea, flu-like symptoms.

- The patient's thiopurine methyltransferase genotype should be determined prior to initiation of therapy to guide proper dosing of the medication.
- A complete blood count and liver biochemical test levels should be monitored during therapy at least every 3 months while the patient is taking the drug.

Biologic agents

- Mandatory tests and considerations prior to initiation of therapy with biologics:
  - A negative test for tuberculosis (Quantiferon, chest X-ray, PPD).
  - Screening for hepatitis B virus (see Chapter 13).
  - Check for measles, mumps, rubella, varicella, hepatitis A virus immunity.
  - Consider vaccination for tetanus, diphtheria, pertussis, human papillomavirus, influenza, *Pneumococcus*, and *Meningococcus*.
- Anti-TNF agents:
  - Available anti-TNF agents include infliximab, adalimumab, certolizumab pegol, a polyethylene-glycosylated Fab′ fragment of a humanized anti-TNF antibody, and golimumab, a human anti-TNF antibody. Infliximab is a chimeric monoclonal antibody against TNF-α, and adalimumab is a human immunoglobulin G1 (IgG1) monoclonal antibody against TNF.
  - Anti-TNF agents bind to and neutralize soluble and receptor-bound TNF. Although the precise mechanism of action is unknown, they inhibit T-cell proliferation and induce apoptosis.
  - UC: used for steroid-refractory moderate-to-severe disease.
  - CD: used for inflammatory and fistulizing disease.
  - Also used for extraintestinal manifestations of IBD.
  - Drug monitoring is available for infliximab and adalimumab; target trough levels are >3 μg ml^{-1} and >7 μg ml^{-1}, respectively; check drug antibodies simultaneously.
  - Side effects include sepsis, reactivation of tuberculosis, fungal infections, and hepatosplenic T-cell lymphoma. Infusion reactions, characterized by chest pain, shortness of breath, rash, and hypotension, are more common with infliximab than with other anti-TNF agents. Delayed hypersensitivity is an uncommon complication that can occur 2–12 days after an infusion of an anti-TNF agent.
  - Patients with moderate-to-severe CD are more likely to achieve glucocorticoid-free remission at 6 months when treated with a combination of infliximab and azathioprine, or infliximab alone, but not azathioprine alone.
  - Additional benefits of combination immunomodulator/biologic therapy: lower rate of infusion reaction, lower rate of anti-biologic antibody formation, higher biologic serum concentrations

- Vedolizumab:
  - Vedolizumab is a humanized monoclonal antibody against α_4/β_7 integrin that inhibits leukocyte adhesion and migration into inflamed tissue.
  - Used for moderate-to-severe CD and UC with evidence of active inflammation refractory to prior treatment, including anti-TNF therapy.
  - Vedolizumab is usually well tolerated in patients with CD and UC. Caution is advised with a history of recurrent infections.
- Ustekinumab:
  - Ustekinumab is a monoclonal antibody to the p40 subunit of interleukin-12 and interleukin-23.
  - Used for moderate-to-severe CD when immunosuppressants or anti-TNF agents have failed or were not tolerated.

Antibiotics

- Ciprofloxacin and metronidazole can be used alone or in combination.
- CD: treatment of mild-to-moderate left-sided colonic and fistulizing disease:
  - Metronidazole: side effects include nausea, irreversible peripheral neuropathy, metallic taste, and a disulfiram effect.
  - Ciprofloxacin: efficacy is similar to that for metronidazole for the treatment of colonic disease, with a more favorable side-effect profile; side effects include nausea, diarrhea, skin rashes, tendinitis, and Achilles tendon rupture.

Surgery

- Surgery is indicated for the treatment of medication-refractory, worsening disease and complications, including severe medication side effects, fistulas, toxic megacolon, and obstruction.
- UC: total or subtotal colectomy with end-ileostomy or an ileal pouch–anal anastomosis; for the latter, the 1-cm residual anorectal segment (cuff) must be surveyed periodically endoscopically to rule out recurrent disease ('cuffitis') or cancer.
- CD: 74% of all patients will require surgery:
  - Fistulectomy.
  - Segmental resection.
  - Diverting ileostomy for distal fistulizing and/or inflammatory disease.

Complications

- Toxic megacolon:
  - Toxic megacolon is a complication of severe UC. It is defined as acute colonic dilatation with a transverse colon diameter of >6 cm (on imaging examination) in a patient with a severe attack of colitis.

- Seen in 5% of patients with severe UC.
- Precipitating factors include hypokalemia, antimotility agents, narcotics, and colonoscopy undertaken during a severe UC flare.
- Medical management includes correction of electrolyte imbalances, empiric antibiotics, discontinuation of antimotility agents and narcotics, intravenous cyclosporine or infliximab, and, in some cases, subtotal colectomy.
- Dysplasia and colorectal cancer:
  - Patients with long-standing UC or colonic CD are at increased risk of colorectal cancer.
  - The most important risk factors include the duration, severity and extent of colitis. Pancolitis is associated with the highest risk. Distal rectosigmoid colitis is not associated with an increased risk above that seen in persons without colitis. Other risk factors include primary sclerosing cholangitis, backwash ileitis, a family history of colon cancer, younger age at diagnosis of disease, and more severe inflammation.
  - The risk of colorectal cancer is estimated to be 7–10% after 20 years of colitis, and as high as 30% after 35 years, although lower rates have been reported.
  - Patients with CD involving more than one-third of their colon are at an increased risk for the development of dysplasia and colon cancer.
  - Annual or biennial colonoscopy with biopsies is recommended for patients with UC or pancolonic CD who have had disease for 8 years.
- Complications in patients with CD include small-intestinal bacterial overgrowth, choledocholithiasis, amyloidosis, metabolic bone disease including osteoporosis, fistulas, nephrolithiasis (due to dehydration or oxalate malabsorption), intestinal malabsorption, and nutritional deficiencies including deficiencies of fat-soluble vitamins, iron, folate, and vitamin B_{12}.

Prognosis

- CD: 75% relapse rate over 5 years after remission is achieved:
  - If the disease is inactive, there is an 80% chance of being relapse free at one year.
  - The rate of relapse is not affected by the segment of bowel involved, patient's age, or severity of disease.
- UC: the behavior of the disease is affected by the extent of colitis, progression proximally in the colon, and associated systemic symptoms.
  - More than 50% of patients have mild disease at the time of initial presentation.
  - Approximately 80% of patients have a disease course characterized by intermittent flares interposed between variable periods of remission.
  - The overall colectomy rate is 24% at 10 years, and 30% at 25 years.

Pearls

- Up to 10% of patients with CD present with proctitis.
- Persistently elevated serum alkaline phosphatase levels may be seen in about 3% of patients with UC or Crohn's colitis, and should prompt further investigation to exclude primary sclerosing cholangitis (see Chapter 13).
- A colonic stricture in a patient with UC is considered malignant until proven otherwise.
- The incidence of *C. difficile* colitis is increased in patients with IBD. Stool samples for *C. difficile* toxin should be obtained during acute flares of IBD, whether or not there is a history of antibiotic use or hospitalization.

Questions

Question 1 relates to the clinical vignette at the beginning of this chapter.

1 Which of the following is the most likely to reveal the diagnosis?
   A Colonoscopy.
   B Computed tomography (CT) of the abdomen and pelvis.
   C Stool culture and examinations for ova and parasites and *Clostridium difficile* toxin.
   D Small-bowel follow-through.
   E Esophagogastroduodenoscopy (EGD).

2 A 56-year-old man with long-standing Crohn's disease (CD) of the cecum and terminal ileum, confirmed by colonoscopy 3 months ago, presents for the third time in a year with a flare characterized by right lower quadrant pain, loss of appetite, and loose stools. Physical examination reveals normal vital signs and right lower quadrant tenderness without rebound tenderness. Besides a slightly elevated white blood cell count, the blood work is unremarkable. He is placed on therapy with prednisone 40 mg daily, which is tapered over the course of 2 months, but he becomes symptomatic again at a dose of 20 mg per day. Which of the following is the appropriate next step?
   A Reassurance.
   B Computed tomography.
   C Colonoscopy.
   D Thiopurine methyltransferase (TPMT) genotype.
   E Magnetic resonance (MR) enterography.

3   A 43-year-old woman with a 10-year history of ulcerative colitis (UC) presents for an annual health examination. Which of the following test(s) would you recommend?
    A Serum alkaline phosphatase level.
    B Colonoscopy.
    C Complete blood count.
    D All of the above.

4   A 23-year-old man with a history of terminal ileal Crohn's disease treated with budesonide presents with nausea, vomiting, and abdominal pain of 2 days' duration. Magnetic resonance enterography reveals a fibrotic stricture approximately 8 inches (20 cm) in length, with proximal dilatation of the small bowel. There is no evidence of an intra-abdominal abscess or fistula. Which of the following is the best treatment option for this patient?
    A Prednisone.
    B Infliximab.
    C Mesalamine.
    D Metronidazole.
    E Surgical resection.

5   A 33-year-old man with a history of ulcerative colitis (UC) presents to the emergency department with a severe flare of UC. Due to work-related activities over the previous 3 weeks, he has not been taking his prescribed medications regularly. On admission, the patient is pale and diaphoretic, with a pulse rate of 120 per minute, blood pressure 90/55 mmHg, and temperature 101 °F (38.3 °C). The white blood cell count is 18 000 mm^{-3}, hematocrit value 15%, and hemoglobin level 6 g dl^{-1}. An intravenous line is started, and fluids and packed red blood cells are administered. Which of the following tests should be ordered next?
    A Colonoscopy.
    B Flexible sigmoidoscopy.
    C Plain X-ray of the abdomen.
    D Barium enema.
    E Small-bowel follow-through.

Answers

1   A
    The symptoms (right lower quadrant pain, weight loss, and diarrhea) and laboratory test results (iron-deficiency anemia) are consistent with a diagnosis of Crohn's disease (CD). Colonoscopy is a reasonable option to

confirm the diagnosis. CT may also be obtained. Because infectious diarrhea is much more common than IBD, it must be ruled out by stool studies prior to embarking on other tests. A small-bowel follow-through and EGD are not indicated in this patient.

2   D

The patient has symptoms consistent with a flare of long-standing CD, but has become glucocorticoid-dependent. Vital signs, physical examination, laboratory test results, and recent endoscopy are all consistent with mild-to-moderate disease. The next step is to prescribe a glucocorticoid-sparing drug, specifically azathioprine or 6-mercaptopurine. Before initiation of this therapy, however, a TPMT genotype should be obtained to determine the appropriate dosing. Patients with low (10% of persons) or absent (0.3% of persons) activity of TPMT are at increased risk for bone marrow toxicity.

3   D

Long-standing UC is associated with an increased risk of colorectal cancer. Therefore, surveillance colonoscopy should be obtained annually or biennially after 8 years of disease. Some 5% of patients with UC may develop primary sclerosing cholangitis, and liver biochemical tests that include a serum alkaline phosphatase level are recommended. A complete blood count should also be obtained annually to evaluate the patient for anemia.

4   E

This patient's symptoms are consistent with small-bowel obstruction secondary to a stricture. Surgical resection of the strictured terminal ileum with primary anastomosis of the small bowel to the colon is the best option for this patient. Medical therapy is not indicated for fibrotic strictures.

5   C

The patient's clinical presentation is concerning for toxic megacolon, a life-threatening complication of severe UC. A colonic diameter of >6 cm on a plain abdominal X-ray (or computed tomography) is suggestive of toxic megacolon. All the other tests listed above are contraindicated in a patient suspected of having toxic megacolon.

Further Reading

Abraham, C. and Cho, J.H. (2009) Inflammatory bowel disease. *New England Journal of Medicine*, **361**, 2066–2078.

Colombel, J.F., Sandborn, W.J., Reinisch, W., *et al.* (2010) Infliximab, azathioprine, or combination therapy for Crohn's disease. *New England Journal of Medicine*, **362**, 1383.

Osterman, M.T. and Lichtenstein, G.R. (2016) Ulcerative colitis, in Sleisenger and Fordtran's Gastrointestinal and Liver Disease: Pathophysiology/Diagnosis/Management, 10th edition (eds M. Feldman, L.S. Friedman, and L.J. Brandt), Saunders Elsevier, Philadelphia, pp. 2023–2061.

Sands, B.E. and Siegel, C.A. (2016) Crohn's disease, in Sleisenger and Fordtran's Gastrointestinal and Liver Disease: Pathophysiology/Diagnosis/Management, 10th edition (eds M. Feldman, L.S. Friedman, and L.J. Brandt), Saunders Elsevier, Philadelphia, pp. 1990–2022.

Weblinks

http://www.clevelandclinicmeded.com/medicalpubs/diseasemanagement/gastroenterology/crohns-disease/

http://www.clevelandclinicmeded.com/medicalpubs/diseasemanagement/gastroenterology/ulcerative-colitis/

http://gi.org/guideline/ulcerative-colitis-in-adults/

http://gi.org/guideline/management-of-crohn's-disease-in-adults/

http://emedicine.medscape.com/article/179037-overview

9

Constipation

Shreya Raja and Shanthi Srinivasan

Clinical Vignette

A 52-year-old woman is seen in the office for difficulty with bowel movements for the past seven to eight years. She reports having one or two bowel movements per week, with effort. Her stools are hard and lumpy. She denies experiencing nausea or vomiting. She has no nocturnal pain, early satiety, abdominal cramps, diarrhea, rectal bleeding, or weight loss. A screening colonoscopy at age 50 was unremarkable. Her past medical and surgical history is unremarkable. She does not take any prescription or over-the-counter medications. Her parents are alive and well. Her two siblings are healthy. Her paternal grandfather died of colon cancer at age 80. She works as a computer analyst. She is married with two children, who were both delivered vaginally. She drinks a glass of wine with dinner and does not smoke. She has no history of illicit drug use. Physical examination reveals a blood pressure of 130/70 mmHg, pulse rate 70 per minute, and body mass index 25; she is afebrile. The remainder of the examination, including an abdominal examination, is unremarkable. Her thyroid is not enlarged. Rectal examination reveals normal sphincter tone, squeeze pressure, and hard stool that is brown and negative for occult blood. Routine laboratory tests show a normal complete blood count and normal levels of blood glucose, serum electrolytes, creatinine, and calcium.

General

- Constipation affects approximately 15% of the general population, but can affect up to 50% of persons over 65 years of age. It is twice as common in women as in men.

Sitaraman and Friedman's Essentials of Gastroenterology, Second Edition.
Edited by Shanthi Srinivasan and Lawrence S. Friedman.
© 2018 John Wiley & Sons Ltd. Published 2018 by John Wiley & Sons Ltd.

- Primary, or functional, constipation is defined by the Rome Foundation as at least two of the following symptoms for a period of 12 weeks, which need not be consecutive, during the preceding 6 months:
  - Infrequent bowel movements (less than three bowel movements per week).
  - Straining during >25% of bowel movements.
  - Lumpy or hard stools in >25% of bowel movements.
  - Sensation of incomplete bowel evacuation in >25% of bowel movements.
  - Sensation of anorectal obstruction or blockade in >25% of bowel movements.
  - Use of manual maneuvers to facilitate defecation in >25% of bowel movements (e.g., digital evacuation, support of the pelvic floor).

Physiology

Colonic Motility

- Coordinated contraction of the colonic muscle is essential to propel colonic contents towards the anus. Peristalsis involves contraction of the colon proximal to an area of distention and relaxation of the colon distal to the area of distention.
- Colonic motility is regulated by intrinsic and extrinsic neuronal innervation. The enteric nervous system is the intrinsic nervous system of the gastrointestinal tract (Figure 9.1) that plays a central role in colonic motility. It is formed by the myenteric plexus, which lies between the circular and longitudinal muscle, and the Meissner's plexus, which is located in the submucosa.

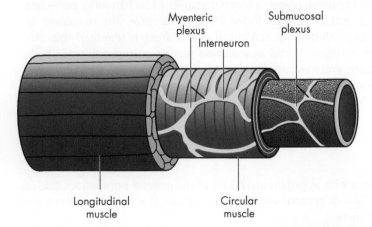

Figure 9.1 Diagram of the colon showing the myenteric plexus located between the circular and longitudinal muscles and the submucosal (Meissner's) plexus located in the submucosa.

- The major extrinsic innervation of the colon includes the sympathetic and the parasympathetic nerves. Sympathetic innervation is through the lumbar colonic nerves that synapse onto the postganglionic neurons in the spinal cord. Sympathetic input results in reduced colonic motility, intestinal secretion, and contraction of the internal anal sphincter. Parasympathetic innervation is through the vagus and pelvic nerves and results in increased colonic contractility and fluid secretion.

Defecation

- The presence of stool in the rectum results in the urge to defecate, and if the social circumstances are appropriate, the process of defecation is initiated.
- The process of defecation involves relaxation of the puborectalis muscle and the internal anal sphincter, accompanied by increased abdominal pressure (Figure 9.2).

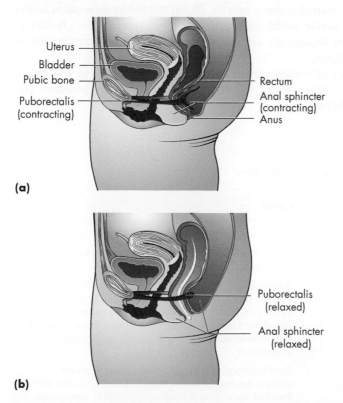

Figure 9.2 Diagram showing the process of defecation. Under normal circumstances (a), the puborectalis is contracted, resulting in an acute anorectal angle. During defecation (b) there is relaxation of the puborectalis with widening of the anorectal angle, thus facilitating the passage of stool.

- Rectal distention results in relaxation of the internal anal sphincter and descent of stool into the anal canal.
- The relaxation of the puborectalis muscle causes a straightening of the anorectal angle and reduction in outflow resistance.
- Voluntary relaxation of the external anal sphincter then results in expulsion of stool.

Etiology

- Constipation can be divided into primary (functional) or secondary.
- Primary, or functional, constipation can be 'simple' constipation associated with insufficient dietary fiber, inadequate fluid intake or decreased physical activity (and reversible by lifestyle modification), or due to irritable bowel syndrome (associated with abdominal pain or distension; see Chapter 7), slow transit (colonic inertia, characterized by infrequent bowel movements), or pelvic outlet obstruction (pelvic dyssynergia, characterized by excessive straining). The most common type of constipation is 'simple' constipation.
- Secondary causes of constipation include structural lesions in the colon, metabolic abnormalities, endocrine diseases, neuromuscular disorders, and medications (Table 9.1).

Table 9.1 Secondary causes of constipation.

Category	Causes
Structural lesions	Anal fissure, colon cancer, colonic stricture, proctitis
Metabolic abnormalities/ endocrine diseases	Diabetes mellitus, heavy metal intoxication, hypercalcemia, hypothyroidism
Neurologic disorders	Autonomic neuropathy, Chagas disease, Hirschsprung's disease, multiple sclerosis, muscular and myotonic dystrophy, Parkinson's disease, pseudo-obstruction, spinal cord lesions (sacral nerves transection or injury to lumbosacral spine, meningomyelocele, spinal anesthesia)
Medications	Anticholinergics, antidepressants, antipsychotics, antispasmodics, calcium channel blockers, cations such as iron and aluminum, 5-hydroxytryptamine$_3$ antagonists, ganglion blockers, opiates, vinca alkaloids

Risk factors for developing constipation include advanced age, female gender, physical inactivity, low income and educational status, and depression.

Clinical Evaluation

History

- A complete history should be obtained. Onset and duration of the complaint should be determined. A recent change in bowel habit is of concern, especially in adults.
  - The medication history should include all medications, including those taken over-the-counter.
  - Typical symptoms include infrequent bowel movements, hard stools, prolonged and excessive straining, and a need for perineal or vaginal pressure or for direct digital manipulation to defecate.
  - Other symptoms may include a sensation of incomplete evacuation, abdominal bloating, abdominal pain, and malaise. The presence of pain or bleeding with defecation should be noted. The presence of fecal and/or urinary incontinence should be noted.
  - An obstetric history should be obtained in women, with particular attention to vaginal deliveries.

Physical Examination

- The physical examination should include a detailed rectal examination (Figure 9.3). This includes inspection of the anus for fissures, hemorrhoids, scars, or fistulas.
  - Pelvic floor function should be evaluated by asking the patient to bear down and examining the descent of the perineum. The normal descent of the perineum is 1–3 cm.
  - The digital rectal examination should be performed to determine the resting sphincter tone, as well as the presence of a stricture, mass, or stool impaction.
  - The appropriate relaxation of the puborectalis (felt posteriorly) and reduction in anal sphincter tone in response to the initiation of defecation is determined by asking the patient to bear down during the digital rectal examination. It should be noted whether the patient finds the examination to be exquisitely painful.
  - The patient should also be asked to squeeze against the examining finger to assess the contractility of the external anal sphincter.

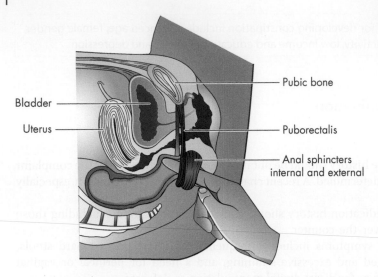

Bladder

Uterus

Pubic bone

Puborectalis

Anal sphincters
internal and external

Figure 9.3 Digital rectal examination and the structures that are palpated, including the internal and external anal sphincters and the puborectalis muscle.

- In female patients, one should look for a rectocele or prolapsed rectum.
- External sensory testing for touch, temperature and pain and perianal wink may be performed on overlying perianal skin.

Laboratory Tests

- These should include a complete blood count, serum thyroid-stimulating hormone (TSH) level, a comprehensive metabolic profile including magnesium, and vitamin D levels.

Colonoscopy

- Colonoscopy (or in some cases flexible sigmoidoscopy) or air contrast barium enema is done to look for structural lesions such as colon cancer or colonic stricture. This is important in patients with 'alarm symptoms' (recent worsening of constipation, blood in the stools, weight loss, anorexia, nausea, or vomiting), or as a screening procedure in patients older than age 50 (in whom colonoscopy is preferred).

Physiologic Tests

- Physiologic tests are used to assess colonic motility (measurement of the colonic transit time) and anal sphincter pressure and function (anorectal manometry). They are usually performed in patients with refractory constipation. In patients who exhibit excessive straining or prolonged or unsatisfactory defecation, with or without anal digitation, it is best to begin with anorectal manometry to assess for a problem in the process of defection (defecatory disorder). If defecation is normal, a colonic transit time can be measured.

– **Colon transit study**. This test determines the colonic transit time, which is measured using radiopaque markers. The patient ingests a gelatin capsule that contains 24 small radiopaque rings (Sitzmark). A plain X-ray of the abdomen is taken 5 days after ingestion of the capsule. The normal colonic transit time is less than 72 hours. If 80% or more (≥19) of the markers are expelled within 5 days, the colonic transit time is considered normal. Slow colonic transit is indicated by the retention of 20% or more (≥5) of the markers in the colon. A scattered distribution of the markers is consistent with colonic inertia, whereas collection of the markers in the pelvis is consistent with pelvic outlet obstruction (Figure 9.4). A wireless

Colonic inertia

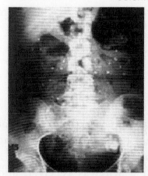 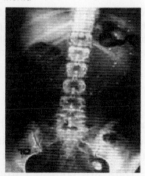

Pelvic floor dysfunction

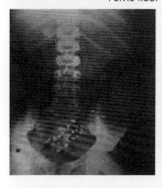 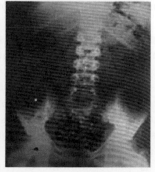

Figure 9.4 Colonic transit study showing plain X-rays of the abdomen taken on day 5 after ingestion of a capsule containing 24 radiopaque markers. The two films at the top from a patient with colonic inertia show markers that are evenly distributed throughout the colon. The two films at the bottom are from a patient with pelvic floor dysfunction and show retention of the markers in the pelvic area (distal colon).

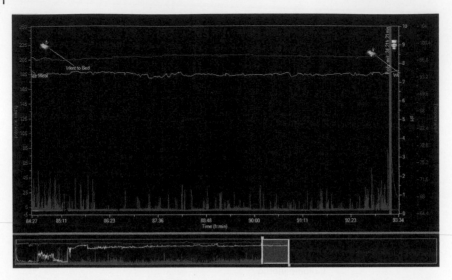

Figure 9.5 Wireless motility capsule tracing showing slow-transit constipation. Temperature tracing is shown in blue, pH tracing is shown in green, and pressure measurements are shown in red. The sharp drop in temperature signals the exit of the capsule from the body shown by the pink vertical bar. In this tracing, whole-gut transit time is 3 days, 21 hours and 21 minutes.

motility capsule (Smartpill; Medtronic, Inc.) has also been developed that can be used to assess regional gastrointestinal transit times, including gastric, small intestine, and colonic transit times, after ingestion with a standardized meal. Data are collected from a wireless receiver, and normal whole-gut transit time is <59 hours (Figure 9.5). Appropriate patient selection is key to avoiding known complications such as capsule retention.

- **Anorectal manometry**. This technique is used to measure internal and external anal sphincter pressures, as well as the anorectal inhibitory reflex. The resting anal canal pressure indicates the tonic activity of the internal and external anal sphincter pressures. The anal pressure measured during maximal voluntary anal contraction indicates the external anal sphincter pressure. The anorectal inhibitory reflex is assessed by the ability of the internal anal sphincter to relax in response to a balloon distended in the rectum. The anorectal inhibitory reflex is reduced in megarectum, and its absence is pathognomonic of Hirschsprung's disease (congenital aganglionosis, usually in a short segment of sigmoid colon). Three-dimensional high-resolution anorectal manometry generates pressure topography images of the anorectal canal during periods of rest, squeeze, and attempted defecation (Figure 9.6).

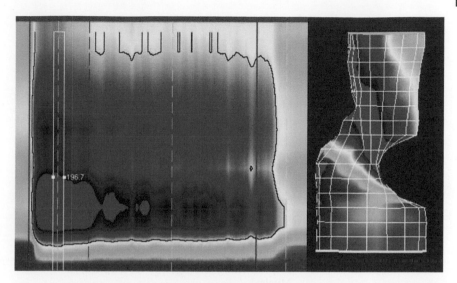

Figure 9.6 High-resolution anorectal manometry images generated during a normal squeeze maneuver. A two-dimensional pressure tracing is shown on the left, and a three-dimensional reconstruction of the same tracing is shown on the right. Warmer colors correspond to areas of higher pressure, and cooler colors correspond to areas of lower pressure.

- **Other methods of assessing the defecatory process.** With defecography, barium is instilled in the rectum, and the patient is asked to defecate on a commode while X-rays are taken. This technique allows the evaluation of the anorectal angle and can detect anatomic abnormalities such as a prolapsed rectum. Increasingly, dynamic magnetic resonance imaging (MRI) has replaced standard barium defecography. In addition, endoscopic ultrasonography of the internal and external anal sphincters can be used to detect tears or scarring of the sphincters.

Treatment

- The first step in the treatment of constipation is to address the underlying cause, such as a structural lesion, metabolic abnormality, or use of a constipation-inducing medication.
- For primary (functional) constipation, the first line of therapy is diet and lifestyle modification:
  - Patients should be encouraged to drink at least 2 liters (8 glasses) of fluid per day, and ingest 20–35 g of fiber per day, preferably in the form of fruits and vegetables.
  - If adequate fruit and vegetable intake is not possible, a fiber supplement (bulk-producing laxative) is recommended (see Table 9.2). It is important to introduce an increasing amount of fiber gradually.

Table 9.2 Laxatives.

Category	Medications	Dose
Bulk-producing agents	Psyllium (Metamucil)	Titrate to 20 g daily
	Methylcellulose (Citrucel)	Titrate to 20 g daily
	Polycarbophil (FiberCon)	Titrate to 20 g daily
Osmotic laxatives		
Saline laxatives	Magnesium hydroxide	15–30 ml daily
	Magnesium citrate	15–30 ml daily
	Sodium phosphate	10–25 ml with 350 ml of water as needed
Poorly absorbed sugars and other compounds	Lactulose	15–30 ml daily
	Sorbitol	15–30 ml daily
	Polyethyelene glycol (e.g., Miralax)	17–36 g daily
Stool softener	Docusate sodium	100 mg daily
Emollient	Mineral oil	5–15 ml orally every night
Stimulant laxatives	Anthraquinones	
	Cascara	325 mg daily
	Senna	187 mg daily
	Castor oil	15–30 ml daily
	Diphenylmethane derivative (Dulcolax)	5–10 mg daily
Rectal enemas and suppositories	Phosphate enema	120 ml daily
	Mineral oil enema	100 ml daily
	Tap water enema	500 ml daily
	Soap suds enema	1500 ml daily
	Glycerin suppository	10 mg daily
	Bisacodyl suppository	One to two 2.4-g suppositories daily
Chloride channel activator	Lubiprostone	24 μg twice daily
Guanylate cyclase activator	Linaclotide	145–290 μg daily
Serotonin receptor agonist (5HT$_4$)	Prucalopride	2–4 mg daily
Mu-opioid receptor antagonists	Methylnaltrexone	0.15 mg kg^{-1} injection every other day
	Naloxegol	12.5–25 mg daily

5HT, 5-hydroxytryptamine.

- Other lifestyle modifications include regular exercise, weight loss, and reserving enough time to have a bowel movement. In addition, patients should be advised not to ignore the urge to have a bowel movement.
- Once fiber and fluid intake is optimized, persistent constipation can be treated with an osmotic laxative such as polyethylene glycol. The dose of osmotic laxative should be adjusted to achieve stools of soft consistency. Stimulant laxatives are used when an osmotic laxative does not produce the desired effect. Lubiprostone is a laxative that stimulates chloride and water secretion into the intestinal lumen. Linaclotide is a laxative that stimulates guanylate cyclase and results in smooth muscle contraction of the colon. Several agents, including methylnaltrexone and naloxegol, have been developed to reverse the effects of opioid-induced constipation after failure of conventional laxative therapies. Agents used in the treatment of constipation are listed in Table 9.2.
- In hospitalized and bed-bound patients, periodic enemas can be given to prevent fecal impaction.

Colonic Inertia

- In patients with colonic inertia, a combination of diet, exercise and medication is the first line of therapy. Usually, these patients require osmotic and stimulant laxatives in addition to enemas. Prucalopride is a serotonin receptor agonist approved in Europe and Canada for the treatment of colonic inertia; however, it is not approved for use in the United States. Colonic resection with anastomosis of the ileum to the rectum (ileorectostomy) is reserved for patients with severe constipation that is refractory to medical treatment.

Pelvic Floor Dysfunction

- Surgical repair of a functionally significant rectocele or a prolapsed rectum can lead to resolution of constipation. Usually, one should demonstrate improvement in defecation when pressure is placed on the posterior wall of the vagina during defecation before proceeding with the repair of a rectocele.
- Biofeedback training is useful in patients with paradoxical puborectalis contraction to retrain muscles involved in the process of defecation. During biofeedback therapy, patients receive visual and auditory feedback on the functioning of the pelvic floor and anal canal muscles. Using these cues, the patient can learn to relax the pelvic floor muscles during straining, thus facilitating evacuation of the rectum.

Pearls

- Constipation is classified as either simple (functional) or secondary to diseases of the colon, metabolic disorders, neurologic disorders, or medications.
- Diagnostic testing for patients with constipation should include a complete blood count and serum TSH, glucose, calcium, vitamin D and creatinine levels. In addition, a colonoscopy to rule out diseases is important, especially in patients with 'alarm' symptoms such as unintentional weight loss, gastrointestinal bleeding, or iron-deficiency anemia.
- Treatment of constipation should be individualized according to the etiology.

Questions

Questions 1 and 2 relate to the clinical vignette at the beginning of this chapter.

1 Which of the following is indicated at this time?
  A Colonoscopy.
  B Defecography.
  C Anorectal manometry.
  D Capsule endoscopy.
  E No additional diagnostic test.

2 The initial approach to the treatment of constipation in this patient is which of the following?
  A Increase dietary fiber and fluid.
  B An osmotic laxative.
  C A stimulant laxative.
  D A rectal phosphate enema.

3 Defecation is associated with which one of the following?
  A Contraction of the external anal sphincter.
  B Contraction of the puborectalis muscle.
  C Widening of the anorectal angle.
  D Ascent of the pelvic floor.

4 A 42-year-old woman presents with constipation that persists despite diet and lifestyle modification. Digital rectal examination shows a large rectocele. Vaginal examination confirms prolapse of the rectum anteriorly into the vagina. A colonic transit study shows markers in the rectosigmoid region 5 days after ingestion. Anal manometry shows normal internal and

external anal sphincter function. A trial of laxatives does not improve symptoms. Which of the following is the best treatment option for this patient?

A Increase fluid intake to 16 glasses of water per day.

B Increase the fiber in her diet to 50 g per day.

C Surgical removal of the colon.

D Surgical repair of the rectocele.

5 All of the following conditions can result in constipation EXCEPT which of the following?

A Anal fissure.

B Excessive fluid intake.

C Colon cancer.

D Colonic stricture.

E Proctitis.

Questions 6–8 refer to the following clinical vignette:

A 25-year-old woman with a recent history of twin gestation presents to the clinic with new difficulty with passing bowel movements following a prolonged vaginal delivery. She is able to pass three bowel movements per week, but admits to frequent straining and having to use her fingers to remove stool at least once a week. She also pushes on her lower abdomen when trying to defecate. She denies rectal bleeding, abdominal pain, pain with defecation and weight loss, and has no family history of colon cancer or inflammatory bowel disease. Polyethylene glycol and fiber have softened the stool, but she continues to feel like stool is still stuck in her rectum. She does not take any other medications or use any herbal supplements. Digital rectal examination shows normal resting sphincter tone and appropriate augmentation of sphincter tone with squeeze. The perineum does not descend with an attempt to bear down, whereas the puborectalis muscle contracts with an attempt to bear down. No obvious rectocele is noted on examination. Laboratory testing shows a normal complete blood count, comprehensive metabolic panel, serum magnesium, calcium, and vitamin D levels, and TSH.

6 What is the most likely cause of this patient's difficulty with passing bowel movements?

A Colonic inertia.

B Irritable bowel syndrome.

C Pelvic floor dysfunction.

D Anal fissure.

E Hypothyroidism.

7 Which of the following tests would confirm the diagnosis?
A Colonoscopy
B Anorectal manometry
C Wireless motility capsule
D Capsule endoscopy
E Flexible sigmoidoscopy

8 Which of the following is most likely to provide long-term relief of the patient's symptoms?
A Stimulant laxatives
B Rectal enemas
C Lubiprostone
D Colectomy with ileorectal anastomosis
E Pelvic floor physical therapy with biofeedback

Answers

1 E

2 A
This patient has constipation (less than three bowel movements a week, and hard, lumpy stool). Her bloating is likely related to constipation. These symptoms do not fit into the criteria for irritable bowel syndrome (see Chapter 7). Her history, physical examination, prior colonoscopy result, and routine blood work do not suggest a secondary cause of constipation. Therefore, she has primary constipation, which is best treated by diet and lifestyle modifications. An oral laxative or a rectal enema (or both) are indicated if her symptoms fail to respond to diet and lifestyle modifications. Additional tests (colonic transit study, anorectal manometry, and defecography) to evaluate her for colonic inertia or anorectal dysfunction should be reserved for refractory constipation.

3 C
The process of defecation involves relaxation (not contraction) of the external and internal anal sphincters and the puborectalis muscle. This results in widening of the anorectal angle, descent (not ascent) of the perineum, and facilitation of the passage of stool.

4 D
This patient has already tried dietary and lifestyle modification with a poor response. A colonic transit test shows accumulation of markers in the anorectal area, indicating pelvic floor dysfunction associated with a large

rectocele. The rectocele is likely secondary to anorectal dysfunction. Repair of the rectocele, in some patients, will improve defecation. Biofeedback therapy may be considered in conjunction with rectocele repair to prevent a recurrent rectocele.

5 B

Proctitis, anal fissures, colonic stricture, and colon cancer cause constipation due to inflammation or obstruction. Reduced (not excessive) fluid intake can be associated with constipation.

6 C

Incomplete evacuation, the need for manual digitation, and frequent straining are suggestive of pelvic floor dysfunction. The recent twin pregnancy with vaginal delivery may have weakened her pelvic floor muscles. The frequency of her bowel movements is not consistent with colonic inertia. The lack of abdominal pain or rectal pain makes irritable bowel syndrome and anal fissure unlikely. The normal TSH excludes hypothyroidism.

7 B

Anorectal manometry is the only option listed which assesses the pelvic floor musculature. Defecography and dynamic pelvic floor MRI may also provide important diagnostic information. A Sitzmark study showing a majority of retained markers clustered in the rectosigmoid would suggest pelvic floor dysfunction. Prolonged or traumatic vaginal deliveries may result in tears or defects in the internal or external anal sphincter muscles; the 'gold standard' for diagnosis of sphincteric defects is endoanal ultrasound.

8 E

Pelvic floor physical therapy with biofeedback is indicated for pelvic floor dysfunction. Stimulant laxatives, enemas, and lubiprostone may be effective for functional constipation but are often ineffective for pelvic floor dysfunction. Colectomy with ileorectal anastomosis is reserved for patients with severe colonic inertia in the absence of pelvic floor dysfunction.

Further Reading

Lembo, A.J. and Ullman, S.P. (2016) Constipation, in *Sleisenger and Fordtran's Gastrointestinal and Liver Disease: Pathophysiology/Diagnosis/Management*, 10th edition, (eds M. Feldman, L.S. Friedman, and L.J. Brandt), Saunders Elsevier, Philadelphia, pp. 259–278.

Rao, S.S., Rattanakovit, K., and Patcharatraukul, T. (2016) Diagnosis and management of chronic constipation in adults. *Nature Reviews Gastroenterology and Hepatology*, **13**, 295–305.

Wald, A. (2010) A 27-year-old woman with constipation: diagnosis and treatment. *Clinical Gastroenterology and Hepatology*, **8**, 838–842.

Weblink

http://www.merckmanuals.com/professional/sec02/ch008/ch008b.html

10

Colorectal Neoplasms

Pruthvi Patel and Vincent W. Yang

Clinical Vignette

A 65-year-old man is seen in the office for increasing fatigue over the past 6 months. He denies abdominal pain, early satiety, nausea, vomiting, or rectal bleeding. His appetite is normal, but he reports an unintentional weight loss of 4.5 kg in the past 6 months. He has never had a colonoscopy. His past medical and surgical history is remarkable only for hypertension. He takes amlodipine, 2.5 mg once a day. He does not take any over-the-counter medications. His family history is unremarkable. He is a schoolteacher, is married, and has one son, who is healthy. He occasionally drinks one or two glasses of wine, and does not smoke cigarettes. He has no history of illicit drug use. Physical examination reveals a blood pressure of 135/85 mmHg, a pulse rate of 72 per minute, and a body mass index of 33. He is afebrile. The abdominal examination is unremarkable. Rectal examination reveals brown stool that is positive for occult blood. Routine laboratory tests show a hemoglobin of 7.9 g dl^{-1}, mean corpuscular volume 65 fl, iron saturation 3%, and ferritin 7 ng ml^{-1}.

General

- The frequency of colorectal cancer (CRC) varies remarkably among different populations and regions. Incidence rates are highest in developed countries of North America and in Australia and Europe.
- The lifetime risk of developing CRC in the US is approximately 1 in 20.
- The number of new cases of CRC in the US was estimated to be approximately 134 500 in 2016.

Sitaraman and Friedman's Essentials of Gastroenterology, Second Edition.
Edited by Shanthi Srinivasan and Lawrence S. Friedman.
© 2018 John Wiley & Sons Ltd. Published 2018 by John Wiley & Sons Ltd.

- CRC is the second leading cause of cancer-related deaths in the US, accounting for approximately 9% of all cancer deaths.
- CRC incidence and death rates have been declining slowly in both sexes since 1998, a result in part of increased screening for CRC.

Definitions

> Colorectal neoplasia refers to either CRC or premalignant adenomas.

> Polyp refers to a discrete mass of tissue that protrudes into the lumen of the bowel. A polyp can be nonadenomatous, adenomatous (premalignant), or malignant (Table 10.1).

- By definition, all colorectal adenomas are dysplastic. Adenomatous epithelium is characterized by hypercellularity of colonic crypts with cells that possess variable amounts of mucin and hyperchromatic elongated nuclei.
- Advanced adenomas are adenomas that have an increased potential for progressing to malignancy. These are tubular adenomas ≥1 cm in size, villous or tubulovillous adenomas, and adenomas with high-grade dysplasia (HGD).

Table 10.1 Classification of colonic polyps.

Based on appearance	Sessile (flat or broad-based)
	Pedunculated (attached to the colonic wall by a stalk)
Based on histology	Neoplastic:
	• Adenoma (benign):
	– Serrated (mixed hyperplastic and adenoma)
	– Tubular (most common)
	– Tubulovillous
	– Villous
	• Carcinoma (malignant)
	– Noninvasive:
	○ Carcinoma-in-situ (confined to the epithelium)
	○ Intramucosal (extends to lamina propria)
	– Invasive: extends to the submucosa and beyond
	Non-neoplastic:
	• Hyperplastic, inflammatory, lymphoid, or hamartomatous

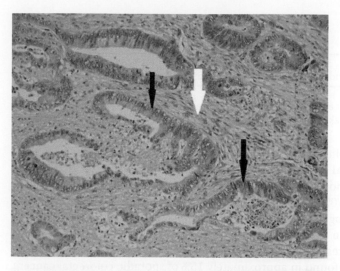

Figure 10.1 Photomicrograph of invasive moderately differentiated colorectal adenocarcinoma. Shown here are the characteristic glandular formation and the characteristic central necrosis (black arrows). There is also stromal desmoplasia with increased fibroblasts surrounding the malignant glands (white arrow). Hematoxylin and eosin staining; original magnification × 10. Illustration courtesy of Stephen Lau, MD, Emory University, Atlanta, GA, USA.

- Because of the lack of lymphatics in the lamina propria in the colonic mucosa, malignant glands that are confined to the colonic mucosa do not have meta-static potential. Therefore, some pathologists refer to carcinoma-in-situ and intramucosal carcinoma as HGD. Labeling noninvasive carcinoma as HGD removes confusion about the need for further work-up or intervention if the lesion is removed completely by endoscopic polypectomy.
- More than 95% of CRCs are adenocarcinomas (Figure 10.1); therefore, the term CRC refers to adenocarcinoma of the colon or rectum unless otherwise specified. Other types of cancers in the colon are lymphoma, carcinoid, leiomyosarcoma, and metastatic lesions.

Molecular Features of CRC

- Most CRCs are considered to develop from adenomas. The transition from normal epithelium to adenoma and carcinoma is associated with acquired molecular alterations that occur in a stepwise fashion and affect multiple genes involved in the regulation of cell growth and differentiation (Figure 10.2).
- A major consequence of molecular alterations is genomic instability.

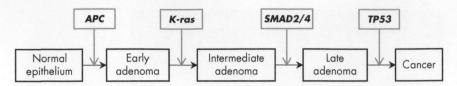

Figure 10.2 Molecular alterations in sporadic colorectal cancer. The transition from normal epithelium to cancer takes approximately 7–10 years. APC, adenomatous polyposis coli.

- Genomic instability can be divided into two categories:
  - **Chromosomal instability** (CIN) is found in 80–85% of CRCs. For example, adenomatous polyposis coli (*APC*), a tumor suppressor gene, is mutated in 70% of colorectal cancers. *K-ras* is the most frequently activated oncogene.
  - **Microsatellite instability** (MSI) refers to changes in tandem repeated DNA sequences secondary to mutations in DNA mismatch repair (MMR) genes. MSI is found in approximately 15% of sporadic colorectal cancers. The most commonly involved genes are *MLH1* and *MSH2*.
- Epigenetic alterations:
  - Epigenetics refers to post-transcriptional silencing of specific genes by a variety of mechanisms, such as methylation. CRCs that have a high frequency of methylation of some CpG (cytosine-phosphodiesterase bond-guanine) islands are referred to as **CpG island methylator phenotype** (CIMP) tumors. These epigenetic alterations in the promoter for the MMR genes can silence their transcription and subsequent protein expression.
  - Activating mutations in the *BRAF* gene occur almost exclusively in sporadic CRCs with high degrees of MSI and CIMP. This group of CRCs is considered to have developed from serrated polyps.

Risk Factors

- Age: 90% of CRCs occur in persons 50 years of age or older.
- Prior personal history of colorectal adenoma or CRC.
- Family history of CRC.
- Inflammatory bowel disease.
- Obesity.
- Potential environmental factors:
  - High-fat and low-fiber consumption.
  - Alcohol.
  - Low dietary selenium.
  - Environmental carcinogens and mutagens (from colonic bacteria and charbroiled meats).
  - Smoking.

- Between 10% and 30% of colorectal cancers occur in persons with a family history of a polyp or CRC.
- A small percentage of CRCs occur as part of an inherited syndrome. Approximately 5% are associated with **Lynch syndrome** (also called hereditary nonpolyposis colorectal cancer; HNPCC), and 1% are associated with **familial adenomatous polyposis** (FAP). Less than 0.1% are associated with other rare CRC syndromes.

> No underlying etiology can be identified in the majority of persons (approximately 75%) with CRC. These cancers are considered 'sporadic' CRCs, and the affected population is termed 'average risk.'

Clinical Features

- Most patients with early CRC are asymptomatic. When symptoms are present, they are nonspecific. The tumors can be distributed throughout the colon.
- Clinical manifestations are often related to tumor size and location.
  - Proximal colon (cecum to splenic flexure) lesions: Common symptoms and signs include ill-defined abdominal pain and occult bleeding. Weight loss is uncommon in the absence of metastatic disease.
  - Distal colon (descending colon to rectum) lesions: Common symptoms and signs include altered bowel habits, decreased stool caliber (sometimes described as 'pencil-thin'), and hematochezia.
- Tumors that are circumferential and large may cause symptoms of bowel obstruction. Patients may present with fatigue (due to anemia from chronic occult blood loss), weight loss, or loss of appetite.
- Up to 5% of patients with colorectal cancer will have a synchronous malignant lesion in the colon or rectum at the time of diagnosis.
- *Streptococcus bovis* bacteremia and *Clostridium septicum* sepsis are associated with colonic malignancies in 10–25% of cases.

Diagnosis and Staging

- **Colonoscopy** is the test of choice to establish a diagnosis when CRC is suspected. It provides a visual inspection of the colonic mucosa, and also the ability to obtain tissue biopsies and often removal of polyps. If a patient is diagnosed with CRC but preoperative obstruction prevents a complete colonoscopy (to the cecum), then a colonoscopy should be done within 3–6 months after surgery to diagnose any synchronous lesion.
- **Computed tomography** (CT) of the abdomen and pelvis (Figure 10.3) and chest radiography are carried out for staging purposes prior to surgery.

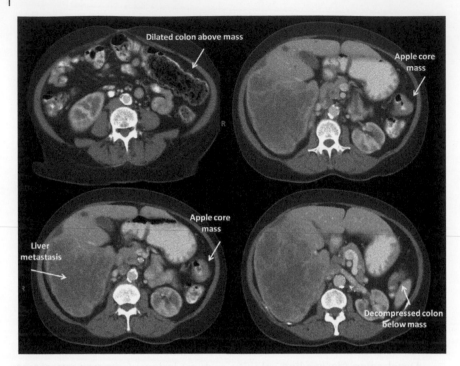

Figure 10.3 Computed tomography in a person with colonic adenocarcinoma. The mass, which has an 'apple-core' appearance, is obstructing the descending colon with resulting dilatation of the colon proximal to the mass. Extensive metastasis in the liver is also seen. Illustration courtesy of Sherif Nour, MD, Emory University, Atlanta, GA, USA.

- In rectal cancer, **endoscopic ultrasonography** (EUS) or **pelvic magnetic resonance imaging** (MRI) is performed to evaluate the depth of tumor invasion and the status of regional lymph nodes. EUS and pelvic MRI both detect regional lymph node metastasis with greater accuracy compared with CT.
- **Carcinoembryonic antigen** (CEA) is a tumor marker for CRC, but has low sensitivity and specificity, and this has limited its use in screening and diagnosis. Elevated serum CEA levels preoperatively may have some prognostic value in advanced colorectal cancer. Patients with stage III disease (see later) have a median time to recurrence of 13 months if CEA preoperative levels are >5 ng ml^{-1} and 28 months if <5 ng ml^{-1}. CEA is used mainly to monitor for recurrent CRC following surgical resection of CRC.

Prognosis

- The American Joint Commission on Cancer (AJCC) system (utilizing the TNM [Tumor Node Metastasis] classification) is commonly used for staging (Table 10.2).

Table 10.2 Colorectal cancer staging.

Stage*	TNM classification	5-year survival rate (%)
0	Tis N0 M0	
I	T1 or T2 N0 M0	92
II	T3 or T4 N0 M0	50–87
III	T1-T4 N1-N2 M0	50–89
IV	Any T Any N M1	11

* This is a simplified staging system. Stage II and III can be further subcategorized, which explains the wide survival rates noted in the table.
Primary tumor (T): Tis, carcinoma-in-situ; T1, tumor invades submucosa; T2, tumor invades muscularis propria; T3, tumor invades through the muscularis propria into the subserosa; T4 tumor invades through the entire colorectal wall to the surface of the visceral peritoneum or directly invades other structures.

- Stage I has a favorable prognosis with a 5-year survival rate of 93%. Stage IV CRC (distant metastases) is associated with a 5-year survival rate of 10%.

Treatment

Surgery is the mainstay of treatment of CRC if no metastatic disease is identified. In selected cases, surgery is performed to resect isolated liver or lung metastases.

Colon Cancer

- **Surgical excision** (usually segmental resection) is recommended for patients without evidence of metastasis (stages I to III) who are medically fit for surgery. **Subtotal colectomy** is performed in patients who have multiple neoplasms. **Proctocolectomy** is reserved for patients with familial cancer syndromes (see below).
- **Postoperative chemotherapy** is recommended for patients with stage III cancer and some patients with stage II cancers.
  - Conventional chemotherapy involves a 5-flurouracil (5FU) plus leucovorin backbone in combination with either oxaliplatin (FOLFOX) or irinotecan (FOLFIRI). Some regimens utilize oral capecitabine in lieu of 5-FU.
  - Targeted biologic agents in combination with conventional chemotherapy are the newest additions to the medical repertoire. These agents include bevacizumab, an antibody to vascular endothelin growth factor (anti-VEGF), and cetuximab, an antibody to epidermal growth factor receptor (anti-EGFR).

Rectal Cancer

- **Low anterior resection** with colorectal anastomosis for middle and upper rectal cancers.
- **Abdominoperineal resection** with a permanent colostomy for lower rectal cancers, or in certain cases a J-pouch can be created by a coloanal anastamosis.
- **Preoperative chemotherapy** with radiation for cancers that are T3 and higher or N1 and higher.
- **Postoperative chemotherapy** for stage II or stage III cancers.

Inherited CRC Syndromes

- Inherited CRC syndromes account for a small percentage of all CRCs. Often, affected patients also have an increased risk of cancers in organs other than the colon. Less common syndromes are listed in Table 10.3.

Familial adenomatous polyposis (FAP)

- FAP is caused by a germline mutation in the *APC* gene and inherited in an autosomal dominant manner.
- The estimated incidence is ~1 in 8000 live births.
- FAP is characterized by multiple (100s–1,000s) adenomas in the colon, first appearing around 15 years of age.
- Almost 100% of patients will have colon cancer at a mean age of approximately 40 years if prophylactic colectomy is not performed before then.
- Patients may have extracolonic manifestations, which include duodenal adenomas and mandibular osteomas.
- Gardner's syndrome is a variant of FAP. In addition to the typical findings of FAP, affected patients have osteomas of the skull and long bones, desmoid tumors, epidermoid cysts, and congenital hypertrophy of the retinal pigmented epithelium.
- Attenuated FAP is also caused by mutations in the *APC* gene. It is associated with fewer colonic adenomas (<100), older age of CRC onset (age of ~55 years), lower cancer penetrance, and greater proximal colonic involvement than seen in classic FAP.

Lynch Syndrome

- Also known as HNPCC, Lynch syndrome is caused by germline mutations in one of the DNA MMR genes, leading to MSI. It is inherited in an autosomal dominant manner.

Table 10.3 Less common inherited syndromes associated with risk of CRC.

Syndrome	Inheritance and genes involved	Additional clinical features
Muir–Torre syndrome	Autosomal dominant; associated with defective DNA MMR	Sebaceous gland tumors and visceral malignancies
MutYH-associated polyposis	Autosomal recessive; biallelic mutations in the *MYH* gene	Similar to attenuated FAP or classic FAP
Turcot's syndrome	Presentation with Lynch syndrome due to *MLH1* or *PMS2* mutation Presentation with FAP due to *APC* gene mutation	Central nervous tumors in association with Lynch syndrome (glioblastoma multiforme) or FAP (often medulloblastoma)
Peutz–Jeghers syndrome	Autosomal dominant; 60% of cases are due to germline mutations in the *LKB1* gene	Hamartomatous polyps involving the epithelium, lamina propria and muscularis mucosa Low risk of CRC Pigmented lesions around mouth, hands, and feet Extracolonic malignancy: small intestine, pancreas, esophagus, ovaries or sex cords, testis, and breast
Juvenile-polyposis syndrome	Autosomal dominant; germline mutations in *PTEN* and *SMAD4*	10 or more juvenile mucous retention polyps in the colon or elsewhere in the gastrointestinal tract Symptoms of colonic obstruction or bleeding during childhood Risk of CRC is not well defined

CRC, colorectal cancer; FAP, familial adenomatous polyposis; MMR, mismatch repair.

- The incidence is 1 in 1000 live births.
- Some 70% of affected persons will develop CRC if surveillance colonoscopy and polypectomy are not performed.
- The adenoma–carcinoma sequence progresses much more rapidly in Lynch syndrome than in sporadic colon cancer. CRC can occur within 2–3 years after a negative colonoscopy.
- The mean age of onset of CRC is 46 years.
- There is an increased risk of extracolonic malignancies, including endometrial, gastric, small bowel, renal pelvic, ureteral, and ovarian neoplasms.

Table 10.4 Revised Bethesda guidelines for testing colorectal cancers for microsatellite instability.

CRC from persons should be tested for MSI in the following situations:

1) CRC diagnosed in a patient who is less than 50 years of age.
2) Presence of synchronous or metachronous colorectal or other HNPCC-related tumors, regardless of age.
3) CRC with MSI-H* histology diagnosed in a patient who is less than 60 years of age.
4) CRC diagnosed in one or more first-degree relatives with HNPCC-related tumors, with one of the persons being diagnosed before age 50 years.
5) CRC diagnosed in two or more first- or second-degree relatives with HNPCC-related tumors, regardless of age.

*MSI-H, microsatellite instability-high refers to changes in two or more of the five National Cancer Institute-recommended panels of microsatellite markers; CRC, colorectal cancer; HNPCC, hereditary nonpolyposis colorectal cancer; MSI, microsatellite instability.

- The Amsterdam II criteria identify high-risk persons for genetic testing ('3-2-1' rule): ≥3 relatives with Lynch syndrome-related cancers, with at least one of them being a first-degree relative of the other two; ≥2 successive generations affected; ≥1 person with a Lynch syndrome-related cancer diagnosed before age 50. FAP should be excluded in cases with CRC.
- The revised Bethesda guidelines for testing colorectal tumors for MSI (Table 10.4) are more inclusive than the Amsterdam II criteria.
- Genetic testing for mutations in the MMR genes is performed to confirm the diagnosis. The tumor can be tested for MSI or the individual for a germline mutation.

Prevention

CRC is preventable through available screening methods, and survival can be improved by early detection. Despite this, approximately 20% of CRC is stage IV at the time of diagnosis. Screening remains underutilized.

Average-Risk Population

- Multiple CRC screening guidelines have been developed, including those by the American Cancer Society in conjunction with gastroenterologic and radiologic societies (Joint Society Guidelines), the US Preventive Services Task Force (USPSTF), and the American College of Gastroenterology (ACG) (Table 10.5).
  - All guidelines recommend CRC screening beginning at age 50.
  - The USPSTF guidelines do not recommend routine screening of adults aged 76–85 years, and do not recommend any screening for adults older than 85 years.

Table 10.5 Screening tests for colorectal cancer in average-risk persons.

Category	Test
Cancer prevention and screening	Colonoscopy every 10 years
	Sigmoidoscopy every 5 years (+ FOBT every 3 years, per USFSTF)
	CT colonography (virtual colonoscopy) every 5 years
Cancer detection	Annual FOBT*, three cards or three specimens:
	Guaiac-based FOBT: detects peroxidase activity of hemoglobin (diet restriction is needed)
	FIT: detects human hemoglobin (diet restriction is not necessary)
	Fecal DNA testing: detects DNA mutations known to be associated with CRC; interval of testing is uncertain
	Barium enema every 5 years

* Only highly sensitive FOBTs are accepted for use in screening by all guidelines (see text). CRC, colorectal cancer; CT, computed tomography; FIT, fecal immunochemical test; FOBT, fecal occult blood test; USPSTF, United States Preventive Services Task Force.

- All the guidelines provide multiple screening options. Colonoscopy every 10 years is included in all the guidelines.
- The Joint Society Guidelines favor 'cancer prevention' screening tests (evaluation of the colon by colonoscopy or imaging that can detect polyps) over 'cancer detection' screening tests (fecal occult blood and stool DNA tests).
- The American College of Physicians recommends colonoscopy as the preferred screening method. CT colonography ('virtual colonoscopy') is reserved for patients who are at high risk to receive anesthesia or in those with incomplete colonoscopic attempts.
- Because up to 46% of lesions are in the right (proximal) colon, sigmoidoscopy with fecal occult blood testing and barium enema tests have largely fallen out of favor.

High-Risk Populations

- Colonoscopy is the preferred screening method for persons who are at increased risk of CRC, such as those with inflammatory bowel disease (IBD), a personal or family history of colonic neoplasms, or hereditary colorectal cancer syndromes.

- The starting age for screening and recommended screening intervals depend on the specific condition.
- For persons who have a family history of CRC or adenomatous polyps in a first-degree relative before age 60, or in two or more first-degree relatives at any age, screening with colonoscopy should begin at age 40, or 10 years before the age at which the youngest family member was diagnosed. The screening interval is every 5 years. For persons with a first-degree relative diagnosed with CRC at age 60 or older, or with two second-degree relatives with cancer, screening should begin at age 40. The screening interval is every 10 years, and screening modalities beside colonoscopy can be used.
- Others:
  - Lynch syndrome: colonoscopy every 1–2 years, beginning at age 20.
  - Peutz–Jeghers syndrome: first colonoscopy in the second decade; subsequent screening interval is based on the findings.
  - IBD: colonoscopy with surveillance biopsies every 1–2 years beginning 8–10 years after the onset of symptoms in those with pancolonic involvement.
- Post-polypectomy surveillance:
  - Advanced adenoma (see earlier) or three or more adenomas: repeat colonoscopy in 3 years.
  - One or two small tubular adenomas (<1 cm): repeat colonoscopy in 5–10 years.
- Post-colorectal cancer resection surveillance:
  - Repeat colonoscopy 1 year after curative resection. If the examination is normal, then the interval before the next examination should be 3 years, and then 5 years thereafter if the examinations remain negative for adenomas.
  - Serum CEA determinations at regular intervals may be cost-effective for detecting recurrent cancers. The National Comprehensive Cancer Network (NCCN) recommends CEA testing every 3 months in the first 2 years and every 6 months for another 3 years.

Pearls

- CRC should be considered when a patient, especially one older than 40 years of age, presents with hypochromic microcytic anemia.
- Screening for CRC should begin at age 50 in average-risk persons, and at an earlier age in high-risk populations.
- Colonoscopy is universally accepted as a preferred modality for CRC screening in the average-risk population. It is the preferred screening modality in high-risk populations and the preferred diagnostic test in patients with any symptom or sign suggestive of CRC.

Questions

Questions 1 and 2 relate to the clinical vignette at the beginning of this chapter.

1　The next step in the management of this patient should be which of the following?

　　A Fecal occult blood test and, if positive, colonoscopy.

　　B Upper endoscopy.

　　C Colonoscopy.

　　D CT of the abdomen and pelvis with oral and intravenous contrast.

　　E Oral iron supplementations and repeat complete blood count in 8 weeks.

2　Colonoscopy revealed a 5-cm mass in the ascending colon and an additional 2-cm mass in the descending colon. Biopsies of both masses were consistent with invasive adenocarcinoma. Chest X-rays and CT of the abdomen and pelvis did not reveal lymphadenopathy or metastasis. The next step in the management of this patient is which of the following?

　　A Right hemicolectomy and endoscopic resection of the colon cancer in the descending colon.

　　B Subtotal colectomy.

　　C Preoperative chemotherapy with radiotherapy, followed by subtotal colectomy.

　　D Chemotherapy only.

3　A 74-year-old man undergoes colonoscopy because of intermittent rectal bleeding and is found to have a 3-cm pedunculated polypoid mass in the sigmoid colon. The mass is ulcerated. A polypectomy is performed. The pathology report shows high-grade dysplasia; no tumor cells are seen in the polyp stalk. What is the appropriate management of this patient?

　　A CT of the abdomen and pelvis.

　　B Positron emission tomography (PET).

　　C Subtotal colectomy.

　　D Repeat colonoscopy in 3 years.

4　Germline mutations in one of the DNA mismatch repair (MMR) genes can lead to which of the following familial cancer syndromes?

　　A Peutz–Jeghers syndrome.

　　B Lynch syndrome.

　　C Familial adenomatous polyposis (FAP).

　　D Gardner's syndrome.

5   A 65-year-old man is seen for a routine physical examination by a new primary care provider. He has no gastrointestinal complaints, and states that a flexible sigmoidoscopy done approximately 5 years ago was normal. Which one of the following tests is **not** recommended as a screening tool for colorectal cancer in this patient?

   A Digital rectal examination and fecal occult blood test (FOBT) performed in the office.

   B A series of three FOBTs.

   C Flexible sigmoidoscopy.

   D Colonoscopy.

Answers

1   **C**

The patient has iron-deficiency anemia in the setting of unintentional weight loss. Occult bleeding from the gastrointestinal (GI) tract, especially from the colon, is the most likely etiology. The patient has not had a prior colonoscopy. In the setting of unexplained iron-deficiency anemia, a fecal occult blood test is not necessary because the patient will require colonoscopy even if the test is negative. Upper endoscopy should be performed if colonoscopy does not reveal a source of blood loss, or if the patient has upper GI symptoms such as nausea, vomiting, early satiety, or epigastric pain. CT should not be done routinely for evaluation of iron-deficiency anemia. CT could be helpful if the patient has signs of colonic obstruction or severe abdominal pain. CT may be helpful to evaluate the patient for metastasis if CRC is found on colonoscopy. Empiric treatment with oral iron is inappropriate in this setting.

2   **B**

The patient has invasive adenocarcinomas of the left and right colon. The most appropriate management is a subtotal colectomy. Endoscopic resection is not recommended for invasive adenocarcinoma. Preoperative chemotherapy with radiotherapy is used to treat locally advanced rectal cancer. Stage II and III rectal cancers and stage III colon cancers also require postoperative chemotherapy.

3   **D**

Malignant polyps in the colon and rectum do not metastasize if cancer is confined to the mucosa. Polypectomy is adequate treatment for a polyp with high-grade dysplasia. This polyp is considered an advanced neoplasm, and the patient should undergo a repeat colonoscopy in 3 years. CT and PET are not indicated because there is no risk of metastasis if dysplasia in the polyp is confined to the mucosa. Subtotal colectomy is not indicated because the polyp has been completely resected endoscopically.

4 B
Peutz–Jeghers syndrome is caused by germline mutations in the *LKB1* gene. Germline mutations of one of the MMR genes lead to Lynch syndrome. FAP is caused by germline mutations in the *APC* gene. Gardner's syndrome is a variant of FAP and is also caused by mutations in the *APC* gene.

5 A
FOBT done on a stool sample (obtained by digital rectal examination) has low sensitivity. Only 4.9% of advanced adenomas and 9% of cancers are detected by this method. Because the accuracy of FOBT done in the office setting is so low, it is not endorsed as a method of CRC screening. The other options are acceptable.

Further Reading

Bresalier, R.S. (2016) Colorectal cancer, in *Sleisenger and Fordtran's Gastrointestinal and Liver Disease: Pathophysiology/Diagnosis/Management*, 10th edition (eds M. Feldman, L.S. Friedman, and L.J. Brandt), Saunders Elsevier, Philadelphia, pp. 2248–2296.

Levin, B., Lieberman, D.A., McFarland, B., *et al.* (2008) Screening and surveillance for the early detection of colorectal cancer and adenomatous polyps, 2008: A joint guideline from the American Cancer Society, the US Multi-Society Task Force on Colorectal Cancer, and the American College of Radiology. *Gastroenterology*, **134**, 1570–1595.

US Preventive Services Task Force (2008) Screening for colorectal cancer: US Preventive Services Task Force recommendation statement. *Annals of Internal Medicine*, **149**, 627–637.

Weblinks

http://www.merckmanuals.com/professional/sec02/ch021/ch021h.html?qt=
   colon%20cancer&alt=sh
http://www.ncbi.nlm.nih.gov/pubmedhealth/PMH0001308/
http://www.gastrojournal.org/article/S0016-5085%2808%2900232-1/fulltext
http://www.cdc.gov/uscs
http://www.cancer.org/cancer/colonandrectumcancer/detailedguide/
   colorectal-cancer-survival-rates

Liver

JP Norvell

11

Liver Anatomy and Histopathology

Joel P. Wedd

Clinical Vignette

A 21-year-old woman with abdominal pain is found on an imaging study to have a large hemangioma in the left lobe of the liver. She wishes to become pregnant, but because estrogen may induce the hemangioma to grow, the obstetrician recommends that she undergo resection of the hemangioma. A partial left lobectomy is performed, and she recovers uneventfully. Follow-up computed tomography 1 month later shows a normal liver size and contour.

Embryonic Development

The endoderm and mesoderm are both involved in liver development. The endoderm gives rise to hepatocytes and cholangiocytes, which line the biliary tree. The mesoderm contributes to the sinusoids and forms the stroma, liver capsule, hematopoietic tissue (including Kupffer cells), connective tissue, and smooth muscle of the biliary tract.

- Weeks 3–4: an endodermal bud appears from the ventral foregut. The bud enlarges and forms a cavity connecting to the foregut, thus creating the hepatic diverticulum. From the hepatic diverticulum comes the epithelial liver cords (hepatocytes) and primordia of the biliary system (epithelial lining of the biliary tract and gallbladder).
- Weeks 4–5: the hepatocytes arrange into a series of branching and anastomosing cords several cells thick in the mesenchyme of the septum transversum. These cords subsequently intermingle with the vitelline and umbilical veins to

Sitaraman and Friedman's Essentials of Gastroenterology, Second Edition.
Edited by Shanthi Srinivasan and Lawrence S. Friedman.
© 2018 John Wiley & Sons Ltd. Published 2018 by John Wiley & Sons Ltd.

form hepatic sinusoids. The hematopoietic cells, Kupffer cells, and connective tissue of the liver are also derived from the septum transversum.

- Week 6: hematopoiesis starts in the liver and gradually subsides during the last trimester as the bone marrow forms and begins to take over hematopoiesis.
- Week 7: the liver accounts for 10% by weight of the fetus. The hepatic artery is formed from the celiac axis, and vitelline veins combine to develop the portal vein.
- Week 12: bile formation begins. At the time of birth, the liver accounts for 5% of the weight of the newborn.
- The major blood supply to the fetal liver is from the umbilical vein.

Liver Regeneration

- In adults, the liver is the only internal organ that can regenerate. The liver regenerates by hepatocyte **hyperplasia** (proliferation of cells resulting in an increased number of cells). Hyperplasia is different from **hypertrophy**, in which the adaptive cell change is an increase in the size of cells, rather than the number of cells.
- Hyperplasia restores the exact same cell mass that was removed so that the liver regenerates to its original size. This principle applies to live donor liver transplantation and hepatic resection.

Anatomy

- The liver is the largest organ in the body and weighs roughly 1500 g when healthy. It extends from the right fifth rib, inferior to the costal margin along the midclavicular line, with a small portion of the left liver extending across the midline. It is separated into lobes and segments. The falciform ligament divides the liver into right and left lobes.
- The right lobe is further divided into the caudate and quadrate lobes. Functionally, the right lobe is divided by a plane through the gallbladder and inferior vena cava, corresponding to different branches of the portal vein, hepatic artery, and bile ducts.
- The liver can be divided further into eight functional segments, each having its own vascular inflow, outflow, and biliary drainage. The importance of the functional anatomy of the liver lies in the planning of anatomic resection.
- The liver has a dual blood supply, which includes the portal vein and the hepatic artery. The **portal vein** provides roughly 80% of the liver's blood supply and carries venous blood rich in nutrients drained from the spleen, gastrointestinal tract, and associated organs. The **hepatic artery** supplies

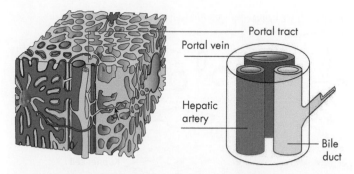

Figure 11.1 Schematic representation of the microscopic anatomy of the normal human liver. The liver consists of a system of anastomosing hepatic plates and sinusoidal spaces. A network of bile duct radicles opens into the portal bile ducts (green). An intralobular artery (red), deriving from a branch of the hepatic artery, bypasses the parenchyma and communicates directly with the sinusoids (blue). The portal vein (blue) drains through the sinusoids into the central vein. Adapted with permission from Dancygier, H. (2010) Springer Images: *Microscopic Anatomy*. Springer, New York.

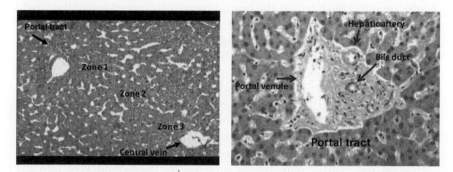

Figure 11.2 Microscopic structure of the liver (Original magnifications: left × 40; right × 100). Photomicrographs courtesy of Charles W. Sewell, MD, Department of Pathology, Emory University, Atlanta, GA, USA.

arterial blood, accounting for the remainder of the liver's blood flow. Oxygen is provided from both sources: approximately half of the oxygen demand of the liver is met by the portal vein, and the other half is met by the hepatic artery. The hepatic artery is the major source of oxygen to the bile ducts.

- Both the portal vein and hepatic artery enter at the liver hilus, where bile ducts are also exiting. Branches of the portal vein, hepatic artery, and bile ducts run together through the liver parenchyma in portal tracts, which can be seen microscopically (Figures 11.1 and 11.2). Branches of the hepatic vein (central vein; Figure 11.2) then collect venous blood to exit the liver and flow back to the right heart.

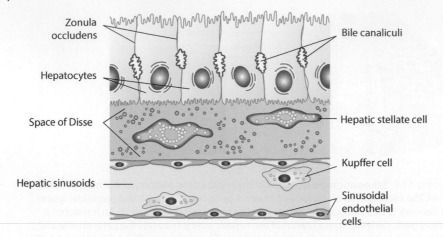

Zonula occludens
Bile canaliculi
Hepatocytes
Space of Disse
Hepatic stellate cell
Kupffer cell
Hepatic sinusoids
Sinusoidal endothelial cells

Figure 11.3 Schematic representation of the microscopic anatomy of the liver.

- The **hepatic lobule** is the functional unit of the liver (Figures 11.1 and 11.2).
  In the center of the lobule is the central vein. At the periphery of the lobule
  are the portal tracts (or portal triads), which consist of a portal venule, bile
  duct, and hepatic arteriole. Connecting the portal tracts with the central vein
  are sheets or cords of hepatocytes (trabeculae) lined by sinusoids on one side
  and biliary canaliculi on the other.
  - The sinusoids are unique structures bordered by blood vessels on one side
    and the space of Disse on the other side. Hepatocyte microvilli project
    into the space of Disse, thus allowing for exchange of particles and
    nutrients between the blood and hepatocytes (Figure 11.3).
  - Blood flows from the hepatic arteriole and portal venule in the portal tract
    toward the central vein. Bile is secreted by the hepatocytes into the
    canaliculi and flows towards the portal tract to drain into the bile ducts
    (see Figure 11.1).
- Alternatively, the liver can be divided into units called **acini**, useful for
  delineating hepatic tissue by oxygen availability and metabolic metabolic
  function. In contrast to the hepatic lobule, which has a central vein in the
  center, the central component of the acinus is the portal tract. Each acinus
  has three zones, based on oxygen and nutrient supply.
  - The periportal zone 1 encircles the portal tracts, where the oxygenated blood
    from hepatic arteries and nutrient-rich blood from the portal vein enter.
  - The centrilobular zone 3 is located around central veins, where oxygena-
    tion is poor. Zone 3 is most susceptible to states of low blood flow such as
    hypotension or heart failure. Therefore, zone 3 is most susceptible to
    necrosis of the liver in such conditions.
  - Zone 2 is located between zones 1 and 3 (see Figure 11.2).

Major Cell Types

The major cell types are illustrated in Figure 11.3 and their details are provided in Table 11.1.

Hepatocyte

- Hepatocytes are the chief functional cells of the liver, and constitute 60–80% of liver mass. They are polarized epithelial cells with distinct apical and basolateral surfaces (the basolateral surface faces the sinusoidal endothelium, whereas the apical surface faces adjacent hepatocytes with enclosure of bile canaliculi).
- Hepatocytes are separated by an intercellular junctional complex (zonula occludens, or tight junction) and organized into sheets of cells. The tight junctions are important for limiting bile leak into the sinusoids, or plasma leakage into bile.
- Hepatocytes perform numerous metabolic and synthetic functions, including gluconeogenesis, glycogenolysis, and the production of cholesterol and bile salts, clotting factors (except factor VIII), and albumin. They also possess enzymatic machinery to metabolize, detoxify, and inactivate exogenous chemicals.

Sinusoidal Endothelial Cell

- Sinusoidal endothelial cells (SECs) line the sinusoidal wall. Along with the Kupffer cells, the SECs constitute the reticuloendothelial system. They are fenestrated and are separated from hepatocytes by the space of Disse (also called the perisinusoidal space). The fenestrae allow small particles and solutes access to the space of Disse for interaction with the hepatocytes.

Table 11.1 Location and function of hepatic cell types.

Cell type	Location	Function
Hepatocyte	Lining one side of the space of Disse	Metabolic/synthetic
Sinusoidal endothelial cell	Lining the sinusoids and the other side of the space of Disse	Transport between sinusoids and the space of Disse; host defense
Kupffer cell	Within the sinusoids	Host defense
Hepatic stellate cell	Within the space of Disse	Regulation of sinusoidal blood flow; fibrotic response to injury

- In cirrhosis, the fenestrations become occluded with extracellular matrix.
- Larger particles, including proteins, glycoproteins, and glycosaminoglycans, are selectively endocytosed.
- SECs are also capable of releasing substances for host defense, such as interleukins and interferon.

Kupffer Cell

- Kupffer cells are specialized macrophages that are anchored along the walls of the hepatic sinusoids and thus are exposed to the blood.
- They are members of the reticuloendothelial system and are the largest population of fixed macrophages in the body.
- Kupffer cells provide the major defense of the liver. They are responsible for endocytosis of cell particles and infectious or toxic elements that come from the intestine via the portal circulation. They are important for antigen presentation, phagocytosis of bacterial products, synthesis and secretion of key cytokines and macromolecules, and host defense against microbes.

Hepatic Stellate Cell

- Hepatic stellate cells (HSCs), previously known as Ito cells, are found in the space of Disse and interact closely with SECs and hepatocytes. In normal liver, they contain fat droplets and store vitamin A and other retinoids.
- HSCs influence differentiation and proliferation of other hepatic cell types during development and regeneration. They also play a role in the regulation of blood flow through the sinusoids.
- When the liver is injured, these cells undergo mitosis and secrete extracellular matrix (e.g., collagen) into the space of Disse.
- HSCs are the cells primarily responsible for the development of hepatic fibrosis through a process of activation in response to signals from damaged hepatocytes and immune cells. When fibrosis regresses, the population of activated HSCs is reduced.

Pearls

- The liver regenerates by hepatocyte hyperplasia, which restores the exact same cell mass as in the liver originally.
- The main blood supply to the liver is provided by the portal vein. Oxygenated blood is provided by both the portal vein and the hepatic artery. The hepatic artery is the major source of oxygen to the bile ducts.
- HSCs play a central role in the development of hepatic fibrosis.

Questions

The following questions relate to the clinical vignette at the beginning of this chapter.

1   The liver regenerates by which of the following mechanisms?
    A Hypertrophy.
    B Hyperplasia.
    C Metaplasia.
    D Dysplasia.

2   In the photomicrograph of the liver below (Figure 11.4), the areas containing the blue double-ended arrows are which of the following?
    A Portal tracts.
    B Hepatocytes.
    C Zonula occludens.
    D Sinusoids.
    E Kupffer cells.

3   In Figure 11.5, match each number with the name of the structure:
    A Space of Disse.
    B Portal blood.
    C Kupffer cell.
    D Bile canaliculi.
    E Tight junction.

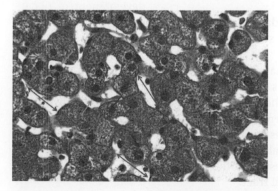

Figure 11.4 See Question 2. Photomicrograph courtesy of Charles W. Sewell, MD, Department of Pathology, Emory University, Atlanta, GA, USA.

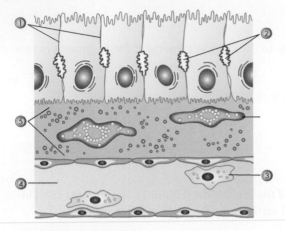

Figure 11.5 See Question 3.

4 Which of the following cell types is associated with facilitating hepatic fibrosis?
A Hepatic stellate cell.
B Hepatocyte.
C Kupffer cell.
D Sinusoidal endothelial cell.

5 Which of the following cells are most responsible for host defense of pathogens?
A Hepatocyte.
B Kupffer cell.
C Hepatic stellate cell.
D Kupffer cell and sinusoidal endothelial cell.
E Hepatocyte and hepatic stellate cell.

6 Which of the following statements regarding oxygen tension and blood flow in the hepatic lobule is correct?
A Oxygen tension is highest near the central vein; blood flows from the portal tract to the central vein.
B Oxygen tension is lowest near the central vein; blood flows from the portal tract to the central vein.
C Oxygen tension is lowest near the central vein; blood flows from the central vein to the portal tract.
D Oxygen tension is highest near the central vein; blood flows from the central vein to the portal tract.
E None of the above statements is correct.

7 In a patient with hepatic ischemia, which zone(s) is most likely to show necrosis on a liver biopsy specimen?
   A Zone 2.
   B Zone 1.
   C Zone 3.
   D Zones 1 and 2.
   E Zone 4.

8 A patient develops hepatic artery thrombosis following liver transplantation. Which of the following structures is most likely to be damaged as a result of the thrombus?
   A Hepatocytes in zone 3.
   B Central veins.
   C Hepatic stellate cells.
   D Bile ducts.
   E Sinusoidal endothelial cells.

9 Which of the following statements regarding embryologic development of the liver is correct?
   A The fetal liver is derived from elements of both the endoderm and the mesoderm.
   B The fetal liver does not have hematopoietic function.
   C Bile flow begins around week 6 of fetal life.
   D The transverse septum is primarily responsible for the development of hepatocytes and biliary tract.
   E Hepatic sinusoids are derived from the hepatic diverticulum.

10 Which of the following statements is true about the space of Disse?
   A It contains Kupffer cells.
   B It is bordered by hepatocytes on one side and sinusoidal endothelial cells on the other.
   C It contains hepatic stellate cells.
   D It is important for exchange between hepatocytes and the sinusoidal blood.
   E B, C, and D.

Answers

1 B
   The liver regenerates by hyperplasia (proliferation of cells, including hepatocytes, resulting in an increase in the number of cells). Hyperplasia restores the same cell mass that was removed so that the

liver regenerates to its original size. This principle applies following hepatic resection, including live liver donation.

2 D

The blue double-ended arrows are in sinusoids, the yellow arrows point to the zonula occludens (intercellular junctions), the red arrows point to hepatocytes, and the green arrows point to Kupffer cells.

3 A5; B4; C3; D2; E1.

4 A

5 D

6 B

7 C

8 D

The principal supply of oxygen to the bile ducts is the hepatic artery, not the portal vein.

9 A

10 E

Further Reading

Dancygier, H. (2010) Microscopic anatomy, in *Clinical Hepatology: Principles and Practice of Hepatobiliary Diseases*, (ed. H. Dancygier), Springer, New York, pp. 15–51.

Eruschenko, V.P. (ed.) (2005) *DiFiore's Atlas of Histology with Functional Correlates*, 10th edition, Lippincott, Williams & Wilkins, Philadelphia.

Golub, R. and Cumano, A. (2013) Embryonic hematopoiesis. *Blood Cells and Molecular Diseases*, **51**, 226–231.

Sanyal, A.J., Boyer, T.D., Terrault, N., and Lindor, K. (eds) (2018) *Zakim and Boyer's Hepatology: A Textbook of Liver Disease*, 7th edition, Elsevier, Philadephia.

Yin, C., Evason, K., Asahina, K., and Stainier, D. (2013) Hepatic stellate cells in liver development, regeneration, and cancer. *Journal of Clinical Investigation*, **123**, 1902–1910.

Weblinks

http://www.anatomyatlases.org/MicroscopicAnatomy/Section10/Plate10214.shtml
http://www.anatomyatlases.org/MicroscopicAnatomy/Section10/Plate10215.shtml
https://embryology.med.unsw.edu.au/embryology/index.php/Gastrointestinal_
   Tract_-_Liver_Development
http://www.siumed.edu/~dking2/erg/liver.htm

12

Liver Biochemical Tests

Nader Dbouk and Samir Parekh

Clinical Vignette

A 39-year-old man is seen in the office for his annual health check-up. He is asymptomatic. His past medical history is remarkable for an appendectomy at age 16. He does not take prescription, over-the-counter, or herbal medications. He has no history of illicit drug use. His family history is unremarkable. He drinks a glass of red wine with dinner and does not smoke cigarettes. He is married and has two children. On physical examination the vital signs are normal. He is overweight with a body mass index of 29. The remainder of the examination is unremarkable. Routine laboratory tests including a complete blood count and a complete metabolic panel are normal except for a serum alanine aminotransferase (ALT) level of 56 U l^{-1} and aspartate aminotransferase (AST) of 42 U l^{-1}.

General

- An estimated 1–4% of persons in the US who are asymptomatic have mildly elevated levels of biochemical tests, specifically, the serum aminotransferases (also called 'liver enzymes' or 'liver function tests,' although liver enzymes do not measure liver function).

Patterns of Liver Biochemical Test Level Elevations

- The standard liver biochemical tests used in assessing hepatobiliary disease include **serum aminotransferases**, **alkaline phosphatase** (ALP), and **bilirubin** (see Chapter 24). Common laboratory tests used to assess synthetic function of the liver include the prothrombin time and serum albumin.

Sitaraman and Friedman's Essentials of Gastroenterology, Second Edition.
Edited by Shanthi Srinivasan and Lawrence S. Friedman.
© 2018 John Wiley & Sons Ltd. Published 2018 by John Wiley & Sons Ltd.

Table 12.1 Patterns of liver injury.

| | Hepatocellular | Cholestatic | |
		Intrahepatic	Extrahepatic
Aminotransferases	+++	0 to +	0 to +
Alkaline phosphatase	0 to +	+++	++ to +++
Bilirubin	0 to ++	0 to ++	+++

- Depending on the predominant liver biochemical test abnormality, two patterns of liver injury can be recognized: hepatocellular and cholestatic (Table 12.1).
  - In **hepatocellular** injury, there is a predominant increase in serum aminotransferase levels compared with ALP. The serum bilirubin level may be elevated.
  - In **cholestatic** disease, the cause may be intrahepatic or extrahepatic (see Chapter 24). Intrahepatic cholestasis is typically associated with an isolated or predominant elevation of the serum ALP level, compared with serum aminotransferase levels; the serum bilirubin level may be normal or elevated. Extrahepatic cholestasis (biliary obstruction) is associated with a predominant increase in the ALP level as well as the serum bilirubin level compared with serum aminotransferase levels.

> Impaired synthetic function in the setting of elevated liver biochemical test levels generally indicates hepatic decompensation, and patients should undergo an expedited evaluation to identify the underlying cause of liver disease.

Aminotransferases

- Aspartate aminotransferase (AST, or serum glutamic oxaloacetic transaminase [SGOT]), and alanine aminotransferase (ALT, or serum glutamic pyruvic transaminase [SGPT]) catalyze the transfer of amino acids from aspartate and alanine to ketoglutaric acid to form oxaloacetate and pyruvate, respectively, during gluconeogenesis.
- ALT is localized predominantly in the cytoplasm of hepatocytes and is more specific to the liver than AST. AST is present in the cytoplasm and mitochondria of hepatocytes, and is also present in various extrahepatic sites, including skeletal muscle, myocardium, kidneys, pancreas, lungs, brain cells, and red blood cells, and is therefore a less specific marker of liver injury than ALT.

- An isolated AST elevation can be seen in various nonhepatic conditions including myocardial ischemia, muscle disorders such as polymyositis, rhabdomyolysis, muscular dystrophy, and strenuous physical exertion. On the other hand, an isolated elevation in the ALT level generally indicates liver injury.
- A transient rise in the ALT level may follow a large, fatty meal or use of acetaminophen 4 g per day for several days.
- The normal range of aminotransferase levels in serum varies among laboratories, but generally accepted values are ≤ 30 U l^{-1} for men and ≤ 19 U l^{-1} for women.
- Mild elevations in serum aminotransferase levels (two- to fivefold the upper limit of normal, or ≤ 150 U l^{-1}) can be seen in 1–4% of seemingly healthy persons in the US.
  - Common causes of mildly elevated serum aminotransferase include:
    - Nonalcoholic fatty liver disease (NAFLD).
    - Chronic hepatitis B or C.
    - Alcoholic liver disease.
    - Medications and toxins (Table 12.2).
    - Hemochromatosis.
  - Less common causes include:
    - Autoimmune hepatitis.
    - Wilson disease.
    - Alpha-1 antitrypsin deficiency.

Table 12.2 Some medications, herbal preparations, and substances of abuse that can result in elevated serum aminotransferase levels.

Prescription medications	Antibiotics: ciprofloxacin, isoniazid, ketoconazole, penicillins, rifampin, trimethoprim–sulfamethoxazole
	Antidepressants: bupropion, fluoxetine, paroxetine, sertraline
	Antiepileptics: carbamezipine, phenytoin, valproic acid
	Antiretroviral therapy drugs
	3-Hydroxy-3-methylglutaryl-coenzyme A (HMG-CoA) reductase inhibitors (statins)
	Oral hypoglycemics: acarbose, glipizide
	Proton pump inhibitors: omeprazole, pantoprazole
	Others: amiodarone, angiotensin-converting enzyme inhibitors, methotrexate, vitamin A
Over-the-counter medications	Acetaminophen
	Nonsteroidal anti-inflammatory drugs (NSAIDs)
Substances of abuse	Anabolic steroids, cocaine, ecstasy, glues, solvents, phencyclidine (angel dust)
Herbal preparations	Chaparral leaf, Chinese herbs (ephedra), gentian, germander, Jin bu huan, kava, shark cartilage, senna, skullcap

- Systemic diseases that can cause mildly elevated serum aminotransferase levels include:
  o Celiac disease.
  o Cytomegalovirus infection.
  o Congestive hepatopathy secondary to passive venous congestion in patients with right-sided heart failure.
  o Hyperthyroidism.
  o Epstein–Barr virus infection.

> Elevated serum aminotransferase levels indicate hepatocellular injury. Levels of 1000 U l^{-1} or more are typical of acute liver injury, such as acute viral hepatitis. ALT is more specific than AST for hepatocellular injury. The level of ALT or AST elevation does not always correlate with the severity of liver injury.

Approach to the Patient with Elevated Serum Aminotransferase Levels

- The first step in evaluating a patient with mildly elevated serum aminotransferase levels is to obtain a careful history and perform a thorough physical examination (Figure 12.1).
  - The history should focus on identifying risk factors for liver disease, including excessive alcohol use or substance abuse; use of medications, including prescription drugs, over-the-counter agents, and herbal supplements (see Table 12.2); prior blood transfusions, tattoos, and promiscuous or unprotected sexual activity; a family history of liver disease; and a history of autoimmune disorders or celiac disease.
  - The physical examination should focus on identifying signs of advanced liver disease such as ascites, splenomegaly, and jaundice as well as cutaneous manifestations of liver disease such as spider telangiectasias, palmar erythema, and palpable purpura, often on the lower extremities, which may be associated with cryoglobulinemia in patients with chronic hepatitis C and occasionally hepatitis B. A careful neurologic examination should also be performed to detect signs of Wilson disease or hepatic encephalopathy (see Chapter 15).
- If the history, physical examination, and tests of liver function or portal hypertension (e.g., prolonged prothrombin time, low serum albumin, low platelet count) indicate decompensated liver disease, an expedited evaluation to identify the cause of liver disease should be performed.
- If potential hepatotoxins (medications, alcohol) are identified in the history and the patient is asymptomatic, the offending agent should be stopped and the liver biochemical tests repeated in 6–8 weeks.

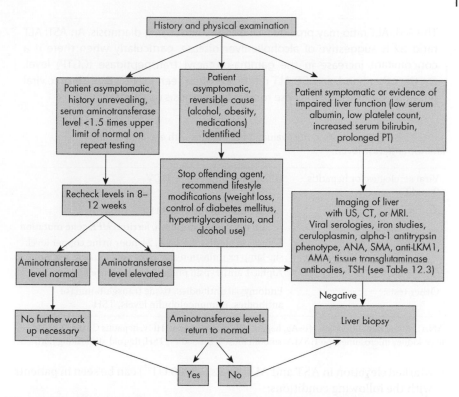

Figure 12.1 Algorithm for the evaluation of patients with mildly elevated serum aminotransferase levels. AMA, antimitochondrial antibodies; ANA, antinuclear antibodies; CT, computed tomography; LKM1, liver-kidney microsome type 1; MRI, magnetic resonance imaging; PT, prothrombin time; SMA, smooth muscle antibodies; TSH, thyroid-stimulating hormone; US, ultrasonography.

- If the history is unrevealing, further laboratory testing to identify common causes of chronic liver disease including chronic hepatitis B and C and hemochromatosis and, if necessary, autoimmune hepatitis, Wilson disease, alpha-1 antitrypsin deficiency, celiac disease, and thyroid disease, should be performed (Table 12.3). A creatine kinase level should be considered, particularly if the AST level is elevated predominantly.
- If the results of biochemical and serologic tests associated with various liver diseases are normal and the patient is asymptomatic and has no evidence of hepatic decompensation, a liver biopsy may be considered. Alternatively, if NAFLD is suspected, lifestyle modifications, including weight loss, limiting alcohol intake, and controlling diabetes mellitus and hypertriglyceridemia should be recommended, followed by regular monitoring of liver biochemical tests.

The AST: ALT ratio may provide a clue to the underlying diagnosis. An AST: ALT ratio ≥2 is suggestive of alcoholic liver disease, particularly when there is a concomitant increase in the gamma-glutamyl transpeptidase (GGTP) level. On the other hand, an AST: ALT ratio <1 is often seen in NAFLD or chronic viral hepatitis, but the ratio may rise to >1 when cirrhosis develops.

Table 12.3 Ancillary tests in the evaluation of persons with elevated serum aminotransferase levels.

Viral serologies for hepatitis B and C	HBsAg and antibody to HCV
Autoimmune markers	ANA, SMA, and anti-LKM1
	Serum iron, iron saturation, ferritin, *HFE* gene mutation
	Serum ceruloplasmin level, 24-hour urine copper level, slit-lamp examination
	Alpha-1 antitrypsin phenotype (protease inhibitor type)
Other tests:	Endomysial antibodies, tissue transglutaminase antibodies, immunoglobulin levels, TSH

ANA, antinuclear antibodies; HBsAg, hepatitis B surface antigen; HCV, hepatitis C virus; LKM1, liver-kidney microsome type 1; SMA, smooth muscle antibodies; TSH, thyroid-stimulating hormone.

- Marked elevation in AST and ALT levels ($>3000 \text{ U l}^{-1}$) can be seen in patients with the following conditions:
  - Ischemic hepatitis (shock liver), a condition often seen in critically ill patients in the intensive care unit. The ALT level may be $>5000 \text{ U l}^{-1}$; the lactate dehydrogenase (LDH) level is also typically high, with an ALT: LDH ratio <1.5, in contrast to viral hepatitis.
  - Toxicity caused by certain medications, especially acetaminophen (values often $>2000 \text{ U l}^{-1}$).
  - Rarely, autoimmune hepatitis or viral hepatitis.
- Marked elevations in serum aminotransferase levels should prompt an expedited evaluation to identify the underlying cause of hepatocellular injury.

NAFLD is the most common cause of asymptomatic, mildly elevated aminotransferase levels in the US and accounts for as many as 67% of cases.

Alkaline Phosphatase (ALP)

- ALP is a catalytic enzyme of uncertain function; it is distributed widely in tissues.
- The liver and bones are the major sources of serum ALP activity. ALP is also present in the placenta, small intestine, kidneys, and leukocytes as well

as some neoplasms. In the liver, ALP is found in the canalicular membrane of hepatocytes.

- Electrophoretic isoenzyme analysis allows fractionation of ALP to determine the tissue origin of an isolated elevation of ALP in serum.
- Alternatively, GGTP or 5′ nucleotidase (5′NT) levels can be measured to verify the hepatobiliary (versus bone) origin of an elevated ALP.
  - GGTP is a microsomal enzyme that is found in hepatocytes and biliary epithelium as well as various extrahepatic organs, including the pancreas, heart, lungs, kidneys, spleen, and brain, but not bone; it is not elevated in pregnancy.
  - Alcohol increases serum GGTP levels. Several medications, including phenytoin, barbiturates, and some antiretroviral therapy drugs, also increase serum GGTP levels.
  - 5′NT is a sensitive test for underlying liver disease and is not elevated in bone disease.

Low serum ALP levels are characteristic of Wilson disease, especially in patients with fulminant hepatitis and hemolysis.

Approach to the Patient with an Elevated Serum Alkaline Phosphatase Level

- ALP may be elevated in liver disease or in nonhepatic diseases (Table 12.4).
- Serum ALP levels can be elevated after a fatty meal due to increased influx of intestinal ALP, and should therefore be measured in the fasting state.
- A two- to threefold rise in serum ALP levels (with normal serum aminotransferase levels) can be seen in physiologic conditions such as pregnancy due to release from the placenta, as well as in adolescents, presumably due to increased bone growth. A gradual rise in serum ALP levels is also seen with increasing age, particularly in women.
- Many drugs can cause a predominant rise in serum ALP levels, with or without elevations in other liver enzymes.
- The first step in the evaluation of a patient with an isolated and asymptomatic elevation in the ALP level is to identify the tissue of origin. This is done most precisely by fractionation of ALP. Alternatively, a serum GGTP or 5′NT level can be measured.
- Some hepatobiliary diseases may be associated with isolated elevation of the ALP or elevation of the ALP that is out of proportion to the elevation in serum aminotransferase levels.
- As with elevated serum aminotransferase levels, a thorough history that includes prescription, over-the-counter, and herbal medication use should be obtained, and a careful physical examination should be performed.

Table 12.4 Common causes of an elevated serum alkaline phosphatase (ALP) level.

Physiologic causes	Adolescence (bone ALP)
	Advanced age, particularly in postmenopausal women
	Fatty meal (intestinal ALP)
	Pregnancy (usually in the third trimester, placental ALP)
Liver disease	Bile duct obstruction (choledocholithiasis, cholangiocarcinoma, pancreatic adenocarcinoma)
	Drug-induced cholestasis
	Infiltrative liver diseases (granulomatous hepatitis, sarcoidosis, amyloidosis, fungal or mycobacterium infections, metastatic cancer, some primary liver tumors such as hepatocellular carcinoma)
	Primary biliary cholangitis
	Primary sclerosing cholangitis
	Primary familial intrahepatic cholestasis and benign recurrent intrahepatic cholestasis
Bone disease	Paget's disease
	Bone metastasis

- If the history is unrevealing for an offending agent, the patient should be evaluated for a cholestatic disorder (see Chapter 24). Abdominal imaging with ultrasonography, CT, or MRI should be performed to look for extrahepatic causes of cholestasis. If the imaging studies show no dilatation of intra- or extrahepatic bile ducts, the patient should be evaluated for intrahepatic causes of cholestasis. The most common causes of intrahepatic cholestasis include primary biliary cholangitis (PBC) and granulomatous disease (e.g., sarcoidosis).
- Intrahepatic cholestasis is typically associated with an isolated elevation in the serum ALP early in the course. PBC is suggested by detection of antimitochondrial antibodies (AMA) in serum (see Chapter 15). An elevated angiotensin-converting enzyme (ACE) level may be seen in patients with sarcoidosis.
- Further evaluation of the patient with cholestasis is summarized in Figure 12.2 and discussed in more detail in Chapter 24.

Albumin

- The majority of proteins circulating in plasma are synthesized by the liver; levels reflect the synthetic capability of the liver.
- Albumin accounts for 10% of hepatic protein synthesis and 75% of protein in the serum; it accounts for 75% of plasma colloid oncotic pressure.

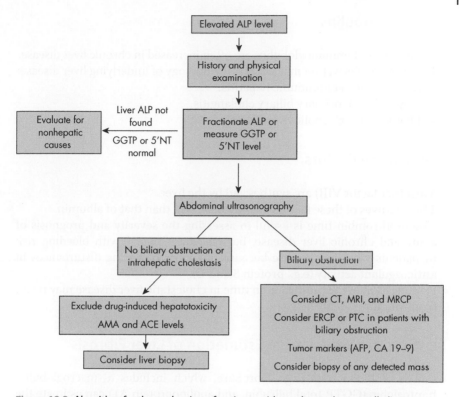

Figure 12.2 Algorithm for the evaluation of patients with an elevated serum alkaline phosphatase level. AMA, antimitochondrial antibodies; ACE, angiotensin-converting enzyme; AFP, alpha fetoprotein; CA, cancer antigen; CT, computed tomography; ERCP, endoscopic retrograde cholangiopancreatography; GGTP, gamma-glutamyl transpeptidase; MRI, magnetic resonance imaging; MRCP, magnetic resonance cholangiopancreatography; 5'NT, 5'nucleotidase; PTC, percutaneous transhepatic cholangiography.

- Albumin has a half-life of about 15 days, and its concentration in blood depends on the synthetic rate (normal = 12 g per day) and plasma volume.
- Hypoalbuminemia:
  - May result from expanded plasma volume or decreased albumin synthesis.
  - Is frequently associated with ascites and expansion of the extravascular albumin pool at the expense of the intravascular pool.
  - Is common in chronic liver disease and an indicator of severity.
- Therapeutic administration of albumin:
  - Intravenous albumin administration has been reported to reduce the risk of hepatorenal syndrome and mortality in patients with cirrhosis and spontaneous bacterial peritonitis (see Chapter 16).
  - An albumin-containing dialysate is sometimes used in the molecular adsorbent recirculating system (MARS) in patients with acute liver failure, because of the ability of albumin to bind toxins.

Immunoglobulins

- Serum levels of immunoglobulins are often increased in chronic liver disease.
- The pattern of elevation may suggest the etiology of underlying liver disease:
  - Elevated IgG: autoimmune hepatitis.
  - Elevated IgM: primary biliary cholangitis.
  - Elevated IgA: alcoholic liver disease.

Coagulation Factors

- Most (not factor VIII) are synthesized by the liver.
- The half-lives of these factors are much shorter than that of albumin.
- The prothrombin time is useful in assessing the severity and prognosis of acute and chronic liver disease, but correlates poorly with bleeding risk in patients with liver disease because of counterbalancing disturbances in anticoagulant activity (e.g., protein S and C).
- Prolongation of the prothrombin time in cholestatic liver disease may result from vitamin K deficiency.

Tests for the Noninvasive Estimation of Liver Fibrosis

- Panels of blood tests (e.g., FibroSure, which includes α_2-macroglobulin, haptoglobin, GGTP, total bilirubin, and apolipoprotein A1) can estimate the degree of hepatic fibrosis. The negative predictive value of the FibroSure test for excluding significant fibrosis is 91%; a high score is accurate for predicting cirrhosis; intermediate scores are less reliable. Combinations of other blood tests are also available.
- Serum hyaluronic acid (and other markers of hepatic extracellular matrix metabolism) show promise.
- Ultrasound elastography: used to measure the elasticity of the liver; magnetic resonance elastography assesses fibrosis by magnetic resonance imaging.

Pearls
- The most common cause of mildly elevated serum aminotransferase levels is NAFLD. - Very high aminotransferase levels (>3000 U l^{-1}) are usually due to ischemic hepatitis or drug-induced liver injury (e.g., acetaminophen toxicity). - An isolated serum alkaline phosphatase elevation may be of hepatic or nonhepatic (usually bone) origin. The former is associated with an elevated GGTP or 5′NT level.

Questions

The following question relates to the clinical vignette at the beginning of this chapter.

1   What is the next best step in the management of this patient's elevated liver biochemical test levels?
    A   Repeat the liver biochemical tests in 8 weeks.
    B   Serologic tests for hepatitis B and C.
    C   Serologic tests for autoimmune hepatitis.
    D   Abdominal ultrasonography.
    E   Liver biopsy.

2   A 15-year-old boy is seen for the evaluation of an upper respiratory tract infection. The history and physical examination are remarkable only for fatigue. Routine laboratory evaluation reveals a normal complete blood count and chemistry tests except for an elevated serum alkaline phosphatase level of 190 U l^{-1}. He is otherwise healthy and does not drink alcohol, smoke cigarettes, or use recreational drugs. He denies the use of prescription drugs, herbal remedies, or over-the-counter medications. There is no family history of liver disease or cirrhosis. Physical examination is unremarkable. The alkaline phosphatase level is repeated 2 weeks later and is 196 U l^{-1}. What is the next best step in evaluating this patient?
    A   Serum gamma-glutamyl transpeptidase (GGTP) level.
    B   Antimitochondrial antibodies (AMA).
    C   Abdominal ultrasonography.
    D   Liver biopsy.

3   A 20-year-old African American college student is referred to the student health clinic for the evaluation of a rash. The patient also complains of the new onset of dyspnea on exertion. He does not smoke cigarettes, drink alcohol, or use recreational drugs. His college performance has deteriorated since the fall term began, and he has become markedly fatigued. At night he occasionally feels warm and has night sweats that require him to change his bed clothes and his pillow case several times per week. He denies nausea, vomiting, diarrhea, or bloody stools. His past medical and surgical history is unremarkable. He has not been sexually active for over 6 months and was vaccinated for hepatitis B as an infant. His mother has a history of ulcerative colitis. His sister and maternal aunt have systemic lupus erythematosus. On physical examination the patient is an asthenic male in no acute distress. The vital signs are within normal limits. He has tender, erythematous nodular lesions on his lower extremities consistent with erythema nodosum. The remainder of the examination, including abdominal and neurologic examinations, is normal. Laboratory tests show

a normal complete blood count. The serum calcium level is $12\,mg\,dl^{-1}$, alkaline phosphatase $360\,U\,l^{-1}$, GGTP $418\,U\,l^{-1}$, ALT $80\,U\,l^{-1}$, AST $110\,U\,l^{-1}$, total bilirubin $2.0\,mg\,dl^{-1}$, and direct bilirubin $1.8\,mg\,dl^{-1}$. A parathyroid hormone level is normal. The titer of antinuclear antibodies titer is <1:20. Serologic tests for hepatitis B and C, cytomegalovirus, and Epstein–Barr virus are negative. A chest X-ray reveals hilar adenopathy. Abdominal ultrasonography demonstrates hepatosplenomegaly but no intra- or extra-hepatic bile duct dilatation. A lymph node biopsy reveals noncaseating granulomas. Which of the following is the most likely diagnosis?

A Autoimmune hepatitis.
B Acute hepatitis B.
C Sarcoidosis.
D Celiac disease.
E Sickle cell disease.

4 A 62-year-old woman is referred for the evaluation of pruritus, which has been progressing over the past several months. She denies weight loss, fatigue, or a history of liver disease. She denies a history of illicit drug or alcohol use and does not take prescription or over-the-counter medications. Her family history is remarkable for thyroid disease in her mother and systemic lupus erythematosus in her sister. Physical examination is remarkable for xanthelasma on her eyelids. Routine laboratory tests including a complete blood count, and comprehensive metabolic panel are normal except for an elevated serum alkaline phosphatase of $280\ U\ l^{-1}$ and GGTP $330\ U\ l^{-1}$. Abdominal ultrasonography reveals a normal liver with no evidence of parenchymal abnormalities. Which of the following is the next best diagnostic step?

A Fractionation of the alkaline phosphatase.
B Antimitochondrial antibodies (AMA).
C Endoscopic retrograde cholangiopancreatography (ERCP).
D Small bowel biopsy.
E Percutaneous liver biopsy.

5 An 80-year-old woman is admitted to the hospital with a urinary tract infection (UTI). She has a history of heart failure, chronic obstructive lung disease, and diabetes mellitus. She takes multiple medications and has been placed on ampicillin–sulbactam for the UTI. Her routine laboratory tests including liver enzymes are normal. Urine and blood cultures grow *Escherichia coli*. Two days after admission her condition worsens, and she is transferred to the intensive care unit and intubated for acute respiratory failure. Following intubation she becomes hypotensive and requires medical therapy to support her blood pressure. Two days after that her serum liver enzymes reveal an aspartate aminotransferase (AST) level of $2570\,U\,l^{-1}$,

alanine aminotransferase (ALT) 2395 U l^{-1}, alkaline phosphatase (ALP) 160 U l^{-1}, and total bilirubin 2.9 mg dl^{-1}. The most likely cause of the abnormal liver biochemical test levels is which of the following?

A Acute viral hepatitis.
B Drug-induced hepatotoxicity.
C Congestive hepatopathy.
D Ischemic hepatitis.
E Transfusion reaction.

6 A 45-year-old man seeking life insurance presents for a physical examination. He is asymptomatic except for fatigue. The physical examination is unremarkable. The body mass index is 25.5. He admits to having used 'recreational' drugs as well as binge drinking on the weekends when he was in college. He is sexually active with several partners. He has been vaccinated against hepatitis A and B. A urine drug screen is negative. Laboratory tests are normal except for ALT 65 U l^{-1} and AST 58 U l^{-1}. What is the most appropriate next step in the evaluation of this patient?

A Recommend weight loss.
B Repeat liver biochemical testing in 3 months.
C Serologic testing for hepatitis C.
D Serum ceruloplasmin level.
E Serologic testing for celiac disease.

Answers

1 **A**
The patient has mild asymptomatic elevations of the ALT and AST levels, with normal bilirubin and ALP levels. The first step is to confirm that the elevations are persistent, and the tests can be repeated in 8 weeks. The most common cause of mildly elevated serum aminotransferase levels in the US is nonalcoholic fatty liver disease (NAFLD). This patient is overweight, making the diagnosis of NAFLD likely. If the elevated aminotransferase levels persist, lifestyle modifications emphasizing weight loss is reasonable. A work-up for other causes of chronic liver disease would also be warranted, including serologic tests for hepatitis B and C and autoimmune hepatitis as well as abdominal ultrasonography. Liver biopsy is not indicated at this time.

2 **A**
Elevation of the serum ALP level can be seen in adolescents due to rapid bone turnover associated with bone growth. This is the most probable cause of an elevated ALP level in this young man. Concurrent elevation of

the GGTP level would prompt a work-up for cholestasis with abdominal imaging; if the GGTP were normal, no further work-up would be necessary. AMA, a marker of primary biliary cholangitis (PBC), is not likely to be useful in a male adolescent in whom PBC would be unlikely. Liver biopsy is not indicated at this time.

3   C

The patient's presentation with dyspnea, hilar adenopathy, erythema nodosum, and hypercalcemia is consistent with a diagnosis of sarcoidosis. This diagnosis is further supported by lymph node biopsy findings of noncaseating granulomas. Hepatic involvement is common in patients with sarcoidosis and is characterized by an elevated serum ALP level that typically is out of proportion to elevation in serum aminotransferase or bilirubin levels.

4   B

This presentation is typical of primary biliary cholangitis (PBC). AMA are detected in 95% of patients with PBC. Ultrasonography does not show evidence of biliary disease, and ERCP is therefore unnecessary. A liver biopsy may be contemplated in order to determine the stage of the patient's disease, but it would not be the appropriate next step in this clinical scenario. A small-bowel biopsy may be considered to diagnose celiac disease, but the clinical presentation and pattern of liver biochemical test abnormalities are not typical of those associated with celiac disease.

5   D

The patient had normal liver enzyme levels on presentation with a UTI and developed markedly elevated aminotransferase levels after a hypotensive episode. This sequence of events suggests ischemic hepatitis. Congestive hepatopathy typically causes an elevated serum bilirubin level, not such a dramatic elevation in aminotransferase levels. Drug-induced hepatotoxicity could potentially cause marked elevations in liver enzymes, but the more likely diagnosis in this clinical scenario is ischemic hepatitis.

6   C

Chronic hepatitis C is prevalent among former intravenous drug users who often are asymptomatic and are found incidentally to have mildly elevated aminotransferase levels on routine laboratory testing. If the patient had no risk factors for hepatitis C, it would be reasonable to stop potentially offending drugs and follow the liver biochemical tests. A serum ceruloplasmin level is helpful in the evaluation of patients with Wilson disease, an uncommon diagnosis after age 40. Celiac disease is often associated with mildly elevated serum aminotransferase levels, but in the setting of prior intravenous drug use, chronic hepatitis C is more likely.

Further Reading

Aragon, G. and Younossi, Z.M. (2010) When and how to evaluate mildly elevated liver enzymes in apparently healthy patients. *Cleveland Clinic Journal of Medicine*, **77**, 195–204.

Pratt, D.S. (2016) Liver chemistry and function tests, in *Sleisenger and Fordtran's Gastrointestinal and Liver Disease: Pathophysiology/Diagnosis/Management*, 10th edition (eds M. Feldman, L.S. Friedman, and L.J. Brandt), Saunders Elsevier, Philadelphia, pp. 1243–1253.

Woreta, T.A. and Algahtani, S.A. (2014) Evaluation of abnormal liver enzymes. *Medical Clinics of North America*, **98**, 1–16.

Weblinks

http://www.clevelandclinicmeded.com/medicalpubs/diseasemanagement/hepatology/guide-to-common-liver-tests/

http://www.med.upenn.edu/gastro/documents/ClinLiverDisoutpatientliverfunctiontestsLFTs2009.pdf

13

Viral Hepatitis

Anjana A. Pillai and Lawrence S. Friedman

Clinical Vignette

A 21-year-old man presents with the insidious onset of anorexia, nausea, and upper abdominal discomfort. His symptoms developed approximately 2 weeks earlier when he returned from a cruise in the Caribbean. For the past 2 days, he has noticed that his urine is darker than usual. He denies illicit drug use, medication (prescription or over-the-counter) use, or other travel outside the US. He received a blood transfusion 6 years ago following a car accident in which he sustained a femoral fracture. His past medical history is otherwise unremarkable. The family history is noncontributory. He smokes six cigarettes a day and drinks two to three beers a day, but has not smoked or had a beer for several days. He is a senior in college, is heterosexual, and has a single partner. He denies high-risk sexual practices. Physical examination reveals a blood pressure of 118/68 mmHg, pulse rate 76 per minute, and body mass index 20. He is afebrile. There are no cutaneous stigmata of liver disease, tattoos, or needle tracks. Conjunctival icterus is present. Chest and cardiovascular examinations are unremarkable. The abdominal examination is notable for a tender liver edge that is palpable 1 cm below the right costal margin. Rectal examination reveals brown stool that is negative for occult blood. Laboratory tests reveal a white blood cell count of 7200 mm^{-3}, hemoglobin 13.1 g dl^{-1}, and platelet count 260 000 mm^{-3}. The serum alanine aminotransferase (ALT) level is 980 U l^{-1}, aspartate aminotransferase (AST) 960 U l^{-1}, alkaline phosphatase 200 U l^{-1}, total bilirubin 14.5 mg dl^{-1}, direct bilirubin 11.2 mg dl^{-1}, prothrombin time (PT) 12.4 seconds, and international normalized ratio (INR) 1.1. Additional testing shows the presence of immunoglobulin M antibody to hepatitis A virus (IgM anti-HAV). He is hepatitis B surface antigen (HBsAg) negative, antibody to HBsAg (anti-HBs) positive, IgG antibody to hepatitis B core antigen (IgG anti-HBc) positive, and antibody to hepatitis C virus (anti-HCV) negative.

Sitaraman and Friedman's Essentials of Gastroenterology, Second Edition.
Edited by Shanthi Srinivasan and Lawrence S. Friedman.
© 2018 John Wiley & Sons Ltd. Published 2018 by John Wiley & Sons Ltd.

Etiology

- There are five major hepatotropic viruses (viruses that have affinity for hepatocytes): hepatitis A virus (HAV); hepatitis B virus (HBV); hepatitis C virus (HCV); hepatitis D virus (HDV); and hepatitis E virus (HEV) (Table 13.1).
  - All hepatitis viruses are RNA viruses except for HBV, which is a partially double-stranded DNA virus.
  - HDV is a defective RNA virus that uses HBsAg as its envelope protein. Therefore, HBV co-infection is necessary for the propagation of HDV virions.
  - Some 90% of cases of viral hepatitis in the US are caused by HAV, HBV, or HCV.
  - Damage to the liver is due primarily to the immune response to the virus rather than to cytopathic effects of the virus.
- Viruses that may affect the liver as a part of a systemic infection include Epstein–Barr virus, cytomegalovirus, herpes simplex virus, varicella-zoster virus, parvovirus B19, adenovirus, and others.

Clinical Features

- Acute infection may result in subclinical (asymptomatic) disease, self-limited symptomatic disease, or acute liver failure (ALF).
- Infections caused by HAV, HBV, and HEV are usually symptomatic in adults but are often asymptomatic in children. Acute infection caused by HCV is usually asymptomatic in both children and adults.
- Following an incubation period that varies with the virus, symptomatic acute hepatitis is characterized by a **prodromal phase** and an **icteric phase**. Typical symptoms in the prodromal phase include flu-like symptoms and are nonspecific: fatigue, anorexia, nausea, vomiting, headache, arthralgias, and myalgias. The icteric phase typically occurs 1–2 weeks after the prodromal phase; symptoms include jaundice, tea-colored urine, pruritus, and right upper quadrant abdominal discomfort.
- In a small number of cases, acute hepatitis may progress rapidly to ALF, marked by markedly abnormal liver enzymes, poor hepatic synthetic function (prolonged PT >16 seconds or INR >1.5), and hepatic encephalopathy in the absence of chronic liver disease.
- Fulminant hepatic failure, defined as ALF that occurs within 8 weeks of the onset of hepatitis, occurs in <2% of patients with acute HAV, HBV, or HEV infection.
- HEV infection is especially dangerous in pregnant women, in whom mortality rates of 15–25% are reported.

Table 13.1 Characteristics of hepatotropic viruses.

	HAV	HBV	HCV	HDV	HEV
Viral type	RNA	DNA	RNA	RNA	RNA
Modes of transmission	Fecal–oral	Parenteral, sexual	Parenteral; infrequent: perinatal or sexual	Parenteral	Fecal–oral
Diagnostic test	IgM anti-HAV	HBsAg, IgM anti-HBc (acute), IgM anti-HBc (chronic) See also Table 13.2	HCV RNA, anti-HCV	Anti-HDV	IgM anti-HEV
Chronic liver disease	No	Yes	Yes	Yes	Rare
Natural immunity	Yes	Yes	No	No	Yes
Vaccine	Yes	Yes	No	No	Yes (experimental)
Treatment options	Supportive care only	Oral nucleoside and/or nucleotide analogs or PEG-IFN-α	DAAs ± ribavirin (genotype dependent); PEG-IFN-α-based therapy	PEG-IFN-α	Supportive care only

Anti-HBc, antibody to hepatitis B core antigen; HAV, hepatitis A virus; HBsAg, hepatitis B surface antigen; HBV, hepatitis B virus; HCV, hepatitis C virus; HDV, hepatitis D virus; HEV, hepatitis E virus; Ig, immunoglobulin; PEG-IFN, peginterferon; DAA, direct-acting antiviral.

> Encephalopathy in ALF is due to cerebral edema and is potentially fatal. Emergent interventions to decrease intracranial pressure are required, and ALF is a clear indication for liver transplant evaluation at a transplant center.

- Typical laboratory test abnormalities in acute hepatitis include elevated serum aminotransferase levels (>500 U l^{-1}) and hyperbilirubinemia, primarily the direct (conjugated) fraction.
- Patients with chronic hepatitis B or C are often asymptomatic. Fatigue is the most common symptom.
- Extrahepatic manifestations associated with HBV infection include the following:
  - Glomerulonephritis.
  - Essential mixed cryoglobulinemia (see later).
  - Palpable purpura and acrodermatitis.
  - Polyarteritis nodosa (rare).
- Extrahepatic manifestations associated with chronic hepatitis C include the following:
  - Essential mixed cryoglobulinemia (most common): Features of cryoglobulinemia include palpable purpura, arthralgias, vasculitis, peripheral neuropathy, glomerulonephritis, and circulating rheumatoid factor.
  - Others: non-Hodgkin's lymphoma, atherosclerosis (cerebrovascular ischemia, cardiovascular ischemia), fatigue/'brain fog,' depression, insulin resistance/diabetes mellitus, membranoproliferative glomerulonephritis, and, polyarteritis nodosa
  - Less well-established extrahepatic manifestations: cognitive decline/ dementia, sexual dysfunction, small-fiber sensory polyneuropathy, autoimmune thyroid disease, sialadenitis/sicca syndrome, porphyria cutanea tarda, lichen planus, and Mooren corneal ulcer.
- HEV infection can be associated with Guillain–Barré syndrome and other neurologic complications and pancreatitis.

Natural History

Hepatitis A Virus and Hepatitis E Virus

- Symptoms related to acute HAV or HEV infection resolve over several days to weeks.
- Acute hepatitis A never and acute hepatitis E rarely (in immunocompromised persons) progress to chronic liver disease.
- Relapsing hepatitis A is an uncommon sequela of acute hepatitis A, more common in elderly persons and characterized by a protracted course with a

relapse of symptoms and signs following apparent resolution. Occasional cases of acute hepatitis A are characterized by marked cholestasis (high serum bilirubin and alkaline phosphatase levels).

- HEV, which is endemic to South, Southeast, and East Asia (especially India), Africa, and Mexico, has a high mortality rate (15–25%) in pregnant women.

Hepatitis B Virus and Hepatitis C Virus

- Age of acquisition is important in HBV infection: approximately 90–95% of neonates, 25–50% of children, and <5% of immunocompetent adults progress from acute hepatitis B to chronic HBV infection.
- Up to 85% of persons with acute HCV infection progress to chronic HCV infection; the remainder are considered to have resolved HCV infection and remain positive for anti-HCV in serum without evidence of viral replication (i.e., HCV RNA is undetectable in serum).
- Cirrhosis ultimately develops in 20% or more of patients with chronic hepatitis B or C.
- Patients with chronic hepatitis B and superimposed HDV infection tend to progress more rapidly to cirrhosis than those with chronic hepatitis B alone.

> Hepatocellular carcinoma is a serious complication of chronic hepatitis B (with or without cirrhosis) and HCV-related cirrhosis.

Diagnosis

Hepatitis A and E

- IgM anti-HAV and IgM anti-HEV are diagnostic of acute hepatitis A and hepatitis E, respectively.

Hepatitis B

- **Acute hepatitis B:**
  - HBsAg is the first serologic marker seen in persons with acute HBV infection. It signifies the presence of HBV virions in serum. The first antibody that appears is IgM anti-HBc.
  - The hallmark of acute hepatitis B is elevation of serum ALT levels and both HBsAg and IgM anti-HBc in serum. Figure 13.1 shows the time course of viral antigens and antibodies in acute self-limiting HBV infection.
  - After acute hepatitis B resolves, >95% of adult patients clear HBsAg, develop antibody to HBsAg (anti-HBs) and recover fully (see Table 13.2).

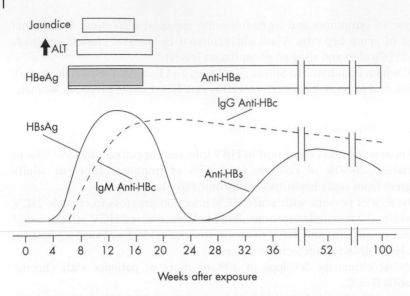

Figure 13.1 Time course of the expression of hepatitis B virus (HBV) antigens and antibodies in acute self-limited HBV infection. ALT, alanine aminotransferase; anti-HBc, antibody to hepatitis B core antigen; anti-HBe, antibody to hepatitis B e antigen; anti-HBs, antibody to hepatitis B surface Ag; HBeAg, hepatitis B e antigen; HBsAg, hepatitis B surface antigen; Ig, immunoglobulin. Redrawn with permission from original figure in Kasper, D.L., Fauci, A.S., Hauser, S.L., *et al.* (2015) *Harrison's Principles of Internal Medicine*, 19th edition, McGraw-Hill, New York.

- **Chronic hepatitis B**:
  - Chronic hepatitis B is defined as persistence of HBsAg in serum for at least 6 months. Persons with chronic hepatitis B are classified based on the presence or absence of active viral replication (HBV DNA $>2 \times 10^3 \, \mathrm{IU \, ml^{-1}}$, HBeAg, elevated serum ALT levels, and active inflammation on a liver biopsy specimen), as outlined below and in Figure 13.2.
    - **Immune-tolerant phase**: Persons who are infected as neonates or as young children may have elevated levels of HBV DNA and detectable HBeAg in serum, but normal serum ALT levels, with minimal histologic evidence of liver damage.
    - **Immune-active phase**: Some persons who are immune-tolerant may enter the immune-active phase of disease. Unresolved acute hepatitis B in an adult can also progress to the immune-active phase of chronic hepatitis B. The HBV DNA and ALT levels remain elevated in serum, and there is histologic evidence of active inflammation.
    - **Inactive carrier state**: Typically, the immune-active phase ends with loss of HBeAg and the appearance of anti-HBe (HBeAg seroconversion). In these patients, the serum HBV DNA level is usually $\leq 2 \times 10^3 \, \mathrm{IU \, ml^{-1}}$, the serum ALT level is normal, and there is minimal inflammation on liver biopsy specimens.

Table 13.2 Interpretation of hepatitis B serologic tests.

	HBsAg	Anti-HBs*	IgG anti-HBc	IgM anti-HBc	HBeAg	Anti-HBe	HBV DNA (IU ml^{-1})	ALT
Acute hepatitis B	+	–	–	+	+	–	$>2 \times 10^3$	Elevated
Natural immunity	–	+	+	–	–	–	Undetectable	Normal
Vaccination	–	+	–	–	–	–	Undetectable	Normal
Chronic hepatitis B (persistence of HBsAg for >6 months)								
Immune-tolerant phase	+	–	+	–	+	–	$>>>2 \times 10^3$	Normal
Immune-active phase	+	–	+	–[†]	+	–	$>2 \times 10^3$	Elevated
Inactive carrier state	+	–	+	–	–	+	$\leq 2 \times 10^3$	Normal
Reactivation phase	+	–	+	–	–	+	$>2 \times 10^3$	Elevated

ALT, alanine aminotransferase; anti-HBc, antibody to hepatitis B core antigen; anti-HBe, antibody to hepatitis B e antigen; anti-HBs, antibody to hepatitis B surface antigen; HBeAg, hepatitis B e antigen; HBsAg, hepatitis B surface antigen; Ig, immunoglobulin; IU, international units.

* Occasionally, anti-HBs is detectable in persons with chronic hepatitis B (who are positive for HBsAg).

[†] Occasionally, IgM anti-HBc is positive during the immune-active phase of chronic hepatitis B.

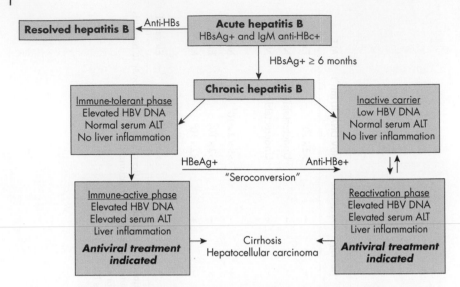

Figure 13.2 Outcomes of HBV infection. ALT, alanine aminotransferase; anti-HBc, antibody to hepatitis B core antigen; anti-HBe, antibody to hepatitis B e antigen; elevated HBV DNA, $>2 \times 10^3\,\mathrm{IU\,ml^{-1}}$; HBeAg, hepatitis B e antigen; HBsAg, hepatitis B surface antigen; Ig, immunoglobulin.

- o **Reactivation phase**: Some persons who have undergone HBeAg sero-conversion may later enter the reactivation phase. These persons often remain HBeAg negative (and anti-HBeAg positive) but have serum HBV DNA levels $>2 \times 10^3\,\mathrm{IU\,ml^{-1}}$, elevated serum ALT levels, and histologic evidence of active inflammation. They presumably were infected with wild-type virus and, over time, acquired mutations in either the pre-core or the core promoter region of the HBV genome, or both. In such patients with pre-core/core mutations, HBV continues to replicate, but HBeAg is not produced. The reactivation phase with pre-core/core mutations is seen in 20% of patients with chronic hepatitis B in the US and 30–50% of patients with chronic hepatitis B in Africa and Asia.
- • Immunity to hepatitis B: The detection of anti-HBs in serum indicates immunity to HBV. When present as the only serologic marker, anti-HBs generally signifies immunity as a result of prior vaccination against HBV. The presence in serum of both IgG anti-HBc and anti-HBs indicates immunity as a result of past infection.

Hepatitis C

- • Anti-HCV in serum, as measured by enzyme-linked immunosorbent assay (ELISA), may indicate active or prior HCV infection. The presence of HCV RNA in serum confirms active infection. All positive anti-HCV test results should be followed by measurement of the HCV RNA level in the serum. In acute hepatitis C, HCV RNA is often present in the absence of anti-HCV. The presence in serum of anti-HCV without detectable HCV RNA represents either spontaneous viral clearance or a false-positive anti-HCV result.

- Six major HCV genotypes have been described (genotypes 1–6). The three HCV genotypes that are most prevalent in the US are 1 (1a and 1b), 2, and 3. Determination of the HCV genotype is recommended after diagnosis of chronic HCV infection because the treatment regimen and response rate to treatment vary with the genotype (see later).

Hepatitis D

- IgM antibody to HDV (IgM anti-HDV) indicates acute infection, and total anti HDV indicates chronic co-infection. If available, HDAg and HDV RNA in serum indicate active infection (acute or chronic).

Treatment and Prevention

Hepatitis A

- Acute hepatitis A is managed with supportive care (e.g., bed rest, fluids, fever-reducing medications), usually guided by symptoms.
- HAV vaccine is recommended for all infants as well as for adults who are at high risk of infection (e.g., travelers to developing countries, persons with human immunodeficiency virus (HIV) infection, patients with chronic liver disease, men who have sex with men, workers at daycare centers). The dose of HAV vaccine (inactivated HAV) is 1 ml and 0.5 ml intramuscularly in adults and children, respectively. A booster dose is recommended at 6 months after the initial dose.
- Postexposure prophylaxis with immune globulin ($0.02 \, \text{ml} \, \text{kg}^{-1}$ intramuscularly) is recommended for household and intimate contacts of persons with HAV infection. In healthy persons aged 1 to 40 years, the HAV vaccine can be administered instead of immune globulin.

Hepatitis B

- Acute HBV infection is managed with supportive care. Nucleoside or nucleotide analogs (see below) are often administered in severe cases of acute HBV infection, especially if there is concern for progression to acute liver failure.

- **Chronic HBV infection**:
  - The agents currently used for the treatment of chronic hepatitis B include oral nucleoside or nucleotide analogs: entecavir, tenofovir, emtricitabine/tenofovir, adefovir, lamivudine, and subcutaneous pegylated interferon alpha. The preferred first-line agents are entecavir and tenofovir.
  - Candidates for antiviral therapy include patients with chronic hepatitis B who have evidence of active viral replication (HBV DNA $>2 \times 10^4 \, \text{IU ml}^{-1}$ (HBeAg positive) or $>2 \times 10^3 \, \text{IU ml}^{-1}$ (HBeAg negative), elevated serum ALT levels, and inflammation or fibrosis on a liver biopsy specimen.
  - The primary goal of antiviral treatment of HBV infection is suppression of viral replication (low or undetectable HBV DNA levels). Ideally, HBeAg seroconversion will also occur. Secondary goals of therapy are amelioration of symptoms and delay in the progression of chronic hepatitis to cirrhosis and/or development of hepatocellular carcinoma.
    - ○ HBsAg clearance is the ultimate treatment endpoint because it improves overall survival and lowers the rate of liver decompensation and development of hepatocellular carcinoma. The rate of HBsAg clearance without treatment is 0.5% to 2% annually, and is increased with antiviral therapy.
    - ○ Currently existing antiviral therapies have no direct effect on the covalently closed circular DNA (cccDNA) of HBV, which is believed to be the viral reservoir in infected hepatocyte nuclei and responsible for persistent HBV infection.
- **Vaccination and prevention**:
  - HBV vaccine: vaccines derived from recombinant HBsAg are used to stimulate the production of anti-HBs in uninfected persons. The available vaccines are highly effective, with seroconversion rates >95%. Vaccine administration is recommended for all infants and for adults who are at increased risk of infection (e.g., persons undergoing dialysis, healthcare workers, persons with high-risk sexual practices). The recommended vaccination schedule for infants is within 12–24 hours of birth, at 1–2 months of age, and at 6–18 months of age. The recommended vaccination schedule for adults is 0, 1, and 6 months.
  - Postexposure prophylaxis: hepatitis B immune globulin (HBIG, 0.5 ml intramuscularly) provides passive immunization for persons who are exposed to blood or body fluids from persons with acute hepatitis B or for contacts of persons who are positive for HBsAg in serum.
  - Recommendations are as follows:
    - ○ Perinatal exposure: HBIG plus initiation of the vaccine series at the time of birth.
    - ○ Sexual contact with an acutely infected patient or chronic carrier: vaccine series.

- o Household contact with an acutely infected person resulting in exposure: HBIG plus vaccine series.
- o Household contact with a chronically infected person: vaccine series.
- o Infants (<12 months) cared for primarily by an acutely infected patient: HBIG plus vaccine series.
- o Inadvertent percutaneous or permucosal exposure: HBIG plus vaccine series.

Reactivation of quiescent HBV infection leading to potentially a life-threatening flare of hepatitis is common in inactive HBV carriers (HBsAg-positive or isolated anti-HBc) who undergo treatment with chemotherapy or immunosuppressant therapy. All candidates for chemotherapy or immunosuppressant therapy should be tested for HBV, and those who are positive for HBsAg or anti-HBc should begin treatment with an antiviral agent prior to initiation of chemotherapy or immunosuppressant therapy and continuing for at least 12 months after completion of such therapy.

Patients with chronic hepatitis B (or with chronic hepatitis C and cirrhosis) should undergo biannual screening with abdominal ultrasonography for hepatocellular carcinoma surveillance; often the serum alpha fetoprotein (AFP) level, a tumor marker for hepatocellular carcinoma, is also measured biannually.

Hepatitis C

- Acute hepatitis C is detected infrequently. When diagnosed at an acute stage, early treatment can be considered.
- **Chronic hepatitis C:**
  - Treatment is with combinations of direct-acting antivirals (DAAs). Ribavirin is used in some treatment regimens. Pegylated interferon alpha-based therapy was used prior to the advent of DAAs, but is rarely used now because of lower rates of efficacy and adverse effects.
  - DAAs target specific nonstructural proteins (NS) of the HCV virus responsible for virus replication and assembly; they specifically inhibit the NS3/4A protease, NS5A protein, and NS5B polymerase (see Table 13.3).
  - The goal of treatment is to achieve a sustained viral response (SVR), defined as the absence of detectable HCV RNA in serum 12 weeks after the completion of treatment. Achievement of an SVR indicates viral eradication, or cure, of HCV infection.

Table 13.3 FDA-approved direct-acting antiviral agents for the treatment of HCV.*

NS3-4A protease inhibitors	NS5A inhibitors	NS5B polymerase inhibitors (nucleoside)	NS5B polymerase inhibitors (non-nucleoside)
Simeprevir	Ledipasvir	Sofosbuvir	Dasabuvir
Paritaprevir	Ombitasvir		
Grazoprevir	Daclatasvir		
Voxilaprevir	Elbasvir		
Glecaprevir	Velpatasvir		
	Pibrentasvir		

* Combinations of agents from different classes are used; the choice of regimen is based on the viral genotype, presence or absence of cirrhosis, and the patient's prior response to therapy.

- The type of DAAs used, doses, and durations depend on the HCV genotype, history of prior therapy, and degree of liver fibrosis and decompensation. DAAs have high rates of cure (>90% in most treated patients), with low rates of adverse events and treatment-emergent resistance.

Hepatitis D

- The treatment of patients co-infected with HBV and HDV is not well studied. HBV/HDV-co-infected patients are less responsive to peginterferon therapy than patients infected with HBV alone. Nucleoside and nucleotide analogs do not suppress HDV.

Pearls

- Hepatitis B and C can lead to chronic liver disease, whereas hepatitis A and E (in immunocompetent persons) do not lead to chronic liver disease.
- Acute hepatitis B progresses to chronic HBV infection in <5% of immunocompetent adults, whereas acute hepatitis B progresses to chronic HBV infection in 90–95% of neonates and 25–50% of children.
- Acute HCV infection progresses to chronic HCV infection in up to 85% of persons.
- Hepatitis A and B can be prevented with the administration of a viral-specific vaccine. A vaccine has not been developed for HCV, and a vaccine for HEV is experimental.
- Chronic hepatitis B and C can be treated with antiviral agents that prevent progression of liver disease.

Questions

Questions 1 to 3 relate to the clinical vignette at the beginning of this chapter.

1   Which of the following is the most likely diagnosis?
   A Acute hepatitis A.
   B Acute hepatitis B.
   C Acute hepatitis A and previous hepatitis B infection.
   D Previous hepatitis A and acute hepatitis B.
   E Acute hepatitis A and previous hepatitis B vaccination.

2   Which one of the following statements is TRUE regarding the patient's acute illness?
   A It is a result of an infection with a DNA virus.
   B He could have avoided the infection if he had been vaccinated prior to travel.
   C Measuring viral DNA levels in serum at the time of infection would have confirmed the diagnosis.
   D He is at risk of cirrhosis.
   E He has an increased risk of developing hepatocellular carcinoma.

3   Appropriate management of the patient includes:
   A Supportive care.
   B Lamuvidine.
   C Peginterferon alfa-2a.
   D Supportive care plus immunoglobulin.
   E Supportive care followed by HAV vaccine.

4   The following hepatitis B serologic profile is found in an asymptomatic 40-year-old man:

HBsAg	Positive
Anti-HBs	Negative
IgG anti-HBc	Positive
IgM anti-HBc	Negative
HBeAg	Positive
Anti-HBe	Negative

Which of the following is the best interpretation of this profile?
   A Past hepatitis B infection.
   B Acute hepatitis B.
   C Inactive HBV carrier.
   D Chronic hepatitis B.
   E Hepatitis B vaccination.

5 Which of the following is a DNA virus?
A Hepatitis A.
B Hepatitis B.
C Hepatitis C.
D Hepatitis D.
E Hepatitis E.

6 Which one of the following antibodies signifies immunity to reinfection?
A Anti-HBs.
B Anti-HBe.
C Anti-HBc.
D Anti-HCV.
E None of the above.

7 A 57-year-old-man is seen in your office for increasing fatigue, anorexia, and jaundice. He was seen in the office 6 months earlier for the same symptoms, and you diagnosed acute hepatitis A based on the results of serologic tests. He says that his symptoms improved gradually during the next month, but he then noticed a recurrence of symptoms over the past month. The patient also has essential hypertension and has taken hydrochlorothiazide, 50 mg daily, for the past 3 years. On examination he appears jaundiced. The liver edge is palpable below the costal margin, and the liver span is 10 cm. There is no splenomegaly or ascites. Laboratory test results are listed below.

AST	872 U l^{-1}
ALT	780 U l^{-1}
Alkaline phosphatase	128 U l^{-1}
Bilirubin:	
Total	6.2 mg dl^{-1}
Direct	4.7 mg dl^{-1}
IgM anti-HAV	Positive
HBsAg	Negative
Anti-HBs	Positive
IgG anti-HBc	Negative
Anti-HCV	Negative

What is the most likely diagnosis of this patient's condition?
A Relapsing hepatitis A.
B Acute hepatitis B.

C Chronic hepatitis B.
D Acute hepatitis C.
E Drug-induced hepatitis.

8 A former intravenous drug user acquired chronic viral hepatitis from sharing needles. He has evidence of chronic hepatitis C and resolved hepatitis B. Which of the following statements is TRUE about his HBV and HCV infections?

A Hepatitis C is more likely to become chronic than hepatitis B in drug users.
B The patient is at risk for hepatocellular carcinoma because of his past history of hepatitis B infection.
C The risk of transmitting HCV to his wife is >20% if the patient does not use condoms.
D The patient is unlikely to respond to antiviral treatment for chronic hepatitis C.

Answers

1 C
The patient is positive for IgM anti-HAV, indicating acute hepatitis A. This diagnosis is consistent with the elevated serum aminotransferase and bilirubin levels. Although the patient reports a history of alcohol use, the serum aminotransferases are not consistent with alcoholic hepatitis. The serum aminotransferase levels in persons with alcoholic hepatitis are typically <500 U l^{-1}, and the AST/ALT ratio is <1 (see Chapter 14). The patient also has anti-HBs and IgG anti-HBc, indicating past infection with HBV (natural immunity).

2 B
HAV vaccine is readily available, and the patient could have avoided HAV infection if he had received the vaccine prior to travel. HAV is an RNA virus. Hepatitis A does not progress to chronic liver disease, and patients are not at risk of cirrhosis or hepatocellular carcinoma.

3 A
Acute hepatitis A is managed with supportive care (bed rest, fluids, and fever-reducing medicines), usually guided by the severity of symptoms. Following recovery, patients develop natural immunity (appearance of IgG anti-HAV in serum) and therefore do not need HAV vaccination. Antiviral medications have no role in the management of acute hepatitis A.

4 D
Chronic hepatitis B is defined by the presence of HBsAg ≥6 months along with a positive IgG anti-HBc. There is no evidence of immunity (negative anti-HBs). The presence of HBeAg indicates active viral replication.

5 B

6 A

7 A

Relapse of acute HAV infection can occur in 3–20% of patients with acute hepatitis A. Following a typical course of acute HAV infection, a remission phase occurs, with partial or complete resolution of clinical and biochemical manifestations. Relapse can occur shortly after symptom resolution and mimics the initial presentation, although it usually is clinically milder. Recrudescence of symptoms and biochemical abnormalities, along with reappearance of IgM anti-HAV in serum, is diagnostic of relapsing hepatitis A. Recovery eventually occurs.

8 A

At least 95% of immunocompetent adults with acute HBV infection recover and do not progress to chronic hepatitis B. However, a majority of patients acutely infected with HCV progress to chronic hepatitis C. In this patient, there is no risk of sequelae from HBV infection, which has resolved. The risk of sexual transmission of HCV is low (<2.5%). Chronic HCV infection is quite responsive to antiviral therapy.

Further Reading

Burgess, S.V., Hussaini, T., and Yoshida, E.M. (2016) Concordance of sustained virologic response at weeks 4, 12 and 24 post-treatment of hepatitis C in the era of new oral direct-acting antivirals: A concise review. *Annals of Hepatology*, **15**, 154–159.

Chhatwal, J., Wang, X., Ayer, T., *et al.* (2016) Hepatitis C disease burden in the United States in the era of oral direct-acting antivirals. *Hepatology* (2016), **64**, 1442–1450.

Sjogren, M.H. and Bassett, J.T. (2016) Hepatitis A, in *Sleisenger and Fordtran's Gastrointestinal and Liver Disease: Pathophysiology/Diagnosis/Management*, 10th edition (eds M. Feldman, L.S. Friedman, and L.J. Brandt), Saunders Elsevier, Philadelphia, pp. 1302–1308.

Terrault, N.A., Bzowej, N.H., Chang, K.M., *et al.* (2016) AASLD guidelines for treatment of chronic hepatitis B. *Hepatology*, **63**, 261–283.

Weblinks

http://www.cdc.gov/hepatitis/
http://www.hcvguidelines.org/
http://digestive.niddk.nih.gov/ddiseases/pubs/viralhepatitis/
http://emedicine.medscape.com/article/185463-overview

14

Alcoholic Liver Disease and Nonalcoholic Fatty Liver Disease

Stephen H. Berger and Ryan M. Ford

Clinical Vignette 1

A 52-year-old man is found unconscious and brought to the emergency department by an ambulance. The patient is unable to provide a history, but his breath smells of alcohol. Physical examination reveals a blood pressure of 160/104 mmHg, pulse rate 120 per minute, respiratory rate 24 per minute, and temperature 101 °F (38.3 °C). The patient is arousable only to painful stimuli, his conjunctivae are icteric, and his mucous membranes are dry. The pupils are reactive to light, and reflexes are 2+ and symmetric. The plantar reflex is flexor bilaterally. The chest is clear and the cardiovascular examination is notable only for tachycardia. Abdominal examination reveals hepatosplenomegaly. He has no edema. His skin is icteric. Laboratory tests show a white blood cell (WBC) count of 19 800 mm^{-3} with 80% neutrophils, 10% band forms, and 8% lymphocytes. The hemoglobin level is 10.0 g dl^{-1}, platelet count 100 000 mm^{-3}, aspartate aminotransferase (AST) 181 U l^{-1}, alanine aminotransferase (ALT) 52 U l^{-1}, total bilirubin 10.8 mg dl^{-1}, direct bilirubin 7.9 mg dl^{-1}, and International Normalized Ratio (INR) 1.8. Computed tomography (CT) of the head without contrast reveals no intracranial hemorrhage. A urine drug screen is negative for cocaine or methamphetamines.

Definition

- Alcoholic liver disease (ALD) and nonalcoholic fatty liver disease (NAFLD) represent a spectrum of liver diseases characterized initially by the accumulation of triglycerides in hepatocytes.

Sitaraman and Friedman's Essentials of Gastroenterology, Second Edition.
Edited by Shanthi Srinivasan and Lawrence S. Friedman.

- The spectrum of ALD and NAFLD include:
  - Bland steatosis (fatty liver): reversible accumulation of triglycerides without inflammation.
  - Steatohepatitis: steatosis with pericellular inflammation and hepatocyte ballooning degeneration.
  - Alcoholic steatohepatitis (ASH), nonalcoholic steatohepatitis (NASH), or both.
  - Cirrhosis: significant fibrosis with regenerating nodules (possibly complicated by portal hypertension or hepatocellular carcinoma); a patient may have compensated or decompensated cirrhosis (see Chapters 15 and 16).
- Histologically, steatosis may be either **macrovesicular**, in which lipid accumulation compresses and displaces the hepatocyte nucleus to the periphery of the cell, or **microvesicular**, in which lipid accumulates in small droplets.
  - ALD and NAFLD typically show macrovesicular steatosis.
  - Microvesicular steatosis occurs as a result of impaired mitochondrial beta-oxidation of free fatty acids. Liver disease associated with microvesicular steatosis is often more severe, with the possibility of multi-organ failure (MOF) and death. Causes of microvesicular steatosis include:
    o Drugs: ethanol, valproic acid, high-dose intravenous tetracycline, amiodarone, aspirin, nevirapine, stavudine, didanosine, and piroxicam.
    o Acute fatty liver of pregnancy.
    o Inborn errors of metabolism affecting beta-oxidation of free fatty acids.
    o Reye's syndrome: a potentially fatal disease that is characterized by encephalopathy and MOF. It is associated with aspirin use in children with a viral illness but may also occur in the absence of aspirin use.

Alcoholic Liver Disease: Overview

- Steatosis typically develops after the consumption of 80 g of alcohol (e.g., six beers or 8 ounces (240 ml) of 80-proof liquor) daily over one to several days. Steatosis is reversible if alcohol consumption is stopped.
- The development of cirrhosis is associated with the consumption of 40–80 g of alcohol daily in men and 20–40 g daily in women for a minimum of 10 years.
- Cirrhosis develops in 10–15% of alcoholics (see definition below).
- Approximately 20% of ingested alcohol is absorbed into the systemic circulation through the stomach and metabolized by hepatocytes through oxidation of alcohol to acetaldehyde by the enzyme alcohol dehydrogenase (ADH) (Figure 14.1).
  - ADH is the rate-limiting enzyme in alcohol metabolism, and its activity varies with race, age, gender, and genetic polymorphisms.

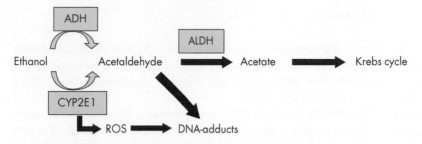

Figure 14.1 Alcohol metabolism. ADH, alcohol dehydrogenase; ALDH, acetaldehyde dehydrogenase; CYP2E1, cytochrome P450 2E1; ROS, reactive oxygen species.

- Women, Native Americans, Asians, and the elderly have lower levels of gastric ADH. This may account in part for the observation that women are more susceptible than men to liver injury for a given dose of alcohol consumed.
- Gastric ADH may account for up to 10% of 'first-pass' metabolism through the oxidation of ethanol before intestinal absorption occurs. The dose of ethanol, concomitant food ingestion, and gastric emptying rate may affect the first-pass gastric metabolism of ethanol.
- Acetaldehyde is an unstable metabolite of ethanol that forms adducts with macromolecules through the Schiff-base reaction. Acetaldehyde can impair mitochondrial function, destroy hepatocyte membranes, and interfere with normal transcriptional activity of the cell. It is more injurious to hepatocytes than ethanol.
- Acetaldehyde is rapidly converted to acetate, an inert and inactive metabolite, by aldehyde dehydrogenase (ALDH). Acetate is eventually converted to CO_2 and H_2O by the Krebs cycle.
- An alternative pathway for hepatic alcohol metabolism involves the microsomal ethanol-oxidizing system and cytochrome P450 (CYP) 2E1. This pathway also produces acetaldehyde and reactive oxygen species that contribute to fatty liver and depletion of glutathione.
  - This pathway is induced in chronic alcoholism and increases susceptibility to drug-induced liver injury from agents such as isoniazid, acetaminophen, or cocaine.

Acetaldehyde is responsible for many of the systemic toxic effects of alcohol, such as nausea, headaches, palpitations, and flushing. The 'Asian flush syndrome' is due to mutations in the *ALDH* gene that result in deficiency of the enzyme, thereby leading to toxic effect of acetaldehyde in persons who consume alcohol.

Alcoholic Steatosis

- In most people, the ingestion of alcohol leads to triglyceride accumulation within the cytoplasm of the hepatocyte. This process is reversible, but persons with chronic alcoholism may develop progressive liver injury (inflammation, fibrosis) over time.
- Patients with steatosis are most often asymptomatic. Physical examination may reveal hepatomegaly. Laboratory tests are frequently normal. If serum aminotransferase levels are elevated, the AST: ALT ratio is typically ≥2.
- The diagnosis of alcohol steatosis is based on imaging or biopsy as well as clinical suspicion. The diagnosis of alcohol abuse is based on history and standardized screening tools such as the Alcohol Use Disorders Identification Test-Consumption (AUDIT-C) questions, and the CAGE (need to cut down, annoyed by criticism, guilty about drinking, need an eye-opener in the morning) questionnaire.
- The mean corpuscular volume (MCV) and serum gamma-glutamyl trans-peptidase (GGTP) level may be elevated in a patient with alcoholism.
- Treatment is abstinence from alcohol, which can lead to reversal of fatty liver. To help maintain abstinence, intensive counseling with or without con-comitant medications (acamprosate, baclofen, naltrexone, disulfiram) and relapse prevention strategies are recommended.

Alcoholic Hepatitis

General

- Alcoholic hepatitis may occur with or without fatty liver. It may occur acutely in a subset of patients with chronic alcohol-induced liver disease, and it ranges in severity from mild to life-threatening.

Clinical and Laboratory Features

- Patients may present with fever, anorexia, nausea, vomiting, jaundice, abdominal pain, or diarrhea.
- The most common finding on examination is tender **hepatomegaly**. Some patients may have prolonged fever, typically >102.2 °F (39 °C). On physical examination, patients with severe alcoholic hepatitis may have spider telangiectasias, splenomegaly, jaundice, ascites, hepatic encephalopathy, and peripheral edema.
- Laboratory tests may reveal an elevated WBC count with neutrophil predominance. Patients may have megaloblastic anemia. Serum AST and

ALT levels are elevated in a ratio of at least 2: 1 and are typically <500 U l^{-1}, even with severe disease. The ALT may be normal or near-normal, in part because of concomitant pyridoxine deficiency. The total bilirubin level can be as high as 40 mg dl^{-1}. The serum albumin level is typically low, often <2 g dl^{-1}. The prothrombin time is markedly prolonged in severe disease.

Diagnosis

- The diagnosis of alcoholic hepatitis is made by history, physical examination, and laboratory tests. Liver biopsy is seldom necessary, but it could be considered for definitive diagnosis or to rule out alternative or additional diagnoses.
- Classic histologic features in the liver include a polymorphonuclear neutrophilic infiltrate, Mallory bodies (or Mallory's hyaline), steatosis, hepatocyte ballooning degeneration, and varying degrees of fibrosis (see Chapter 28).

Prognosis

- Estimating the prognosis is important in determining the need for specific therapy. The 28-day mortality rate may be as high as 75% in patients with severe disease, who often have underlying cirrhosis. The systemic inflammatory response syndrome (SIRS) and subsequent MOF contributes to the high mortality. Serum lipopolysaccharide levels can be predictive of MOF.
- Five clinical tools may help predict mortality:
  - The Maddrey Discrimination Function (DF) is calculated as 4.6 × (the patient's prothrombin time – control prothrombin time in seconds) + total bilirubin (mg dl^{-1}). A DF >32 indicates severe disease and is associated with a mortality rate of up to 50% at 4 weeks.
  - The Model for End-Stage Liver Disease (MELD) and MELD-Na scores utilize the serum bilirubin, INR, serum creatinine, and serum sodium (see Chapter 16).
  - The Glasgow alcoholic hepatitis score utilizes the patient's age, WBC count, blood urea nitrogen level, prothrombin time ratio (ratio of the patient's prothrombin time to the control value), and serum bilirubin level.
  - The Lille Model score incorporates age, serum bilirubin level on presentation, bilirubin level at day 7, serum creatinine, serum albumin, and prothrombin time. Failure of the serum bilirubin to decline by day 7 with medical therapy is a negative prognostic sign.
  - The ABIC score is calculated as (age × 0.1) + (serum bilirubin × 0.08) + (serum creatinine × 0.3) + (INR × 0.8). The higher the score, the higher the risk of death.

Treatment

- The most important therapy is complete abstinence from alcohol.
- Nutritional support improves long-term survival. It is not considered necessary to restrict the patient's protein calories, and enteral feedings are preferred, even if a nasogastric feeding tube is required. A high-calorie diet with multivitamins, thiamine, and folic acid supplementation is recommended.
- Medical treatments for patients with severe disease include:
  - Glucocorticoids:
    o Recommended regimen is prednisolone 40 mg daily for 28 days, followed by a taper.
    o Contraindications include gastrointestinal bleeding requiring blood transfusion and systemic infection.
    o Prednisolone has not been shown to be effective in patients in whom hepatorenal syndrome has developed (see Chapter 16).
  - Pentoxifylline:
    o An alternative agent used in patients with a contraindication to the use of glucocorticoids or in patients with renal failure. The recommended dose is 400 mg orally three times daily for 28 days.
- A large randomized trial (STOPAH) analyzed over 1000 patients with severe alcoholic hepatitis. Although treatment with prednisolone was associated with a trend towards an improved 28-day mortality rate, it had no effect on long-term outcomes and was associated with an increased rate of serious infections compared with placebo. Pentoxifylline appeared to have no effect on survival.
- Early liver transplantation can improve survival in carefully selected patients with a first episode of severe alcoholic hepatitis not responding to medical therapy.

Alcoholic Cirrhosis

General

- Cirrhosis is, for the most part, an irreversible complication of ALD and other forms of chronic liver disease (see Chapter 15).
- Histopathologic findings of alcoholic cirrhosis do not correlate reliably with clinical findings.

Clinical and Laboratory Features

- Patients with compensated cirrhosis are often asymptomatic or may have nonspecific constitutional symptoms such as fatigue, anorexia, or weight loss.
- Patients with decompensated cirrhosis may present with jaundice, weakness, abdominal pain, or complications of portal hypertension, such as ascites, encephalopathy, or variceal bleeding (see Chapter 16).

- The physical examination may reveal hepatosplenomegaly; however, the examination is often normal in patients with well-compensated cirrhosis.
- Patients with decompensated cirrhosis may show muscle wasting, jaundice, spider telangiectasias, palmar erythema, gynecomastia, a small liver, ascites, caput medusae, asterixis, and fetor hepaticus (a distinct odor to the breath that is caused by volatile aromatic substances that accumulate in the setting of cirrhosis).
- Findings on laboratory tests may include mildly to moderately elevated serum aminotransferase and bilirubin levels, an increased INR, a low serum albumin level, anemia, an increased mean corpuscular volume, a low platelet count, and evidence of renal insufficiency.

Diagnosis

- The diagnosis of alcoholic cirrhosis is based on history, physical examination, laboratory tests, and imaging.
- Abdominal imaging by ultrasonography, CT, or magnetic resonance imaging (MRI) may show a nodular and shrunken liver, in addition to signs of portal hypertension (ascites, varices, and/or splenomegaly).

Patients with alcoholic cirrhosis are susceptible to sudden decompensation. Factors that contribute to decompensation in an otherwise stable person with cirrhosis include drug-induced liver injury, infection, portal vein thrombosis, and hepatocellular carcinoma (HCC). Once the diagnosis of cirrhosis is established, a patient is at risk of developing decompensated liver disease and HCC, even if he or she abstains from alcohol or has no symptoms of chronic liver disease.

Prognosis

- The overall 5-year survival rate for patients with alcoholic cirrhosis is 50–75%. The survival rate decreases dramatically with the development of ascites, spontaneous bacterial peritonitis, bleeding varices, hepatorenal syndrome, or hepatic encephalopathy (see Chapter 16).
- The clinical tools used most widely to determine prognosis in patients with alcoholic cirrhosis are the Child–Turcotte–Pugh (CTP) score (Child–Pugh classification) and the MELD score (see earlier). The CTP score is based on the serum bilirubin, ascites, serum albumin, INR, and encephalopathy.

Chronic hepatitis C virus (HCV) infection, obesity, and smoking are independent risk factors for the progression of ALD to cirrhosis.

Treatment

- The treatment of patients with alcoholic cirrhosis involves abstinence from alcohol, which is beneficial even in patients with decompensated cirrhosis.
- Nutritional supplementation with thiamine, folic acid, vitamin B_{12}, and magnesium is often necessary.
- The management of portal hypertension is discussed in Chapter 16.
- Liver transplantation is definitive treatment for patients with decompensated cirrhosis; the MELD score is an important determinant for the eligibility for transplantation (see Chapter 16). Given the dramatic benefits of abstinence from alcohol, a period of abstinence is recommended prior to transplantation.

Nonalcoholic Fatty Liver Disease (NAFLD)

Clinical Vignette 2

A 55-year-old woman was found to have elevated serum aminotransferase levels when she applied for life insurance. She presents to her primary care physician for evaluation. She is asymptomatic. Her past medical history is significant for type 2 diabetes mellitus, hypertension, hypercholesterolemia, obesity, and osteoarthritis. She has never used alcohol or tobacco and denies use of illicit drugs. She works as a bank teller. Her mother died from cirrhosis of unknown cause. There is a strong family history of obesity and type 2 diabetes mellitus; an older brother died of a myocardial infarction at age 58. She notes that weight-loss programs and diet pills have not worked for her. Chronic back and knee pain prohibit her from participating in vigorous exercise. Medications include pioglitazone, glyburide, metformin, enalapril, simvastatin, and a generic over-the-counter nonsteroidal anti-inflammatory drug. Physical examination reveals an obese woman in no distress. The blood pressure is 150/94 mmHg, pulse rate 88 per minute, respiratory rate 18 per minute, and temperature 99.3 °F (37.4 °C). Her body mass index (BMI) is 44. An S_4 gallop is heard on auscultation of the heart. The abdomen is obese, precluding palpation of the liver or the spleen. Neurologic examination reveals decreased sensation in her toes, and the extremities demonstrate 2+ pitting edema. The remainder of the examination is unremarkable. Laboratory tests reveal a fasting total cholesterol of 312 mg dl^{-1}, low-density lipoprotein (LDL) cholesterol 172 mg dl^{-1}, high-density lipoprotein (HDL) 28 mg dl^{-1}, triglycerides 230 mg dl^{-1}, glucose 298 mg dl^{-1}, AST 100 U l^{-1}, ALT 150 U l^{-1}, and hemoglobin Alc 9.8%. Tests for viral hepatitis, human immunodeficiency virus, hereditary hemochromatosis, Wilson disease, autoimmune hepatitis, and alpha-1 antitrypsin deficiency are unremarkable. Ultrasonography of the right upper quadrant reveals a few gallstones in the gallbladder; the liver is echogenic and heterogeneous.

General

- The estimated prevalence of NAFLD in the US is 30–46% (80–100 million Americans).
- NAFLD is typically diagnosed in adults; however, the frequency of NAFLD is increasing among obese children and adolescents.
- NAFLD affects men and women equally. Hispanics have the highest frequency of NAFLD (45%) compared with whites (33%) and African Americans (24%). Familial clustering of NAFLD has been observed.
- Many drugs and conditions are associated with NAFLD (Table 14.1), but NAFLD occurs most commonly with the metabolic syndrome, a constellation of clinical disorders that include obesity, type 2 diabetes mellitus, essential hypertension, low serum levels of HDL, and elevated fasting serum triglycerides levels.
- NAFLD has also been linked to polycystic ovarian syndrome (PCOS), pituitary disorders, and hypothyroidism.
- The spectrum of NAFLD includes fatty infiltration of the liver without inflammatory changes (nonalcoholic fatty liver; NAFL) and fatty infiltration of the liver with inflammatory changes and ballooning degeneration on biopsy (nonalcoholic steatohepatitis; NASH). NASH may lead to hepatocyte cell death and fibrosis and ultimately cirrhosis.

NAFLD is the most common liver disease in the US and the most common reason a patient is evaluated for elevated serum aminotransferase levels. NASH cirrhosis is the second leading indication for liver transplantation in the US after hepatitis C cirrhosis.

Pathophysiology

- Insulin resistance, particularly hepatic insulin resistance, is the hallmark of NAFLD. Hepatocytes of affected persons do not have a normal response to insulin, and accumulate excess free fatty acids.
- Genetic variation in the patanin-like phospholipase domain-containing protein 3 (PNPLA3) enzyme has been linked to the development of NASH. Like most chronic medical conditions, NASH involves a complex interplay between genetics and the environment.
- Investigations have revealed an interplay between the liver, innate immune system, gut, and adipose tissue. Dysregulation of the gut-liver axis has been implicated via alterations in the intestinal microbiome. Chemokines, such as adiponectin and tumor necrosis factor-alpha, may be mediators of some of the systemic changes.

Table 14.1 Causes of nonalcoholic fatty liver disease.

Metabolic syndrome	Diabetes mellitus
	Hypertension
	Hypertriglyceridemia
	Low high-density lipoprotein levels
	Obesity
Other disorders of lipid metabolism	Abetalipoproteinemia
Surgical procedures:	Extensive small bowel resection
	Gastric bypass
	Jejuno-ileal bypass
Drugs:	Amiodarone
	Glucocorticosteroids
	Hormonal therapy (e.g., tamoxifen, high-dose estrogen)
	Methotrexate
Others:	Hepatitis C genotype 3
	Hypothyroidism
	Lysosomal acid lipase deficiency
	Pituitary disorders
	Polycystic ovarian syndrome
	Total parenteral nutrition
	Wilson disease

Clinical and Laboratory Features

- Most patients with NAFLD are asymptomatic. Some patients may have vague right upper quadrant discomfort or fatigue. Patients with NAFLD-associated cirrhosis may have stigmata of chronic liver disease (see Chapter 15).
- The past medical history is important and may reveal risk factors for NAFLD including obesity, diabetes mellitus, hyperlipidemia, and hypertension. Physical examination is nonspecific; hepatomegaly may be present in up to 75% of patients but may be difficult to appreciate due to obesity.
- Results of laboratory studies are nonspecific and most commonly show elevated serum ALT and AST levels (ALT usually greater than AST) and occasionally elevated alkaline phosphatase levels.
- Antinuclear antibodies and smooth muscle antibodies, which typically are associated with autoimmune hepatitis, may be present in low titers.
- NAFLD is often found incidentally on imaging studies and can be seen on ultrasonography (increased echogenicity, seen as a 'bright liver'), CT (lower density than spleen), or MRI (bright on T1-weighted imaging; see Figure 14.2).
- Histologic features of NAFL and NASH are indistinguishable from those of alcoholic fatty liver and alcoholic hepatitis, respectively.

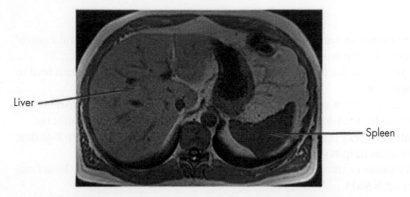

Figure 14.2 Magnetic resonance imaging (MRI) showing hepatic steatosis. On this T1-weighted image, the liver is brighter than the spleen because of fat in the liver.

Diagnosis

- ALD must be excluded before a diagnosis of NAFLD can be made.
- NAFLD is often a clinical diagnosis and requires the exclusion of other causes of chronic liver disease. Laboratory testing, including antibody to hepatitis C virus, hepatitis B surface antigen, iron indices, ceruloplasmin, alpha-1 antitrypsin level, antinuclear antibodies, smooth muscle antibodies, antimitochondrial antibodies, and transglutaminase antibodies, should be conducted to exclude other causes of liver disease.
- Hepatomegaly may be observed on imaging (ultrasonography, CT, or MRI); ultrasonography may show increased echogenicity if >30% of the liver is involved by steatosis.
- A variety of tests are available for the noninvasive estimation of liver fibrosis (see Chapter 12), but are unable to distinguish bland steatosis from steatosis with inflammation (NASH).
- Liver biopsy may be performed in select patients to distinguish bland steatosis (NAFL) from NASH, assess degree of fibrosis, and rule out other hepatic disorders.

Prognosis

- The long-term prognosis of patients with NAFLD is unknown. Approximately 20% of persons with NAFLD have NASH, and 30–40% of those with NASH are at risk of developing advanced fibrosis and cirrhosis. Although NASH and alcoholic hepatitis are similar histologically, the short-term prognosis of NASH is substantially better.
- NASH is more concerning than NAFL in terms of overall prognosis; however, it is difficult to predict which patients with NAFLD will progress to NASH or cirrhosis.

Treatment

- The mainstay of treatment for NAFLD is lifestyle modification and control of metabolic syndrome risk factors:
  - A 10–15% reduction of body weight through diet and exercise can lead to improvement.
  - A carbohydrate-restricted or Mediterranean diet should be considered.
- Pharmacotherapy for obesity has proved challenging due to side effects.
- Bariatric surgery (gastric sleeve, laparoscopic banding, or Roux-en-Y gastric bypass) can help reverse steatosis in morbidly obese patients.
- Pioglitazone is used to treat diabetes mellitus and may have a beneficial effect on NASH.
- Lipid-lowering agents such as a 3-hydroxy-3-methylglutaryl [HMG]-coenzyme A reductase inhibitor (statin) or fibrate should be considered.
- Vitamin E 800 IU daily may be considered in some patients, and has been shown to have some histologic benefit on steatohepatitis.
- Moderate coffee consumption may be of benefit in this population.
- Liver transplantation may be considered in persons who develop cirrhosis or hepatocellular carcinoma.

Pearls

- The metabolic syndrome is a group of risk factors (obesity, elevated triglycerides, low HDL, hypertension, insulin resistance, diabetes mellitus) that portends an increased risk of NAFLD.
- Weight loss can reverse NAFL and NASH and can prevent the development of cirrhosis.
- Insulin resistance, particularly hepatic insulin resistance, is the hallmark of NAFLD. Hepatocytes of affected persons escape the normal response to insulin (e.g., glycogen synthesis and storage) and paradoxically synthesize excess glucose and free fatty acids.
- Prompt recognition of and institution of treatment for severe alcoholic hepatitis will reduce mortality.

Questions

Question 1 relates to clinical vignette 1 at the beginning of this chapter.

1 What is the most likely diagnosis?
   A Acetaminophen-induced acute liver failure.
   B Acute viral hepatitis.
   C Budd–Chiari syndrome.

D Acute alcoholic hepatitis.

E Wilson disease.

Questions 2 and 3 relate to clinical vignette 2 earlier in this chapter.

2 Which of the following is the likely cause of the patient's elevated serum aminotransferase levels?
 A Primary biliary cholangitis.
 B NAFLD.
 C Alcoholic hepatitis.
 D Acute cholecystitis.
 E Drug-induced hepatotoxicity.

3 Which of the following would you recommend to this patient?
 A Lifestyle modification including a weight-loss program.
 B Cholecystectomy.
 C Discontinue simvastatin.
 D Oral cholestyramine.
 E Liver biopsy.

4 A patient with acute alcoholic hepatitis has a Maddrey Discriminant Function >32. Which of the following statements regarding treatment is true?
 A Pentoxifylline is superior to glucocorticoid therapy.
 B Prednisolone may improve 28-day mortality but carries an increased risk of infectious complications.
 C Pentoxifylline and prednisolone in combination provides a greater mortality benefit than either alone.
 D Total parenteral nutrition is preferred over enteral nutrition.
 E Liver transplantation is too risky in this patient.

5 Which of the following causes macrosteatosis?
 A Acute fatty liver of pregnancy.
 B Alcohol.
 C High-dose intravenous tetracycline.
 D Reye's syndrome.
 E Valproic acid.

Answers

1 **D**
 This case has many of the classic features of acute alcoholic hepatitis. The patient has an odor of alcohol on the breath, hypertension, tachycardia,

a moderate elevation of serum aminotransferase levels (with an AST: ALT ratio of over 2:1), a neutrophil-predominant leukocytosis, low-grade fever, hepatomegaly, decreased platelet count (which may be due to alcohol-induced bone marrow suppression), a mildly prolonged prothrombin time, and jaundice. Acetaminophen overdose and severe acute viral hepatitis usually present with serum aminotransferase levels above 1000 U l^{-1}, and do not generally present with deep jaundice until later in the course of disease. Acute viral hepatitis is associated with a lymphocyte-predominant leukocytosis. Wilson disease is a chronic liver disease that may present as acute liver failure in younger patients and is usually associated with a low serum ceruloplasmin level. Budd–Chiari syndrome may present as acute abdominal pain with hepatomegaly, ascites and, in some cases, liver failure. Imaging studies generally show hepatic vein thrombosis, and there is often a history of or risk factors for a hypercoagulable state.

2 B

This patient has metabolic syndrome and many of the classic features of NAFLD, and more specifically NASH. The serum ALT level is greater than the AST level, and abdominal ultrasonography shows bright echoes of fat within the liver. Primary biliary cholangitis causes a cholestatic pattern of liver biochemical tests and is typically associated with antimitochondrial antibodies. Although alcoholic liver disease and drug-induced liver injury cannot be entirely ruled out, the history, physical examination, and laboratory findings are more consistent with NAFLD. Gallstones are an incidental finding and commonly found in obese women. The patient has no clinical (e.g., right upper quadrant pain, fever) or imaging (thickened gallbladder wall with pericholecystic fluid) features of acute cholecystitis.

3 A

The mainstay of treatment for NAFLD is lifestyle modification (diet, exercise, weight loss) and control of risk factors such as hypertension, diabetes mellitus, and hyperlipidemia. Simvastatin should be continued to treat hypercholesterolemia. Cholecystectomy is not indicated for asymptomatic gallstones in this patient. Cholestyramine is a bile acid-binding agent and has no role in the management of NAFLD. Liver biopsy may be considered in the future but is not the next step in the management of this patient.

4 B

In patients with alcoholic hepatitis who have a high mortality rate as predicted by a Maddrey Discriminant Function >32, medical therapy can be considered. Glucocorticoids are contraindicated if the patient has a severe infection, such as sepsis, but they otherwise may improve short-term mortality. Combining pentoxifylline with glucocorticoids has shown no additional benefit to either drug alone, and pentoxifylline alone has shown no benefit. Nutritional support has been shown to improve long-term survival, but enteral, not parenteral, nutrition is the preferred method of feeding. There have been some reports of successful liver transplantation in patients with severe alcoholic hepatitis, but only in a highly select group of patients.

5 B

Alcohol is associated with predominantly macrovesicular steatosis. The other choices are associated with microvesicular steatosis, in which smaller fat droplets are seen on liver biopsy specimens. In general, microvesicular steatosis is more toxic to hepatocytes than macrovesicular steatosis.

Further Reading

Mathurin, P., Moreno, C., Samuel, D., *et al.* (2011) Early liver transplantation for severe alcoholic hepatitis. *New England Journal of Medicine*, **10**, 790–800.

O'Shea, R.S., Dasarathy, S., McCullough, A.J., *et al.* (2010) Alcoholic liver disease. Practice Guideline Committee of the American Association for the Study of Liver Diseases and the Practice Parameters Committee of the American College of Gastroenterology. *Hepatology*, **51**, 307–328.

Rinella, M.E. (2015) Nonalcoholic fatty liver disease: a systematic review. *Journal of the American Medical Association*, **313**, 2263–2273.

Sanyal, A.J., Chalasani, N., Kowdley, K.V., *et al.* (2010) Pioglitazone, vitamin E, or placebo for nonalcoholic steatohepatitis. *New England Journal of Medicine*, **362**, 1675–1685.

Thursz, M.R., Richardson, P., Allison, M., *et al.* (2015) Prednisolone or pentoxifylline for alcoholic hepatitis. *New England Journal of Medicine*, **23**, 1619–1628.

Wong, R.J., Aguilar, M., Cheung, R., *et al.* (2015) Nonalcoholic steatohepatitis is the second leading etiology of liver disease among adults awaiting liver transplantation in the United States. *Gastroenterology*, **148**, 547–555.

Weblinks

http://pubs.niaaa.nih.gov/publications/aa64/aa64.htm

http://www.acg.gi.org/physicians/guidelines/AlcoholicLiverDisease.pdf

http://www.aasld.org/practiceguidelines/Documents/Practice%20 Guidelines/ position_nonfattypg.pdf

http://www.aasld.org/sites/default/files/guideline_documents/ NonalcoholicFattyLiverDisease2012.pdf

http://www.digestive.niddk.nih.gov/ddiseases/pubs/nash/

15

Chronic Liver Disease

Preeti A. Reshamwala

Clinical Vignette

A 59-year-old woman is seen in the office for complaints of fatigue, increasing abdominal girth, pruritus, and diarrhea for the past 4 months. The pruritus is diffuse and is most bothersome at night. She has four to five watery stools each day that usually occur after a meal. She denies blood in the stool, rectal urgency, or tenesmus. She denies recent travel, sick contacts, antibiotic use, or recent hospitalization. Her husband notes that she is often forgetful and repetitive. She has a history of diabetes mellitus and hypertension, but currently takes no medications. She has no history of alcohol, tobacco, or illicit drug use. The family history is unremarkable. Physical examination reveals a blood pressure of 90/60 mmHg, pulse rate 98 per minute, and respiratory rate 16 per minute. She is afebrile, alert, and oriented, but with slow responses to questions. She has mild conjunctival icterus, bitemporal wasting, and multiple spider telangiectasias on the face and torso. A fluid wave, shifting dullness, and bulging flanks are noted on abdominal examination. She has 2+ lower-extremity pitting edema. Rectal examination shows scant brown stool that is negative for occult blood. Laboratory tests show a serum alkaline phosphatase level of 345 U l^{-1}, total bilirubin 3 mg dl^{-1}, alanine aminotransferase (ALT) 48 U l^{-1}, aspartate aminotransferase (AST) 65 U l^{-1}, and International Normalized Ratio (INR) 2.8. Abdominal ultrasonography shows a cirrhotic-appearing liver with normal intra- and extrahepatic bile ducts. Serologic tests are negative except for antimitochondrial antibodies (AMA).

Sitaraman and Friedman's Essentials of Gastroenterology, Second Edition.
Edited by Shanthi Srinivasan and Lawrence S. Friedman.
© 2018 John Wiley & Sons Ltd. Published 2018 by John Wiley & Sons Ltd.

General

- Chronic liver disease is a process of progressive destruction and regeneration of the liver parenchyma. Although multiple pathophysiologic mechanisms of injury exist (see later), the final common pathway is hepatic fibrosis that replaces damaged hepatocytes and that ultimately results in cirrhosis. Although the process may initially be reversible, the continued deposition of dense extracellular matrix can lead to irreversible end-stage liver disease and portal hypertension (see Chapter 16).
- Chronic liver disease may be caused by a number of conditions (Table 15.1). The most common causes of chronic liver disease worldwide are excessive alcohol intake (see Chapter 14), chronic hepatitis B and C (see Chapter 13), and nonalcoholic fatty liver disease (see Chapter 14).

Clinical Features

- Most patients with chronic liver disease are asymptomatic. When present, symptoms and signs depend on the etiology, degree of parenchymal damage, and presence of cirrhosis, which may be compensated or decompensated.

Table 15.1 Causes of chronic liver disease.

Viral	Autoimmune	Metabolic	Other pediatric	Miscellaneous
Hepatitis B	Autoimmune hepatitis	Alpha-1 antitrypsin deficiency	Biliary atresia	Alcoholic liver disease
Hepatitis C	Primary biliary cholangitis	Wilson disease	Alagille syndrome	Nonalcoholic fatty liver disease
Hepatitis D	Primary sclerosing cholangitis	Hemochromatosis	Congenital biliary cysts	Medications and toxins
		Disorders of amino acid metabolism (e.g., tyrosinemia)	Cystic fibrosis	Granulomatous liver disease (e.g., sarcoidosis)
		Disorders of carbohydrate metabolism (e.g., fructose intolerance, galactosemia, glycogen storage diseases)		Cryptogenic chronic liver disease/cirrhosis
		Disorders of lipid metabolism (e.g., abetalipoproteinemia)		
		Porphyria		
		Urea cycle enzyme defects (e.g., ornithine decarboxylase deficiency)		

- Patients with well-compensated cirrhosis may remain asymptomatic or can present with anorexia, weight loss, weakness, and fatigue. From 80–90% of the liver parenchyma must be destroyed before decompensated cirrhosis manifests clinically. Persons with decompensated cirrhosis may present with ascites, spontaneous bacterial peritonitis, hepatic encephalopathy, and variceal bleeding from portal hypertension (see Chapter 16).
- A thorough history is the first step in identifying the etiology of chronic liver disease. Risk factors that predispose patients to liver disease should be elicited; these include alcohol consumption, risk factors for hepatitis B and C transmission (e.g., birth in endemic areas, high-risk sexual behaviors, intravenous drug use, body piercing, tattooing, prior blood transfusions), and a personal or family history of liver, autoimmune, or metabolic diseases.

> Cirrhosis is an often irreversible and potentially fatal consequence of untreated chronic liver disease.

Diagnosis

- If liver disease is suspected, a complete blood count and comprehensive metabolic panel should be obtained. Further diagnostic work-up should be dictated by the pattern of elevated serum aminotransferase, alkaline phosphatase, and bilirubin levels, as outlined in Table 15.2 and in Chapters 12 and 24.

Autoimmune Hepatitis

- Autoimmune hepatitis (AIH) is a chronic inflammatory condition of the liver characterized by elevated serum autoantibodies, interface hepatitis (periportal inflammation) on histologic examination, and hypergammaglobulinemia.
- Women are more likely to be affected with AIH than men and often are diagnosed in the fifth to sixth decade of life.
- The pathogenesis of AIH is unknown. It is believed to involve a robust immune response to foreign or self antigen resulting in the destruction of hepatocytes by a combination of cell- and antibody-mediated cytotoxicity.
- AIH can present as a chronic smoldering disease, cirrhosis without prior documentation of AIH, or acute hepatitis (including acute liver failure).
- The elements of diagnosis of AIH include the following:
  - Elevated serum aminotransferase levels: serum aminotransferases may be as high as 10 or more times the upper limit of normal.
  - Hypergammaglobulinemia with an elevated serum immunoglobulin G level.
  - Circulating serum autoantibodies, which include antinuclear antibodies (ANA) and/or smooth muscle antibodies (SMA), or rarely (in the US) anti–liver-kidney microsomal antibodies (anti-LKM) type 1.

Table 15.2 Characteristic laboratory test and imaging abnormalities in common chronic liver diseases.

Disease	Abnormalities
Alcoholic liver disease	AST:ALT ratio ≥2; elevated serum GGTP level
Alpha-1 antitrypsin deficiency	Decreased serum alpha-1 antitrypsin level; gene test available
Autoimmune hepatitis	ANA and/or SMA, elevated IgG level
Chronic hepatitis B	HBsAg, HBeAg, HBV DNA
Chronic hepatitis C	HCV antibody, HCV RNA
Hereditary hemochromatosis	Transferrin saturation ≥45% or unsaturated iron-binding capacity ≥155 µg dl^{-1}; serum ferritin >200 ng ml^{-1} (women) and >300 ng ml^{-1} (men); *HFE* gene mutation
Nonalcoholic fatty liver disease	Elevated serum AST and/or ALT level; ultrasonography suggestive
Primary biliary cholangitis	Elevated serum ALP level, AMA
Primary sclerosing cholangitis	Abnormal MRCP and/or ERCP
Wilson disease	Serum ceruloplasmin <20 mg dl^{-1} (normal: 20–60 mg dl^{-1}) or low serum copper level (normal: 80–160 µg dl^{-1}); basal 24-hour urinary copper excretion >100 µg (normal: 10–80 µg); gene test available

ALP, alkaline phosphatase; ALT, alanine aminotransferase; AMA, antimitochondrial antibodies; ANA, antinuclear antibody; AST, aspartate aminotransferase; ERCP, endoscopic retrograde cholangiopancreatography; GGTP, gamma-glutamyl transpeptidase; HBeAg, hepatitis B e antigen; HBsAg, hepatitis B surface antigen; HCV, hepatitis C virus; MRCP, magnetic resonance cholangiopancreatography; SMA, smooth muscle antibodies.

- Interface hepatitis (inflammation of the portal tracts extending into the hepatic lobules) on histologic examination of the liver (Figure 15.1): the infiltrate is often predominantly plasmacytic. The bile ducts are generally spared from inflammatory destruction. There may be varying degrees of fibrosis depending on the chronicity of the condition.
- Exclusion of other causes of chronic liver disease, such as chronic hepatitis B, chronic hepatitis C, alcoholic liver disease, Wilson disease, and hemochromatosis.
- A slowly tapering course of prednisone is usually prescribed initially to decrease inflammation, and can be used in combination with azathioprine for maintenance therapy. Budesonide is an alternative glucocorticoid to prednisone in selected cases. Patients who present with acute liver failure may be treated with intravenous glucocorticoids.

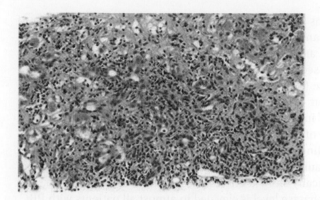

Figure 15.1 Photomicrograph of the liver in autoimmune hepatitis. Note severe interface hepatitis and an intense plasma cell infiltrate. Hematoxylin and eosin staining, original magnification × 10. Illustration courtesy of S. Sharma, MD, Emory University, Atlanta, GA, USA.

- Alternative treatment options for patients with severe side effects or intolerance to standard therapy include immunosuppressants such as mycophenolate mofetil, tacrolimus, and cyclosporine; these drugs often require monitoring of serum levels and are also associated with side effects.
- Liver transplantation is an effective treatment and may be considered in patients with decompensated cirrhosis or acute liver failure due to AIH.

> Characteristic features of AIH include elevated serum aminotransferases levels, elevated serum IgG levels, serum autoantibodies, and interface hepatitis with plasma cells on histologic examination of the liver.

Primary Biliary Cholangitis

- Primary biliary cholangitis (PBC, formerly primary biliary cirrhosis) is an autoimmune disorder characterized by granulomatous destruction of small intrahepatic bile ducts with resulting chronic cholestasis and cirrhosis in up to one-third of patients.
- The disease affects women and men in a ratio of 9 : 1.
- The pathogenesis of PBC is unknown. Over 95% of patients with PBC have detectable antimitochondrial antibodies (AMA). AMA target a family of enzymes, including the pyruvate dehydrogenase complex, that are found on the inner membrane of mitochondria.

- A majority of persons with PBC are asymptomatic. Typical symptoms of PBC include fatigue and pruritus. Other symptoms include jaundice, right upper quadrant pain, and anorexia.
- Patients are at increased risk for fat-soluble vitamin deficiency (vitamins A, D, E, K), bone disease (hepatic osteodystrophy), and hypercholesterolemia. Steatorrhea can occur in the late stages of PBC. These clinical problems develop as a result of impaired enterohepatic circulation of bile salts, which are deficient because of chronic cholestasis (see Chapter 20).
- Other physical findings may include xanthomas, xanthelasma, spider telangiectasias, and jaundice.
- Laboratory tests typically show a cholestatic picture (see Chapter 20). The serum alkaline phosphatase level is elevated in almost all patients with PBC. The bilirubin level is normal in early stages of the disease and may increase as the disease progresses. Serum aminotransferase levels are mildly elevated; levels more than fivefold the upper limit of normal should raise suspicion of other diseases, or of a PBC–AIH 'overlap' syndrome.
- Other serologic markers, including ANA, SMA, rheumatoid factor, and antithyroid antibodies, may be detected in up to 50% of patients with PBC.
- An important characteristic histopathologic finding is granulomatous biliary injury, also called the florid duct lesion (see Chapter 28). Florid duct lesions are seen in only a small number of patients. 'Ductopenia,' defined as a reduced number of bile ducts in >50% of portal tracts visualized under high-power microscopy, is seen in more advanced stages of PBC.
- Treatment generally includes ursodeoxycholic acid, a fat-soluble bile acid (see Chapter 20), which has been shown to delay both histologic progression of the disease and the time to liver transplantation. Obeticholic acid, a derivative of chenodeoxycholic acid, may be effective in reducing alkaline phosphatase in patients who do not have an adequate response to ursodeoxycholic acid, but it can cause pruritus in some patients.
- The prognosis of PBC has improved greatly since the 1990s due to diagnosis at earlier stages and widespread treatment with ursodeoxycholic acid.

Due to impaired enterohepatic circulation, patients with advanced PBC are at increased risk of fat-soluble vitamin deficiency (vitamins A, D, E, K), bone disease (hepatic osteodystrophy), and hypercholesterolemia with a predominant elevation of plasma high-density lipoprotein (HDL) levels. Patients are generally not at increased risk of cardiovascular disease; therefore, treatment of hypercholesterolemia in patients with PBC is usually not necessary. Patients with PBC should be screened regularly for osteoporosis by dual-energy X-ray absorptiometry (DEXA) scan.

Primary Sclerosing Cholangitis

- Primary sclerosing cholangitis (PSC) is a chronic inflammatory condition of the intra- and extrahepatic bile ducts resulting in strictures (or narrowing) of the biliary tract and consequent cholestasis.
- PSC is primarily a disease of large ducts, in contrast to PBC, which is primarily a disease of the bile ductules in the portal tracts.
- Symptoms can be vague and may include right upper quadrant pain, pruritus, and weight loss.
- Patients with PSC are at risk of bacterial cholangitis due to biliary stasis and bacterial overgrowth. Acute cholangitis, a suppurative infection of the bile duct, is a medical emergency and should be treated in consultation with a gastrointestinal endoscopist (see Chapter 21).
- Up to 90% of patients with PSC also have concomitant inflammatory bowel disease, usually ulcerative colitis.
- No specific autoantibody is diagnostic of PSC. The diagnosis of PSC is made when patients have a cholestatic pattern of liver biochemical test abnormalities (elevated serum alkaline phosphatase and bilirubin levels disproportionate to the serum aminotransferase levels) and a cholangiogram that shows characteristic biliary strictures alternating with areas of dilatation. Typically, the bile ducts appear 'beaded' and the radicles are pruned or truncated on a cholangiogram (Figure 15.2).
- Magnetic resonance cholangiopancreatography (MRCP) is the preferred diagnostic test (Figure 15.2), with a high sensitivity and specificity. Endoscopic

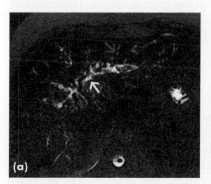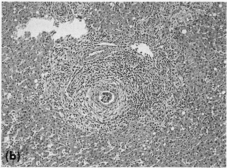

Figure 15.2 Primary sclerosing cholangitis. (a) Magnetic resonance cholangiopancreatography showing irregular appearance of the intrahepatic ducts with areas of dilatation (white arrow) and small strictured ducts (red arrow). Illustration courtesy of D. Martin, MD, Emory University, Atlanta, GA, USA; (b) Liver biopsy specimen showing the typical 'onion skin' appearance of periductular fibrosis. Hematoxylin and eosin staining, original magnification × 20. Illustration courtesy of S. Sharma, MD, Emory University, Atlanta, GA, USA.

retrograde cholangiopancreatography (ERCP) is often deferred due to the risk of procedure-related complications such as pancreatitis, but it can be used as a therapeutic procedure to dilate and place a stent across a significant (dominant) bile duct stricture to permit drainage of bile, decrease the risk of acute cholangitis, and reduce morbidity.

- A liver biopsy is not required to make a diagnosis of PSC. The typical finding on histologic examination of the liver is onion-skin fibrosis surrounding a bile duct. About 10% of patients have onion-skin fibrosis of only small intrahepatic bile ductules with no abnormalities on cholangiography, a condition often referred to as 'small-duct PSC', which appears to have a better prognosis than PSC associated with strictures involving the extrahepatic bile duct.

- No effective medical therapy exists for PSC; management is aimed at treating the symptoms and monitoring the patient for acute cholangitis. Like PBC, PSC is also a cholestatic liver disease and can result in fat-soluble vitamin deficiency and osteodystrophy. Ursodeoxycholic acid does not appear to affect the course of PSC, but is often prescribed.

- Liver transplantation is an effective treatment and should be considered in patients with advanced PSC.

- A dominant stricture in the bile duct or the major hepatic ducts should raise concern for cholangiocarcinoma, for which patients with PSC may have a 10% lifetime risk.

Hemochromatosis

- Hereditary hemochromatosis (HH) comprises several inherited disorders of iron homeostasis characterized by increased intestinal absorption of iron that results in the deposition of iron in the liver, pancreas, heart, and other organs.

- HH is the most common genetic abnormality in Caucasians, with a gene carrier frequency of approximately 1 in 200 persons. HFE-related HH is an autosomal recessive disorder most common in persons of northern European ancestry. Most patients with HH are homozygous for the C282Y mutation of the *HFE* gene. Some patients are compound heterozygotes (C282Y/H63D).

- Causes of secondary iron overload include iron-overload anemias (e.g., aplastic anemia, thalassemia major, sideroblastic anemia), parenteral iron overload (e.g., red cell transfusions, hemodialysis), and chronic liver diseases (e.g., alcoholic liver disease, chronic hepatitis B and C, nonalcoholic steatohepatitis).

- The pathophysiologic mechanisms leading to iron overload in HH are not fully understood. Increased intestinal absorption of dietary iron, decreased expression of the iron-regulatory hormone hepcidin, altered function of the HFE protein, and iron-induced tissue injury and fibrogenesis have been implicated. The predominant mechanism is thought to be related to dysregulated expression of hepcidin by the mutated HFE protein. Hepcidin is a hormone synthesized by the liver that regulates iron absorption from enterocytes.

- Most persons with HH remain asymptomatic. When present, symptoms include weakness and lethargy, arthralgias, abdominal pain, and loss of libido or potency in men. In symptomatic patients, hepatomegaly is a common finding on examination. Although rare now, a pathognomonic finding on physical examination includes bronzed or slate-gray skin pigmentation. Other signs of chronic liver disease such as splenomegaly, ascites, jaundice, and peripheral edema may be present. Diabetes mellitus usually occurs in patients who have developed cirrhosis.
- Other clinical manifestations include cardiomyopathy, arrhythmias, heart failure, and a characteristic arthropathy that involves the second and third metacarpophalangeal joints.
- The diagnosis of HH should be considered in any patient with typical symptoms, a positive family history, or (most commonly) abnormal screening iron test results. Measurements of the serum iron level and total iron-binding capacity or transferrin, with calculation of the transferrin saturation (TS), and a serum ferritin level should be obtained.
- The diagnosis of HH is based on identification of increased iron stores with elevated serum ferritin levels and TS. If the TS is >45% in women and >50% in men, the serum ferritin level is elevated, or an unsaturated iron-binding capacity $\geq 155 \mu g \, dl^{-1}$, genetic testing should be considered.
- Siblings of persons who are homozygous for the C282Y mutation or a compound heterozygote (C282Y/H63D) should undergo genetic screening for the *HFE* mutation.
- A liver biopsy is indicated for histopathologic evaluation (see Chapter 28) and quantification of hepatic iron content in affected patients with a serum ferritin >1000 ng ml^{-1} or elevated serum aminotransferase levels.
- Imaging of the liver can reveal hepatomegaly or evidence of cirrhosis, and magnetic resonance imaging (MRI) may detect hepatic iron overload (but is not yet sensitive enough to be used as a screening test).
- Patients with HH are treated with phlebotomy, initially 1 unit and occasionally 2 units weekly, to deplete iron stores in the body. The goal is to achieve a serum ferritin level of 50–100 ng ml^{-1} and a TS <50%. Then, maintenance phlebotomies, one unit three or four times a year, are continued. Iron desaturation in a patient who does not have cirrhosis will prevent progression to cirrhosis. Each unit of blood removed contains 250 mg of iron; many patients with genetic HH have a hepatic iron burden of 50 g.
- Intravenous chelation therapy with desferoxamine may be offered to patients who do not tolerate phlebotomy.
- For patients who develop cirrhosis as a consequence of HH, liver transplantation can be considered.

Up to 30% of patients with cirrhosis due to HH develop hepatocellular carcinoma (HCC). Screening for HCC with imaging of the liver every 6 months is recommended in these patients.

Wilson disease

- Wilson disease (WD) is a chronic hepatic and neurologic condition that results from excessive copper deposition.
- WD is an autosomal recessive disorder. The genetic defect is a mutation in the *ATP7B* (also called Wilson adenosine triphosphatase, [ATPase]) gene. *ATP7B* is expressed predominantly in hepatocytes, the placenta, and the kidney. The gene encodes a P-type (cation transport enzyme) ATPase that transports copper into bile. Mutations lead to the accumulation of copper within hepatocytes, thereby causing oxidative damage.
- WD commonly presents in persons under age 40. Patients may present with chronic or fulminant liver disease, a progressive neurologic disorder without clinically prominent hepatic dysfunction, or acute hemolysis. A neurologic presentation occurs in the third or fourth decade of life, and symptoms may include depression, tremor, movement disorders, dystonia, and even psychosis. The classic Kayser–Fleischer ring is caused by copper deposition in Descemet's membrane of the cornea. A careful slit-lamp examination is mandatory in patients with suspected WD. Sunflower cataracts may be seen in some patients with WD.
- Genetic testing is expensive and often unavailable; therefore, patients with unexplained liver disease and a low or low–normal ceruloplasmin level should have a 24-hour urine collection to detect elevated copper concentrations and a slit-lamp examination for Kayser–Fleischer rings.
- Liver biopsy for histology (see Chapter 28) and copper quantification is generally performed. A hepatic copper concentration $>250\,\mu g\,g^{-1}$ liver is typical of Wilson disease; a concentration $\leq 40\,\mu g\,g^{-1}$ excludes the diagnosis.
- Copper chelation with D-penicillamine or trientine is an effective treatment for WD. Oral zinc may be considered in asymptomatic or pregnant patients or as maintenance therapy. If treatment is initiated early, most patients live a normal healthy life.
- Liver transplantation, when indicated, is curative.

Alpha-1 Antitrypsin Deficiency

- Alpha-1 antitrypsin deficiency (A1ATD) is the second most common metabolic disease affecting the liver. It is an autosomal recessive disorder that predominantly affects the liver and the lung.

- Alpha-1 antitrypsin (A1AT) is a protease inhibitor that promotes the degradation of serine proteases in the serum and tissues. Neutrophil elastase is one of the most important serine proteases that is inhibited by A1AT. A1ATD is a consequence of a mutation in the *SERPINA1* gene that results in deficiency of the protein product, thereby leading to uninhibited neutrophil elastase activity and the development of pulmonary emphysema in affected patients.
- Emphysema occurs due to the destruction of normal lung tissue. Precocious emphysema is often a clue to the diagnosis. With the most common phenotype (ZZ), liver disease occurs as a result of the inability of the abnormal protein to be secreted from the endoplasmic reticulum and Golgi, because the protein is misfolded and has an abnormal tertiary structure; it accumulates in the hepatocytes and results in hepatocyte destruction, which may lead to cirrhosis.
- A liver biopsy specimen in a patient with A1ATD can be stained with a periodic acid-Schiff (PAS) stain to demonstrate the excess abnormal proteins (see Chapter 28).
- A1ATD can be diagnosed in the neonatal period or can manifest later in life with jaundice, liver dysfunction, or cirrhosis.
- The diagnosis is based on a decreased serum level of A1AT and phenotype testing for the genetic defect; the A1AT level alone is not sufficient to confirm the diagnosis.
- Treatment of A1ATD liver disease is aimed at management of portal hypertension and complications associated with end-stage liver disease. A1AT replacement therapy does not improve the liver disease.
- Liver transplantation is curative because the donor liver will synthesize normal A1AT protein.

Vascular Disorders of the Liver

Portal Vein Thrombosis

- Portal vein thrombosis (PVT) is the most common vascular disorder of the liver. It occurs most commonly in patients with cirrhosis and results from sluggish portal blood flow and a possible prothrombotic state associated with cirrhosis. PVT is not a cause of cirrhosis *per se*.
- PVT can also occur in noncirrhotic patients with malignancy, infection, trauma, or a hereditary prothrombotic state (e.g., factor V Leiden mutation, prothrombin 20210A mutation, deficiencies of protein C, protein S, or antithrombin, sickle cell disease, hyperhomocysteinemia).
- Acute PVT can present with severe abdominal pain and fever, and occasionally with possibly bloody diarrhea. With extensive thrombosis, intestinal ischemia and infarction can ensue.
- Chronic PVT may result in cavernous transformation of the portal vein (portal cavernoma).
- Doppler ultrasonography, computed tomography, or MRI may reveal PVT.

- Most patients with acute PVT can be treated with anticoagulation to restore blood flow.
- Anticoagulation for chronic PVT is generally not recommended.

Budd–Chiari Syndrome

- Budd–Chiari syndrome (BCS) refers to hepatic venous outflow tract obstruction. BCS can result from thrombosis or other secondary causes of outflow obstruction. Chronic BCS can result in cirrhosis.
- BCS can present with acute abdominal pain, ascites, and hepatomegaly; often it is associated with a prothrombotic state.
- Investigation for underlying malignancy or a prothrombotic state (e.g., a myeloproliferative disorder associated with the V617F mutation of the *JAK2* gene, factor V Leiden mutation, prothrombin 20210A mutation, deficiencies of protein C, protein S, or antithrombin, sickle cell disease, hyperhomocysteinemia) should be performed.
- MRI or venography is generally diagnostic (Figure 15.3).
- The clinical features are similar to those for sinusoidal obstruction syndrome (veno-occlusive disease).

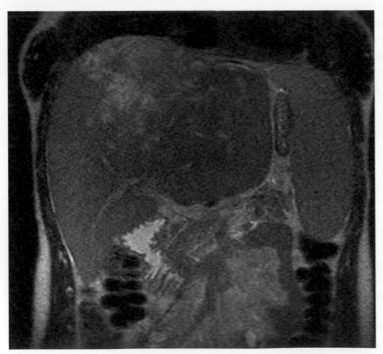

Figure 15.3 Magnetic resonance imaging in a patient with Budd–Chiari syndrome. A characteristic spider-web pattern of venous collaterals is seen at the dome of the liver. Illustration courtesy of B. Kalb, MD, Emory University, Atlanta, GA, USA.

- Anticoagulation therapy should be considered in patients with BCS, especially in patients who present acutely.
- A transjugular intrahepatic portosystemic shunt (TIPS) is indicated in patients with portal hypertension, and liver transplantation can be considered for those patients with progressive symptoms and evidence of liver failure or when TIPS is ineffective.

Pearls

- Chronic liver disease may be caused by a number of conditions. Multiple pathophysiologic mechanisms of injury exist, but the final common pathway is hepatic parenchymal fibrosis and cirrhosis.
- A thorough history and physical examination can often narrow down the potential etiology of chronic liver disease.
- A variety of biochemical and serologic tests can aid in the determination of the cause of chronic liver disease.
- Abdominal ultrasonography is a noninvasive, fast, and cost-effective test that should be used for first-line imaging of the liver; however, it is insensitive for detecting cirrhosis.
- Liver transplantation can be offered as a final therapeutic option for patients who have progressed to liver failure due to chronic liver disease.
- Screening for hepatocellular carcinoma should be performed for all patients who have chronic liver disease with advanced fibrosis.

Questions

Questions 1 and 2 relate to the clinical vignette at the beginning of this chapter.

1 Which of the following is the most likely diagnosis?
   A Autoimmune hepatitis.
   B Primary biliary cholangitis (PBC).
   C Heart failure.
   D Chronic hepatitis C.
   E Drug-induced liver injury.

2 The patient asks you about potential implications of her diagnosis to her overall health. You inform her that she is at risk for which of the following?
   A Fat-soluble vitamin deficiencies.
   B Osteoporosis.
   C Hypercholesterolemia.
   D Hepatocellular carcinoma.
   E All of the above.

3   A 21-year-old man presents for evaluation of jaundice and pruritus that has been worsening over the previous 8 weeks. He has ulcerative colitis that is being treated with mesalamine, and is in remission. He denies abdominal pain, fever, chills, or weight loss. He does not drink alcohol, smoke cigarettes, or use illicit drugs. Physical examination shows jaundice. Laboratory tests show a serum alkaline phosphatase level of 693 U l^{-1}, total bilirubin 7 mg dl^{-1}, ALT 65 U l^{-1}, and AST 83 U l^{-1}. Serologic tests for viral hepatitis, antimitochondrial antibodies, smooth muscle antibodies, and antinuclear antibodies are negative. Serum ceruloplasmin and alpha-1 antitrypsin levels are normal. Ultrasonography of the abdomen shows mildly dilated intra- and extrahepatic bile ducts. Magnetic resonance cholangiopancreatography (MRCP) shows a beaded pattern with multiple biliary strictures and focal areas of ductal dilatation proximal to the strictures. A long 'dominant' stricture is noted in the mid bile duct. The most likely diagnosis is which of the following?

A   Autoimmune hepatitis.

B   Primary biliary cholangitis.

C   Viral hepatitis.

D   Nonalcoholic fatty liver disease.

E   Primary sclerosing cholangitis (PSC).

4   A 16-year-old girl presents to the emergency department with obtundation. There is no history of drug or alcohol use. Her parents note that she has become increasingly withdrawn at home and school; there is no report of suicide attempts. Physical examination reveals an unresponsive young woman with conjunctival icterus. Laboratory evaluation is remarkable for a hemoglobin level of 9 g dl^{-1} (normal 20–50 mg dl^{-1}), International Normalized Ratio 3.8, total bilirubin 11.6 mg dl^{-1} with an indirect fraction at 9 mg dl^{-1}, and ceruloplasmin 8 mg dl^{-1}. A toxicology screen is negative. Which of the following should be the next step in management this patient?

A   24-hour urine copper measurement.

B   Administer intravenous glucocorticoids.

C   Immediate transfer to a liver transplant center.

D   Urgent phlebotomy.

E   Begin copper chelation therapy.

5   A 55-year-old woman with Graves' disease is evaluated in the office for a persistently elevated serum alkaline phosphatase level. Physical examination is unremarkable except for shiny deposits over her eyelids. Laboratory testing reveals a serum alkaline phosphatase level of 355 U l^{-1}, ALT 35 U l^{-1}, AST 25 U l^{-1}, and total cholesterol 500 mg dl^{-1}. Other tests including complete blood count, prothrombin time, platelet count, serum electrolytes, serum creatinine, and total bilirubin are within normal limits. Ultrasonography of the abdomen is unremarkable. Which of the following is the next best test to identify the cause of the elevated serum alkaline phosphatase level?

A Liver biopsy.

B Antineutrophil cytoplasmic antibodies (ANCA).

C Magnetic resonance cholangiopancreatography (MRCP).

D Antimitochondrial antibodies (AMA).

E Serum immunoglobulins.

6 A 45-year-old man is referred for evaluation of increased abdominal girth. He has chronic shortness of breath and has been started on two inhalers to help with his symptoms. He has no history of tobacco, drug, or alcohol use. His father died at an early age from emphysema, and was also a lifelong nonsmoker. Physical examination shows a thin man with expiratory wheezes on lung examination, shifting dullness of the abdomen, and spider telangiectasias. Laboratory evaluation reveals a serum ALT of 88 U l^{-1}, AST 65 U l^{-1}, ALP 138 U l^{-1}, and total bilirubin of 2 mg dl^{-1}. A hepatitis C antibody is negative. Abdominal ultrasonography reveals a shrunken nodular appearing liver with moderate ascites in the abdomen. Which of the following tests will help confirm the cause of this patient's liver disease?

A Hepatitis C viral RNA.

B Magnetic resonance cholangiopancreatography (MRCP).

C Alpha-1 antitrypsin level and genotype.

D Urine alcohol screen.

E Serum ferritin level.

Answers

1 B

The most likely diagnosis is PBC, as evidenced by the patient's clinical presentation with fatigue and pruritus (and symptoms of advanced liver disease), cholestatic liver biochemical test pattern (elevated serum alkaline phosphatase and bilirubin levels disproportionate to the serum aminotransferases), and antimitochondrial antibodies.

2 E

Patients with PBC are at increased risk for fat-soluble vitamin deficiencies (vitamins A, D, E, K), bone disease (hepatic osteodystrophy), and hypercholesterolemia due to impaired enterohepatic circulation. In addition, they are at increased risk of developing hepatocellular carcinoma.

3 E

This is a classic presentation of PSC. PSC is a chronic inflammatory condition of the intra- and extrahepatic bile ducts resulting in strictures (or narrowings) of the biliary tract, with resulting cholestasis. The diagnosis of PSC is made when patients have a cholestatic pattern of liver biochemical test abnormalities and cholangiography reveals biliary strictures and intervening areas of dilatation. Up to 90% of patients with PSC also have inflammatory bowel disease. The clinical picture does not fit the other choices.

4 C

This patient has acute Wilson disease and should be referred immediately to a liver transplant center. This is a classic presentation in a young patient with altered mentation preceded by neurocognitive changes (depression and withdrawal) that is seen when copper is deposited in the central nervous system. She also has evidence of hemolytic anemia (elevated indirect hyperbilirubinemia) and a low serum ceruloplasmin level. Slit-lamp examination may reveal Kayser–Fleisher rings or rarely sunflower cataracts. Liver transplantation is curative.

5 D

The next step in the evaluation of this middle-aged woman with evidence of cholestatic liver disease should be a serum AMA. AMA are present in 95% of patients with PBC. Additionally, total cholesterol levels are often elevated in patients with cholestatic liver disease due to impaired enterohepatic circulation. The patient has thyroid disease, which is prevalent in patients with PBC. ANCA and serum immunoglobulins are not useful in the diagnosis of PBC. MRCP would be considered if there were evidence of extrahepatic biliary obstruction, but ultrasonography is normal.

6 C

This patient has evidence of early chronic obstructive pulmonary disease (COPD) and a family history of COPD. He has no history of drug or alcohol use. Given the lung findings in a young patient with a family history of precocious COPD, alpha-1 antitrypsin deficiency should be considered. The serum A1AT level will be low, and genetic testing can confirm the presence of common gene mutations.

Further Reading

Gatselis, N.K. and Dalekos, G.N. (2016) Molecular diagnostic testing for primary biliary cholangitis. *Expert Review of Molecular Diagnostics*, **16**, 1001–1610.

Larson, A.M. (2014) *Diagnosis and Management of Chronic Liver Diseases, Medical Clinics of North America*, Volume **98**, No. 1 (ed. A.M. Larson), Elsevier, Philadelphia.

Leonis, M.A. and Balistreri, W.F. (2016) Other inherited metabolic disorders of the liver, in *Sleisenger and Fordtran's Gastrointestinal and Liver Disease: Pathophysiology/Diagnosis/Management*, 10th edition (eds M. Feldman, L.S. Friedman, and L.J. Brandt), Saunders Elsevier, Philadelphia, pp. 1280–1301.

Pinto, R.B., Schneider, A.C., and da Silveira, T.R. (2015) Cirrhosis in children and adolescents, an overview. *World Journal of Hepatology*, **3**, 392–405.

van Bokhoven, M.A., van Deursen, C.T., and Swinkels, D.W. (2011) Diagnosis and management of hereditary haemochromatosis. *British Medical Journal*, **342**, c7251.

Weblinks

http://digestive.niddk.nih.gov/ddiseases/pubs/cirrhosis/
http://www.aafp.org/afp/2006/0901/p756.html

16

Portal Hypertension

JP Norvell

Clinical Vignette

A 58-year-old man presents to the emergency department with a 2-month history of increasing abdominal girth and diffuse abdominal pain, fatigue, lower extremity edema, and fever for the past week. He denies confusion, diarrhea, melena, hematemesis, or rectal bleeding. Physical examination reveals a blood pressure of 90/50 mmHg, pulse rate 106 per minute, respiratory rate 18 per minute, and temperature of 101.5 °F (38.5 °C). Conjunctival icterus is present. Abdominal examination reveals a tense abdomen with a fluid wave and shifting dullness. The abdomen is diffusely tender to palpation. Normal bowel sounds are present. The liver edge is not palpable. Laboratory tests are significant for a serum sodium 125 mmol l^{-1}, creatinine 1.8 mg dl^{-1}, aspartate aminotransferase 68 U l^{-1}, alanine aminotransferase 58 U l^{-1}, total bilirubin 6.8 mg dl^{-1}, platelet count 80 000 mm^{-3}, white blood cell (WBC) count 14 000 mm^{-3}, hemoglobin 10.2 g dl^{-1}, hematocrit 33%, and International Normalized Ratio (INR) 1.7.

Definition

- Portal hypertension can result from increased resistance in the portal venous system or increased portal blood flow.
- When caused by hepatic sinusoidal damage from liver disease, portal hypertension is defined as an increase in the pressure gradient between the portal vein and hepatic vein as measured by the hepatic venous pressure gradient (HVPG).
- Portal hypertension is a key consequence of cirrhosis and can result in a number of life-threatening complications.

Sitaraman and Friedman's Essentials of Gastroenterology, Second Edition.
Edited by Shanthi Srinivasan and Lawrence S. Friedman.
© 2018 John Wiley & Sons Ltd. Published 2018 by John Wiley & Sons Ltd.

Pathophysiology

Normal Portal Circulation

- The portal venous system delivers blood directly to the liver from the organs involved in nutrient digestion, including the esophagus, stomach, pancreas, small and large intestine, and spleen. The portal vein is formed by the confluence of the splenic vein and the superior mesenteric vein (see also Chapter 11).
- The portal venous system is normally a high-compliance, low-resistance system that has the ability to accommodate high blood-flow volumes, as occurs after a meal, without increasing portal venous pressure.
- The hepatic artery converges with the portal vein to flow into the hepatic sinusoids, thus providing a dual blood supply to the liver, and constitutes nearly 30% of the total cardiac output.

Hemodynamic Changes that Lead to Portal Hypertension

- Portal hypertension results from an increase in portal resistance (R) and/or portal blood flow (F), and can be represented by Ohm's law, $\Delta P = F \times R$, where ΔP represents the pressure gradient across the portal circulation, F is a function of blood flow, and R is resistance to portal blood flow.
- In cirrhosis, portal hypertension and its complications are a key consequence of the synergistic effect of intrahepatic (sinusoidal) resistance to portal blood flow and increased portal blood flow from the splanchnic circulation:
  - **Intrahepatic resistance**: the resistance to portal flow consists of both fixed and functional components.
    - The fixed component results in distortion of the intrahepatic microcirculation by sinusoidal fibrosis and compression by regenerative nodules.
    - The functional, or dynamic, component is intrahepatic vasoconstriction and is thought to be due to contraction of activated hepatic stellate cells and myofibroblasts. There is increased production of vasoconstrictors such as endothelins and reduced intrahepatic production of the vasodilator nitric oxide (NO), resulting in enhanced intrahepatic vasoconstriction.
  - **Increased portal blood flow**: Increases in portal pressures trigger endothelial nitric oxide synthase (eNOS) expression and subsequent overproduction of NO in splanchnic endothelial cells. This leads to progressive splanchnic vasodilatation and increased portal inflow.
- Portal hypertension leads to a hyperdynamic circulatory syndrome characterized by decreased systemic vascular resistance (SVR), decreased mean arterial pressure (MAP), and increased cardiac index (CI).
- The reduction in pressure detected at the carotid and renal baroreceptors induced by cirrhotic vasodilatation activates sodium-retaining

neurohormonal mechanisms in an attempt to restore perfusion. This leads to the activation of the renin–angiotensin–aldosterone axis, as well as increased levels of norephinephrine and antidiuretic hormone (ADH). These hormones are activated to cause an increase in effective arterial blood volume via avid renal reabsorption of sodium and increased afferent arteriolar resistance in the nephron. These are important steps that can lead to complications of portal hypertension such as ascites and hepatorenal syndrome.

- Portosystemic collateral vessels develop to decompress the increased portal pressure and can lead to potentially fatal complications such as hemorrhage from gastroesophageal varices.

Classification and Causes of Portal Hypertension

- In North America and Europe the most common cause of portal hypertension is **cirrhosis**. Other common causes of portal hypertension worldwide include extrahepatic portal vein thrombosis and schistosomiasis (the deposition of eggs in presinusoidal portal venules causes presinusoidal fibrosis).
- Classification of portal hypertension is based on the site of increased resistance (Table 16.1).

Measurement of Portal Pressure

- The HVPG is a measurement of portal pressure, and is an independent predictor of variceal hemorrhage and death.
- Measurement of the HVPG via a transjugular or femoral approach is the most commonly used method to measure portal pressure.
- The HVPG is obtained by first measuring the wedged hepatic venous pressure (WHVP). A balloon catheter is wedged into a branch of the hepatic vein and then inflated, thereby occluding the vessel; this provides an

Table 16.1 Classification of portal hypertension.

Site of resistance	Causes
Prehepatic	Portal vein thrombosis
Hepatic	
Presinusoidal	Schistosomiasis, early primary biliary cholangitis
Sinusoidal	Alcoholic cirrhosis, alcoholic hepatitis
Postsinusoidal	Sinusoidal obstruction syndrome
Posthepatic	Budd–Chiari syndrome, constrictive pericarditis

estimation of the sinusoidal pressure. The pressure reading obtained (WHVP) must be corrected for increases in abdominal pressure (such as ascites) by subtracting the free hepatic vein pressure (FHVP). The difference in pressures (WHVP – FHVP) represents the HVPG.

- The normal range of HVPG is 3–5 mmHg. HVPG ≥6 mmHg defines sinusoidal portal hypertension.
- Elevated HVPG levels (above 10–12 mmHg) are predictive of the development of complications of portal hypertension.

- Measurement of the HVPG is only valid for sinusoidal and postsinusoidal causes of portal hypertension. For example, portal hypertension caused by extrahepatic portal vein thrombosis is not reflected in an increased HVPG.

Variceal Hemorrhage

- Gastroesophageal varices are present in approximately 50% of patients with cirrhosis, and their presence corresponds with the severity of liver disease.
- Aggressive and early management of cirrhotic patients presenting with suspected variceal hemorrhage is critical, given mortality rates of 15–20%.

Pathophysiology

- Portosystemic collateral vessels develop to decompress the increased portal pressure, either by opening pre-existing vessels or by angiogenesis. Additionally, in pre-existing low-flow collaterals, blood flow may reverse so that the direction is out of the portal circulation toward the systemic venous circulation. Although it usually is an ineffective means to decompress the portal vein, collateral formation can lead to potentially fatal complications such as hemorrhage from varices in the esophagus or stomach.
- Variceal wall tension is the primary factor determining the risk of variceal hemorrhage and correlates with the vessel diameter and the pressure within the vessel. Esophageal varices may hemorrhage when the HVPG is ≥12 mmHg.

Clinical and Laboratory Features

- Patients with variceal bleeding present most commonly with large-volume hematemesis and/or melena. Varices should be considered as a possible etiology for gastrointestinal hemorrhage in a patient with stigmata of chronic liver disease (i.e., jaundice, ascites, splenomegaly).
- Variceal hemorrhage is commonly associated with hypovolemic shock.
- In addition to anemia, laboratory studies are usually consistent with chronic liver disease and portal hypertension, as reflected by a prolonged prothrombin time, thrombocytopenia, and hypoalbuminemia.

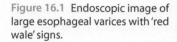

Figure 16.1 Endoscopic image of large esophageal varices with 'red wale' signs.

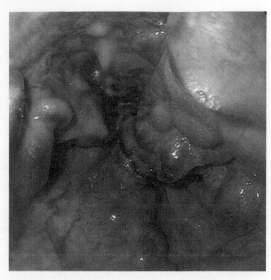

Diagnosis

- The diagnosis of esophageal and gastric varices is made by esophagogastroduodenoscopy (EGD). EGD will reveal esophageal or gastric varices and identify active bleeding and/or stigmata of a high risk for hemorrhage. Such stigmata include pigmented spots (cherry red spots) and 'red wale' signs (longitudinal red streaks) on a varix (see Figure 16.1).
- All patients diagnosed with cirrhosis should undergo variceal screening by EGD to assess for the presence of varices and to predict the risk of bleeding based on variceal size and the presence of stigmata that suggest a high risk for bleeding.

> Portal hypertension should be suspected in all patients with gastrointestinal bleeding and peripheral stigmata of liver disease (e.g., jaundice, ascites, splenomegaly, spider angiomas, and encephalopathy).

Treatment

- Patients with **acute variceal bleeding** should be admitted to an intensive care unit and should be stabilized hemodynamically (see Chapter 22). Transfusion of red blood cells with goal of achieving a hemoglobin concentration of $7-9\,g\,dl^{-1}$, thus avoiding overtransfusion, which can increase the HVPG and the risk of further bleeding.
  - **Pharmacologic therapy**:
    - Octreotide (a somatostatin analog), which causes splanchnic vasoconstriction and reduces portal blood flow, is a beneficial adjunct to endoscopic therapy (see below) in achieving hemostasis.

- o Administration of an antibiotic reduces the risk of bacterial infections including spontaneous bacterial peritonitis (see later). Ceftriaxone or a fluoroquinolone is recommended for 5–7 days.
- **Endoscopic therapy**:
  - o Emergent EGD should be performed as soon as the patient is hemodynamically stable, preferably within 12 hours of hospital admission.
  - o Once esophageal varices are identified as the bleeding source, the preferred endoscopic therapeutic modality is endoscopic variceal ligation (EVL), in which a varix is suctioned into a cap on the tip of the endoscope and a rubber band is applied around the varix to strangulate it, thereby causing thrombosis of the varix.
- **Balloon tamponade**:
  - o When EVL is not successful in achieving hemostasis, balloon tamponade is an effective way to achieve short-term hemostasis until more definitive therapy can be applied.
  - o A tube (i.e., Sengstaken–Blakemore tube) with gastric and esophageal balloons is inserted through the mouth into the esophagus with subsequent inflation of the gastric balloon and esophageal balloon sequentially to tamponade the varices.
  - o This procedure is associated with substantial morbidity and should be used only as a temporizing measure until definitive treatment is performed.
- **Transjugular intrahepatic portosystemic shunt (TIPS)**:
  - o TIPS should be considered for uncontrolled esophageal variceal hemorrhage after failed pharmacologic and endoscopic therapy, to prevent re-bleeding in patients at high risk, or for gastric variceal hemorrhage. Gastric varices can bleed independently of HVPG, and TIPS with embolization of gastric varices can be an effective treatment.
  - o A TIPS dramatically reduces elevated portal pressure by creating a communication between the hepatic vein and an intrahepatic branch of the portal vein.
  - o A TIPS is placed via transjugular hepatic vein cannulation with subsequent advancement into the portal vein with placement of a stent between a hepatic vein branch and portal vein branch with the goal of reducing the portal pressure below 12 mmHg (or by at least 20%).
  - o Contraindications to TIPS placement include severe right-sided heart failure, severe hepatic failure, polycystic liver disease, a history of severe hepatic encephalopathy, and occlusive portal vein thrombus.
  - o Complications of TIPS include an increased risk of hepatic encephalopathy, hepatic failure, pulmonary hypertension, heart failure, and stent occlusion (less likely with a polytetrafluroethylene-covered than an uncovered stent).

Endoscopic treatment of varices (EVL) is generally performed as first-line interventional therapy for acute bleeding esophageal varices. A TIPS is used as first-line interventional therapy for bleeding gastric varices that do not respond to pharmacologic treatment. (In some countries, injection of gastric varices with 'glue' (cyanoacrylate) via endoscopy is another option for the treatment of bleeding gastric varices.)

Prevention of Variceal Hemorrhage

- Primary prophylaxis: Patients at risk for bleeding (moderate or large esophageal varices) should undergo primary prophylaxis with either a nonselective beta-receptor antagonist (beta-blocker, NSBB) or EVL to decrease the risk of hemorrhage. An NSBB decreases portal venous inflow via unopposed alpha-adrenergic-mediated vasoconstriction in the mesenteric arterioles.
- Secondary prophylaxis (following control of an acute variceal bleed): Combination therapy with both an NSBB and serial EVL is recommended. TIPS can be effective to prevent recurrent bleeding in selected patients.

Hepatic Encephalopathy

Definition

- Hepatic encephalopathy (HE), or portosystemic encephalopathy, refers to potentially reversible neurologic and psychiatric symptoms usually seen in patients with end-stage liver disease and/or portosystemic shunting. Up to 70% of patients with cirrhosis will develop HE.
- HE is a poor prognostic indicator with 3-year survival rates approximating 20% without liver transplantation.

Pathophysiology

- The pathophysiology of HE is poorly understood. The best-characterized neurotoxin involved in the development of HE is ammonia, which leads to astrocyte swelling, alterations in neurotransmitters, and brain edema.
- Ammonia is produced by enterocytes from glutamine and from colonic bacterial catabolism of nitrogenous sources, such as dietary proteins. Ammonia enters the circulation via the portal vein, and the liver normally converts it into glutamine. Impaired hepatic function, portosystemic shunting, and muscle wasting (an important site of extrahepatic ammonia removal) all lead to increases in serum ammonia levels.

- Elevated serum ammonia levels are seen in 90% of patients with HE, but serum levels of ammonia do not correlate well with symptoms. Therefore, the measurement of venous ammonia in clinical practice is an expensive test with little clinical value for patient management.
- There are likely other poorly understood mechanisms in the development of HE. There may be a role for inhibitory neurotransmission through gamma-aminobutyric acid (GABA) receptors in the central nervous system.

> Although elevated ammonia levels are seen in 90% of patients with HE, serum levels of ammonia do not correlate with symptoms. Therefore, the measurement of venous ammonia in clinical practice is an expensive test with little clinical value in managing the patient with HE.

Clinical Features

- Typically, early changes are subclinical (also designated covert, or minimal, hepatic encephalopathy) and may only be identified by abnormal results on psychometric or neurophysiologic testing.
- The onset of asterixis and/or disorientation marks overt HE.
- There is a wide spectrum of symptoms and signs of HE. The presentation may range from subtle changes such as a disruption in the sleep–wake cycle, to inability to perform activities of daily living, forgetfulness, and lethargy, to frank coma. Neuromuscular manifestations may include hyperreflexia, myoclonus, and asterixis. Reversible focal neurologic findings are present in a minority of patients.
- HE is often precipitated by an inciting event such as gastrointestinal bleeding, infection, electrolyte abnormalities, and sedating medications.
- The West Haven criteria grade HE on a scale of I–IV based on varying levels of consciousness, intellectual function, and behavior (Table 16.2).

Table 16.2 Grading of hepatic encephalopathy based on the West Haven criteria.

Grade	Clinical features
I	Decreased attention span/concentration; abnormal sleep pattern; mildly slowed mentation; mild confusion; minimal changes in memory
II	Lethargy; inappropriate behavior; slurred speech; personality changes
III	Somnolence; disorientation; marked confusion; incomprehensible speech
IV	Coma; unresponsive to verbal or noxious stimuli

Diagnosis

- The diagnosis of HE requires a high level of suspicion and careful attention to the cognitive and neurologic examination. A low threshold for intracranial imaging is necessary if focal neurologic findings are found on examination to rule out other causes of altered mental status.
- HE in chronic liver disease is clinically and pathophysiologically different from HE associated with acute liver failure. In acute failure, encephalopathy is a consequence of cerebral edema and is a medical emergency.
- Elevated serum ammonia levels in a patient with cirrhosis and altered mental status support the diagnosis of HE; however, the serum ammonia level is neither sensitive nor specific for the diagnosis and does not confirm the diagnosis alone.
- Patients with covert HE or mild degree of symptoms may require psychometric and electrophysiologic testing to confirm the diagnosis.

Treatment

- The cornerstone of treatment of HE includes prompt identification and correction of precipitating factors, including the following:
  - Gastrointestinal bleeding.
  - Infection (including spontaneous bacterial peritonitis [see later]).
  - Acid–base and electrolyte disturbances.
  - Dehydration and acute kidney injury.
  - Constipation.
  - Medications (e.g., sedatives, tranquilizers, narcotics).
  - Medication nonadherence (e.g., lactulose).
- Patients with acutely worsening or high-grade encephalopathy (e.g., coma) should be admitted to an intensive care unit, with a low threshold for elective intubation to protect the airway. In such patients, computed tomography (CT) of the brain is important to rule out other causes of altered mental status including hemorrhage, prior infarcts, or a space-occupying lesion (e.g., tumor, abscess).
- General supportive care includes nutritional support, correction of electrolyte derangements, and providing a safe environment with frequent orientation. Reinforce good 'sleep hygiene' and avoid sedating medications often used for insomnia, because these may worsen HE.
- Dietary protein restriction is not necessary for most patients with HE.
- Pharmacologic therapy:
  - Lactulose, a nonabsorbable disaccharide, has long been a first-line pharmacologic agent used to treat and to prevent the recurrence of HE.

- o Lactulose decreases colonic transit time and reduces ammonia production by acidifying colonic contents, thereby converting NH_3 to the less-absorbable NH_4^+.
  - o Lactulose is administered orally; however, in patients who are at risk for aspiration, it may be given as an enema.
  - o Side effects of lactulose include abdominal cramping, flatulence, diarrhea, and electrolyte imbalance.
  - o The dose should be titrated so that patients have two to three soft bowel movements per day. Overuse of lactulose may lead to dehydration and metabolic alkalosis, which paradoxically can worsen HE.
- – Antibiotics:
  - o Antibiotics have been used as second-line agents after lactulose or in patients who are intolerant of lactulose. Antibiotics are thought to modify the intestinal flora and lower stool pH, thereby decreasing ammonia production and enhancing its excretion.
  - o Rifaximin 550 mg twice daily has been shown to reduce the frequency of episodes of HE. Rifaximin is largely non-absorbed and therefore has relatively few side effects. Its efficacy and safety make rifaximin more conducive to long-term patient compliance compared with other antibiotics, although it can be expensive.
- – Other agents:
  - o Zinc has been used for patients with recurrent HE, because zinc deficiency is common in patients with HE and may modulate neurotransmission; however, there is little evidence for its efficacy.
  - o Oral L-ornithine-L-asparate (LOLA) enhances metabolism of ammonia to glutamine. It is not currently available in the US.

Lactulose, a nonabsorbable disaccharide, is the mainstay of treatment for HE. The dose of lactulose should be titrated so that patients have three soft bowel movements per day. Overuse of lactulose may lead to dehydration and metabolic alkalosis and may worsen HE or precipitate hepatorenal syndrome. Rifaximin is an important addition to the armamentarium for the treatment of HE.

Ascites

Definition

- Pathologic accumulation of fluid within the peritoneal cavity. There are numerous causes of ascites; cirrhosis is the cause in 80% of cases in the US.
- Ascites is the most common complication of cirrhosis.

Pathophysiology

- In the setting of cirrhosis, portal hypertension with a portal pressure >12 mmHg is required for ascites to develop. Sinusoidal hypertension leads to increased hydrostatic pressure, leading in turn to transudation of fluid into the peritoneal space in excess of the capacity of the lymphatic system to remove the fluid.
- Progressive peripheral vasodilatation in cirrhosis leads to a reduction in pressure measured at carotid and renal baroreceptors, resulting in activation of sodium-retaining neurohormonal mechanisms to attempt to restore perfusion pressures. Activated systems include the rennin–angiotensin–aldosterone system, sympathetic nervous system, and ADH. The net effect of activation of these pathways is avid sodium and water retention, despite increased plasma volume and excess total body sodium.

Clinical Features

- Patients usually present with increased abdominal girth and distention. They may have shortness of breath.
- Physical examination may reveal dullness to percussion, particularly in the flanks, shifting dullness, and a fluid wave.

Diagnosis

- All patients who present with the new onset of ascites in an outpatient or inpatient setting, as well as those with ascites admitted to the hospital, should undergo a diagnostic paracentesis.
- Ascitic fluid should be sent for cell count, including a differential count of the white blood cells (WBCs), albumin concentration, and total protein concentration. A Gram stain and bacterial culture are indicated if initial analysis of the fluid is consistent with infection.
- In uncomplicated (uninfected) cirrhotic ascites, the WBC count is <500 cells mm^{-3}, and the polymorphonuclear (PMN) neutrophil count is <250 mm^{-3}. A PMN count ≥250 mm^{-3} suggests a bacterial infection.
- The serum–ascites albumin gradient (SAAG) is used to categorize ascites and help determine the etiology. The SAAG is calculated by subtracting the ascitic fluid albumin concentration from the serum albumin concentration. A SAAG ≥1.1 $g\,dl^{-1}$ indicates portal hypertension as the etiology. Other causes of ascites with a SAAG ≥1.1 $g\,dl^{-1}$ include alcoholic hepatitis, Budd–Chiari syndrome, portal vein thrombosis, and cardiac ascites.
- A SAAG ≥1.1 $g\,dl^{-1}$ with an ascitic total protein level >2.5 $g\,dl^{-1}$ suggests cardiac ascites. Classically, the SAAG may narrow with diuresis in patients with heart failure, but not in cirrhotic patients.

- The most common condition associated with a low SAAG ($<1.1\,g\,dl^{-1}$) is peritoneal carcinomatosis. Other causes of a low-SAAG ascites include biliary or pancreatic leaks, nephrotic syndrome, and tuberculous peritonitis.

Treatment

- Because of the avid renal retention of sodium in cirrhotic ascites, dietary sodium restriction to $\leq 2\,g$ per day is essential. Because fluid follows sodium passively, fluid restriction is generally not required unless patients have severe hyponatremia ($<125\,mEq\,l^{-1}$).
- Treatment of the underlying cause of cirrhosis, such as alcohol abstinence in a patient with alcoholic cirrhosis, can be beneficial. Nonsteroidal anti-inflammatory drugs (NSAIDs), angiotensin-converting enzyme inhibitors, and angiotensin II receptor blockers should be avoided.
- Pharmacotherapy:
  - Spironolactone and furosemide in a ratio of 100 : 40 mg once daily can be increased gradually (every 3–5 days) to a maximum of 400 mg and 160 mg per day, respectively, as needed to achieve diuresis. The spironolactone and furosemide regimen in this ratio maintains normokalemia and achieves diuresis in >90% of patients with cirrhotic ascites.
  - The patient's weight and serum electrolyte and creatinine levels should be monitored closely.
  - Diuretics should be discontinued in patients who develop encephalopathy, a serum sodium concentration $<120\,mEq\,l^{-1}$ despite fluid restriction, or acute kidney injury.
- Large-volume paracentesis (LVP) may be performed in patients who have tense ascites or are refractory to diuretics. LVP should be avoided in patients with diuretic-sensitive cirrhotic ascites. Intravenous albumin (6–8 g per liter of fluid removed) should be administered to prevent circulatory dysfunction if >5 liters of ascitic fluid is removed.
- Refractory ascites is defined as ascites not responsive to dietary sodium restriction and maximal diuretic therapy or serial paracentesis. In such cases, TIPS placement and liver transplantation should be considered in appropriate candidates.

Spontaneous Bacterial Peritonitis

Definition

- Spontaneous bacterial peritonitis (SBP) is defined as acute infection of ascitic fluid without an apparent intra-abdominal source, e.g., perforated viscus.

- SBP typically occurs only in the setting of advanced cirrhosis and is associated with high mortality; it is a known precipitant of hepatorenal syndrome (HRS) (see later) and hepatic encephalopathy (see earlier).
- Bacterial translocation in the gut is increased in patients with advanced cirrhosis and is likely the source of SBP.

Clinical Features

- Patients may present with fever, abdominal pain and tenderness, or mental status changes. However, symptoms and signs of infection may be subtle or even absent, and, therefore, a high index of suspicion and low threshold to perform paracentesis are required to make a timely diagnosis.

> All hospitalized patients with cirrhosis and known ascites or new-onset ascites should undergo a diagnostic paracentesis.

Diagnosis

- The diagnosis of SBP is made by the demonstration of an ascitic fluid absolute PMN count ≥250 cells mm^{-3} in the absence of known peritonitis of other etiologies. The diagnosis cannot be made clinically without ascitic fluid analysis from a paracentesis.
- The most common pathogens are *Escherichia coli, Klebsiella pneumonia,* and *Streptococcus pneumoniae.*

Treatment

- Third-generation cephalosporins such as cefotaxime or ceftriaxone given intravenously for 5–7 days.
- Antibiotic coverage can be tailored once culture results are available, but the yield of cultures is low.
- Intravenous administration of albumin on days 1 and 3 (in addition to antibiotics) has been shown to decrease renal impairment and mortality rates.
- Antibiotic prophylaxis is recommended in cirrhotic patients with ascites at high risk for SBP. High-risk characteristics include an ascitic fluid protein concentration <1.5 g dl^{-1}, renal dysfunction, and active variceal bleeding. Secondary prophylaxis for those who have had SBP is also recommended. Oral fluoroquinolones or trimethoprim–sulfamethoxazole are commonly used.
- The liver transplant-free survival rate one year after an episode of SBP is approximately 40%.

Hepatorenal Syndrome

Definition

- Hepatorenal syndrome (HRS) is defined as functional acute kidney injury that occurs in the setting of portal hypertension usually due to cirrhosis or alcoholic hepatitis. By definition, instrinsic kidney disease is absent.
- Histologically, the kidneys are typically normal in HRS, and their function may be restored by correction of portal hypertension, as with liver transplantation.
- HRS occurs in 25% of patients hospitalized with cirrhosis and carries a high mortality rate.

Classification

- Type I HRS:
  - Defined as an increase in the baseline serum creatinine level of at least $0.3\,\mathrm{mg\,dl}^{-1}$ and by $\geq 50\%$ within 7 days. In many cases, renal function declines more substantially, and the serum creatinine level may be $>2.5\,\mathrm{mg\,dl}^{-1}$ within 2 weeks.
  - Rapidly progressive and potentially fatal. If untreated, the median survival is 2 weeks.
- Type II HRS:
  - Serum creatinine rises more gradually and typically reaches $1.5\,\mathrm{mg\,dl}^{-1}$ to $2.5\,\mathrm{mg\,dl}^{-1}$.
  - This often occurs in patients on chronic diuretic therapy with refractory ascites.
  - The course is more indolent than that of type I HRS, with an increase in serum creatinine level occurring over weeks to months. The median survival without liver transplantation is 6 months.

Pathophysiology

- The kidneys perceive decreased arterial blood volume resulting from decreased systemic vascular resistance in the setting of late-stage portal hypertension and attempt to compensate by activating sodium retention mechanisms including the renin–angiotensin–aldosterone system. This results in enhanced renal vascular constriction and avid sodium reabsorption. The persistence of an ineffective arterial blood volume resulting from enhanced renal vasoconstriction further reduces the glomerular filtration rate, and oliguric renal failure ensues.

Diagnosis

- The diagnosis of HRS requires a high index of clinical suspicion and exclusion of other causes of acute kidney injury. It occurs in up to 25% of patients with SBP. It can be associated with acute tubular necrosis, but can also be precipitated by it. HRS is classically seen in patients with end-stage liver disease with ascites, hyponatremia, and a 'spot' urinary sodium concentration $<10\,mEq\,l^{-1}$, reflecting avid sodium retention.

- Diagnostic criteria for HRS include:
  - Presence of portal hypertension from cirrhosis, alcoholic hepatitis, or acute hepatic disease.
  - Acute kidney injury as defined by increase in serum creatinine of $\geq0.3\,mg\,dl^{-1}$ within 48 hours or an increase from baseline of $\geq50\%$ within 7 days.
  - Lack of improvement in renal function despite volume expansion with intravenous albumin ($1\,g\,kg^{-1}$ of body weight up to 100 g per day) for 2 days and withdrawal of diuretics.
  - Absence of other apparent causes of acute kidney injury, including urinary tract obstruction, intrinsic renal parenchymal disease, hemodynamic shock, or recent treatment with a nephrotoxic medication.
  - Bland urinary sediment, protein excretion $<500\,mg$ per day, and normal renal imaging.

HRS is seen in up to 25% of patients with SBP. SBP may not be accompanied by overt symptoms or signs, and all patients with HRS should be evaluated for SBP.

Treatment

- Any potentially nephrotoxic medications, diuretics, angiotensin-converting enzyme inhibitors, angiotensin-receptor blockers, and NSAIDs should be discontinued.
- Pharmacologic agents targeted at producing splanchnic vasoconstriction should be initiated:
  - Octreotide 100 μg subcutaneously three times daily; increase to a maximum dose of 200 μg subcutaneously three times daily or as continuous intravenous infusion at $50\,\mu g\,h^{-1}$.
  - Midodrine, an alpha-adrenergic agonist, 5–10 mg orally three times daily, titrated to a mean arterial pressure increase of at least 15 mmHg.
  - For critically ill patients in an intensive care unit, an infusion of norepinephrine infusion (0.5–$3\,mg\,h^{-1}$) or vasopressin to raise mean arterial pressure along with intravenous administration of albumin.
- On recognition of acute kidney injury, a 'fluid challenge' consisting of intravenous albumin, $1\,g\,kg^{-1}$ per day for 2 days (up to 100 g), followed by 25–50 g per day until midodrine and octreotide therapy is discontinued, should be administered.
- Outside the US, intravenous terlipressin is commonly used instead of midodrine, octreotide, and norepinephrine.

- Because HRS is associated with a high mortality rate, the following prophylactic measures to prevent HRS are recommended:
  - Albumin should be administered intravenously before all large-volume paracenteses (>5 liters removed).
  - Administration of albumin on days 1 and 3 of the treatment of SBP has been shown to decrease the incidence of HRS.
- Liver transplantation is curative. The transplant-free survival rate is <20% of patients with Type I HRS treated with albumin, midodrine, and octreotide. Renal replacement therapy (e.g., dialysis) can be used as a bridge to liver transplantation.

> HRS is associated with a high mortality rate and should be identified expeditiously and treated promptly. Precipitating factors should be identified and corrected.

Hepatic Hydrothorax

Definition

- Transudative pleural effusion (usually >500 ml) in a patient with portal hypertension without any other underlying cardiopulmonary source.
- Occurs in approximately 5–10% of cirrhotic patients.
- Hepatic hydrothorax may become infected (*spontaneous bacterial empyema*).

Pathophysiology

- Thought to result from the passage of ascites to the pleural space via small diaphragmatic defects.
- Increased abdominal pressure due to ascites and thinning of the diaphragm due to malnutrition may increase gaps between diaphragmatic muscle fibers and lead to pleuroperitoneal blebs. These blebs can rupture and allow free passage of intraperitoneal fluid preferentially into the pleural space, given the negative intrathoracic pressure.
- Hepatic hydrothorax occurs when the rate of fluid accumulation exceeds the rate of reabsorption.

Clinical Features

- Dyspnea, cough, hypoxia, and pleuritic chest pain are typical symptoms. Patients usually present with ascites.
- If severe, hepatic hydrothorax can lead to severe respiratory distress.
- Hepatic hydrothorax typically occurs on the right side (85%), although it may occur on the left (13%) or bilaterally (2%).

Diagnosis

- Hepatic hydrothorax:
  - Pleural fluid analysis in hepatic hydrothorax is transudative with cell count <500 cells mm^{-3} and total protein concentration <2.5 g dl^{-1}.
  - Thoracentesis should be performed to rule out infection and other causes of pleural effusion.
- Spontaneous bacterial empyema:
  - Total fluid PMN count ≥250 mm^{-3} with a positive fluid culture; or
  - Fluid PMN count ≥500 mm^{-3} with a negative fluid culture; and
  - No evidence of pneumonia/parapneumonic effusion on imaging.

Treatment

- Medical management of hepatic hydrothorax should focus on treating ascites (see earlier), and includes diuretics, dietary sodium retention, and nutritional repletion.
- Therapeutic thoracentesis and paracentesis should be performed in dyspneic and/or hypoxic patients.
- Spontaneous bacterial empyema is treated with intravenous antibiotics, as for SBP.
- Placement of a chest tube is, in general, contraindicated in cirrhotic patients due to poor outcomes because of renal failure from fluid depletion, protein loss, and infection.
- There have been studies assessing the utility of video-assisted thoracoscopy with pleurodesis for the treatment of hepatic hydrothorax. Success rates are limited by a lack of apposition between the visceral and parietal pleura. Additionally, any surgical procedure in a patient with decompensated liver disease may increase mortality.
- Patients who are refractory to medical management and thoracentesis should be considered for TIPS placement. Up to 75% of patients with refractory hepatic hydrothorax may respond to TIPS placement, but careful patient selection is key.
- Liver transplantation should be considered in patients with refractory hepatic hydrothorax.

Hepatopulmonary Syndrome

Definition

- Hepatopulmonary syndrome (HPS) is a pulmonary complication characterized by the triad of impaired oxygenation (with an increased alveolar–arterial gradient), pulmonary vascular vasodilatations, and portal hypertension (with or without cirrhosis).

- HPS occurs in up to 30% of patients with cirrhosis, resulting in arterial hypoxemia. Patients with mild HPS may be asymptomatic.

Pathophysiology

- Capillary vasodilatation results from increased circulating vasodilators (i.e., NO) primarily at the lung bases.
- Pulmonary vasodilatation causes intrapulmonary shunting, leading to hyperperfusion of the lungs and reduced oxygenation of venous blood transported via the pulmonary arteries and returned to the heart. Consequently, there is rapid blood flow through the dilated pulmonary circulation that leads to inadequate oxygenation of erythrocytes and clinical hypoxia.
- The degree of hypoxemia does not correlate with the severity of underlying liver disease, but HPS does increase mortality.

Clinical Features

- **Platypnea** is defined as dyspnea that worsens when the patient sits upright but improves when the patient is lying down. Platypnea occurs because of **orthodeoxia**, or a decrease in arterial oxygen tension >4 mmHg when the patient moves from the supine to upright position because increased blood circulating at the lung bases is shunted away from alveoli. There are more arteriovenous shunts (intrapulmonary vascular dilatations) in the lower than upper lung fields in cirrhotic patients who have HPS.
- Other symptoms and signs include shortness of breath, cyanosis, digital clubbing, and hypoxia.
- Multiple spider telangiectasias on the face and chest may be markers of intrapulmonary vascular dilatations.

Diagnosis

- Hypoxia in the absence of coexisting cardiopulmonary disease. In severe cases, the PaO_2 is below 60 mmHg on a room air blood gas measurement.
- Increased arterial–alveolar gradient without CO_2 retention.
- A contrast-enchanced (or 'bubble') echocardiogram may reveal delayed appearance of air bubbles in the left side of the heart within three to six beats after visualization in the right heart. Such a finding suggests trapped air bubbles in newly developed pulmonary shunts.
- A ^{99m}Tc macro-aggregated albumin lung perfusion scan can confirm the diagnosis.

Treatment

- Supplemental oxygen.
- Liver transplantation will reverse HPS.

Portopulmonary Hypertension

Definition

- Pulmonary arterial hypertension in the setting of portal hypertension with elevated pulmonary resistance and a normal pulmonary artery wedge pressure.
- Portopulmonary hypertension is a rare but serious complication of portal hypertension that, if untreated, can result in right-sided heart failure and death.

Pathophysiology

- The mechanisms are incompletely understood. Theories include increased vascular flow causing shear stress that may trigger remodeling of the vascular endothelium and portosystemic shunting. A decrease in the phagocytic capacity of the cirrhotic liver may allow circulating bacteria and toxins to enter the pulmonary circulation, thereby causing cytokine release, which triggers vascular inflammatory changes.

Clinical Features

- Dyspnea on exertion (the most common presenting symptom), orthopnea, and signs of volume overload are typical. Physical examination may reveal a loud second pulmonary valve heart sound, murmurs of tricuspid and pulmonary regurgitation, and a right ventricular heave. In contrast to HPS, hypoxemia is uncommon.

Diagnosis

- Screening with echocardiography may reveal an elevated right ventricular pressure systolic pressure or right-sided heart failure.
- Right-sided heart catheterization is necessary to confirm the diagnosis and determine the severity. Typical findings are a mean pulmonary artery pressure >25 mmHg, normal pulmonary wedge pressure, and elevated pulmonary vascular resistance >125 dynes s^{-1} ·cm^{-5}.
- Histopathology of the lung may show intimal fibrosis, smooth muscle hypertrophy, and characteristic plexiform lesions in small arteries and arterioles.

Treatment

- Liver transplantation for patients with mild portopulmonary hypertension (mean pulmonary artery [PA] pressure <35 mmHg) is curative.
- Patients with moderate or severe (mean PA pressure ≥35 mmHg) portopulmonary hypertension are at risk of acute right heart failure from increased preload at the time of reperfusion during liver transplantation.
- Patients with moderate or severe portopulmonary hypertension are often placed on pharmacologic pulmonary vasodilator therapy with the primary goals of reducing the mean pulmonary artery pressure to <35 mmHg and then considering liver transplantation.

Cirrhotic Cardiomyopathy

Definition

- As cirrhosis progresses, the loss of a hyperdynamic circulation and decreased cardiac output occurs in parallel with diastolic dysfunction. Other findings include electrophysiologic repolarization changes such as a prolonged QT interval, enlargement or hypertrophy of the cardiac chambers, and a blunted ventricular response to physiologic, pathologic, or pharmacologic stress.

Pathophysiology

- The pathophysiology of cirrhotic cardiomyopathy is unknown. Abnormal beta-adrenergic receptor function, altered levels of cytokines, endogenous cannabinoids, and NO, and cardiomyocyte plasma membrane changes have been reported.

Clinical Features

- Patients are usually asymptomatic or have mild shortness of breath or chest pain.
- Overt heart failure can be precipitated by a TIPS, liver transplantation, or major surgery.

Treatment

- Liver transplantation reverses cirrhotic cardiomyopathy.

Prognostic Scoring Systems for Cirrhosis

- Once complications of cirrhosis develop, mortality rates are high. Various scoring systems have been developed to determine the prognosis and the need for transplantation.

Child–Turcotte–Pugh Score

- This scoring system uses five variables (serum bilirubin, INR, serum albumin, ascites, and encephalopathy), each of which is allocated a score of 1–3, to compute an overall score and three Child–Pugh classes (A, B, and C).
- Major limitations of this scoring system include the subjective evaluation of the degree of ascites and encephalopathy and the classification into just three classes. Thus, its use in clinical practice has largely been replaced by the Model for End-stage Liver Disease (MELD) score.

MELD Score

- This is a prospectively developed and validated scoring system that uses a patient's laboratory values to predict 3-month mortality. It has been modified by the United Network for Organ Sharing to facilitate objective allocation of donor organs for patients in need of liver transplantation, with the severity of liver disease guiding prioritization.
- The MELD score predicts 3-month mortality for patients with end-stage liver disease.
- The score ranges from 6 to 40 based on three variables – INR, serum creatinine, and serum bilirubin – plus the need for renal replacement therapy. Because hyponatremia is an independent marker of mortality in end-stage liver disease, serum sodium levels are now incorporated into the MELD score for organ allocation purposes in the United States.
- 3-month mortality rates according to MELD score are as follows:
  - <9: 1.9%
  - 10–19: 6.0%
  - 20–29: 19.6%
  - 30–39: 52.6%
  - 40 or more: 71.3%
- Patients with a MELD score >15 have been shown to have improved survival with liver transplantation.

Liver Transplantation

- Liver transplantation offers patients with acute or chronic liver disease improved survival and quality of life.
  - Indications: acute liver failure, end-stage liver disease of any cause with complications of portal hypertension and a MELD score of ≥15, hepatocellular carcinoma (single lesion 2–5 cm or no more than three lesions each <3 cm), and liver-based metabolic deficiency (e.g., ornithine transcarbamylase deficiency).
- Outcomes: The 5-year survival rate in adults post-transplantation is approximately 70% in the United States.

> **Pearls**
>
> - Approximately 50% of all patients with cirrhosis have gastroesophageal varices. All patients with cirrhosis should be screened for the presence of varices by EGD. Those with large esophageal varices at risk for bleeding should be started on an NSBB or undergo EVL for primary prevention.
> - A majority of patients with cirrhosis will develop HE, which is a prognostic indicator of poor survival (3-year survival rate 20% without liver transplantation).
> - Patients with SBP are often asymptomatic. All hospitalized patients with cirrhosis and ascites should undergo a diagnostic paracentesis.

Questions

Questions 1 and 2 relate to the clinical vignette at the beginning of this chapter.

1 The next step in the management of the patient is which of the following?
   A Magnetic resonance imaging of the liver.
   B Diuretic therapy with spironolactone and furosemide.
   C Large-volume paracentesis.
   D Diagnostic paracentesis.
   E Echocardiogram.

2 The patient is admitted to the hospital, and a diagnostic paracentesis is performed. The peritoneal fluid analysis should include which of the following?
   A Albumin.
   B Cell count with differential.
   C Bacterial culture.
   D All of the above.
   E None of the above.

3 A 58-year-old man with cirrhosis due to hepatitis C virus is admitted to the intensive care unit for hemorrhage from esophageal varices that continue to bleed soon after EVL. Prior to TIPS placement, the radiologist obtains the following venous pressure measurements: right atrial pressure: 5 mmHg, free hepatic vein: 7 mmHg and WHVP: 10 mmHg. Which of the following conditions would best explain these findings?
   A Constrictive pericarditis.
   B Portal vein thrombosis.
   C Hepatocellular carcinoma.
   D Budd–Chiari syndrome.
   E Hepatopulmonary syndrome.

4 Which of the following regarding portal hypertension is true?
  A It results in an increase in effective arterial blood volume to the nephron.
  B It results from increased intrahepatic resistance and an increase in portal blood flow.
  C It is measured by calculating the difference between the central venous pressure and the portal vein pressure.
  D It is mediated by carbon dioxide released from endothelial cells.
  E It is associated with increased peripheral vasomotor tone.

5 Which of the following variables correlate **least** with a patient's risk of hemorrhage from esophageal varices?
  A Size of varices.
  B Number of varices.
  C HVPG >12 mmHg.
  D Presence of stigmata of bleeding.
  E Child–Pugh class C decompensated cirrhosis.

Answers

1 D
  This clinical scenario is suspicious for SBP. Given the high mortality rate of SBP, timely diagnosis and initiation of appropriate antibiotics are essential. Imaging studies are not necessary prior to paracentesis. Diuretics in general should be avoided in patients with SBP. A large volume paracentesis is not necessary and can precipitate circulatory dysfunction.

2 D
  Newly diagnosed ascites requires a paracentesis with ascitic fluid analysis to determine the etiology of the ascites and rule out infection. Fluid albumin, cell count, total protein, and culture should be obtained.

3 B
  HVPG measurement is accurate only for determining sinusoidal and postsinusoidal causes of portal hypertension. Causes of prehepatic portal hypertension, such as portal vein thrombosis, may indicate a normal sinusoidal gradient, as in this case. Constrictive pericarditis has elevated right atrial pressures. The hepatic vein usually cannot be cannulated in Budd–Chiari syndrome.

4 B
  Portal hypertension results from intrahepatic resistance to blood flow and increased portal venous blood inflow. The increased intrahepatic

resistance is mediated by sinusoidal fibrosis and compression by regenerative nodules. Increased portal venous blood flow is caused by decreased release of nitric oxide in the intrahepatic sinusoids coupled with increased release of nitric oxide and vasodilatation in both the splanchnic and systemic circulation.

5 B

The number of columns of varices in the esophagus is the least important variable in predicting a patient's risk of future hemorrhage. The risk of bleeding correlates best with the size of varices, degree of HVPG, presence of bleeding stigmata, and underlying severity of liver disease.

Further Reading

Angeli, P., Gines, P., Wong, F., *et al.* (2015) Diagnosis and management of acute kidney injury in patients with cirrhosis: revised consensus recommendations of the International Club of Ascites. *Gut*, **64**, 531–537.

Ra, G., Tsien, C., Renner, E.L., and Wong, F.S. (2015) The negative prognostic impact of a first ever episode of spontaneous bacterial peritonitis in cirrhosis and ascites. *Journal of Clinical Gastroenterology*, **49**, 858–865.

Shah, V.H. and Kamath, P.S. (2016) Portal hypertension and variceal bleeding, in *Sleisenger and Fordtran's Gastrointestinal and Liver Disease: Pathophysiology/Diagnosis/Management*, 10th edition (eds M. Feldman, L.S. Friedman, and L.J. Brandt), Saunders Elsevier, Philadelphia, pp. 1524–1552.

Villanueva, C., Colomo, A., Bosch, A., *et al.* (2013) Transfusion strategies for acute upper gastrointestinal bleeding. *New England Journal of Medicine*, **368**, 11–21.

Weblinks

http://www.turner-white.com/pdf/brm_Gast_pre10_1.pdf

http://www.med.upenn.edu/gastro/documents/Gastroenterologyportal hypertensionandcomplications.pdf

http://www.aafp.org/afp/2006/0901/p767.html

http://www.jefferson.edu/gi/education/documents/ComplicationsChronicLiver DiseaseHerrine-06.pdf

Pancreas and Biliary System

Stephan Goebel and Lisa Cassani

17

Pancreatic Anatomy and Function

Field F. Willingham

> **Clinical Vignette**
>
> A 36-year-old woman presents to the emergency department with a one-day history of epigastric pain radiating to the back. She has had several similar episodes, but the current episode is the most severe. She complains of nausea and has had three episodes of non-bloody emesis. She denies diarrhea, constipation, melena, hematemesis, fatigue, and weight loss. Her past medical and surgical history is unremarkable. Her only medication is an oral contraceptive pill. She drinks one to two glasses of wine per month. She does not smoke. Physical examination reveals a blood pressure of 144/85 mmHg, pulse rate 89 per minute, and temperature 100.2 °F (37.9 °C). She has mild tenderness to palpation in the epigastrium and right upper quadrant. There is no rebound tenderness or guarding. Bowel sounds are normal. The remainder of the examination is unremarkable. Abdominal ultrasonography reveals a normal gallbladder with no wall thickening, pericholecystic fluid, or gallstones. There is fluid around the pancreas. Laboratory tests including liver enzymes are normal. The serum lipase level is 269 U l^{-1}, and the amylase level is 223 U l^{-1}.

Anatomy

- The pancreas is a retroperitoneal organ that lies posterior to the stomach.
- The head of the pancreas lies in the curvature of the duodenum and to the right of the portal vein confluence (formed by the union of the superior mesenteric vein and splenic vein) (Figure 17.1).

Sitaraman and Friedman's Essentials of Gastroenterology, Second Edition.
Edited by Shanthi Srinivasan and Lawrence S. Friedman.
© 2018 John Wiley & Sons Ltd. Published 2018 by John Wiley & Sons Ltd.

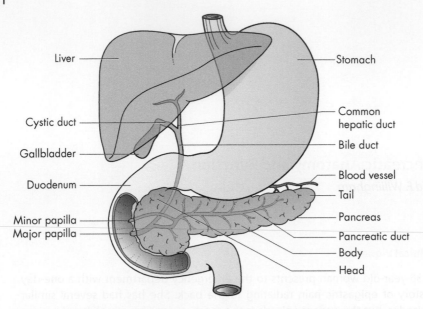

Figure 17.1 The anatomy of the pancreas, pancreatic ducts, and the bile duct.

> Tumors in the head of the pancreas may cause compression of the duodenum leading to gastric outlet obstruction.

- The neck of the pancreas lies anterior to the portal vein.
- The body of the pancreas lies between the portal confluence and the abdominal aorta.

> Due to its proximity to the local vasculature, pancreatic adenocarcinoma frequently invades the portal vein, celiac axis, and/or superior mesenteric artery early in the course. Therefore, pancreatic cancer is often advanced and unresectable at the time of presentation.

- The splenic vein and artery course along the length of the pancreas. Splenic vein thrombosis can occur in patients with pancreatitis and pancreatic tumors.
- The tail of the pancreas terminates in the superior portion of the splenic hilum.
- The uncinate process of the pancreas is tucked in posteriorly behind the superior mesenteric artery and vein.

> Tumors in the head of the pancreas may cause dilatation of the bile duct and pancreatic duct, resulting in the 'double-duct sign.' The sensitivity of the double-duct sign for detecting pancreatic cancer is 77–85%.

- The midline portion of the pancreatic body lies anterior to the lumbar spine.

> Blunt severe force in the anterior–posterior direction of the abdominal cavity, as in a motor vehicle collision, is most likely to cause injury to the body of the pancreas as it crosses anterior to the lumbar spine.

- The distal portion of the bile duct runs through the pancreatic parenchyma in the head and joins with the pancreatic duct.

> Mass lesions in the head of the pancreas may present with painless jaundice resulting from extrinsic compression of the distal bile duct.

- The common channel formed by the union of the bile duct and pancreatic duct terminates at and drains through the major papilla.

> Gallstones that pass from the gallbladder may obstruct biliary and pancreatic outflow, resulting in elevated liver biochemical test levels and/or gallstone pancreatitis.

- The accessory pancreatic duct, called the duct of Santorini, drains through the minor papilla and usually communicates with the main pancreatic duct, the duct of Wirsung.
- The pancreatic duct is typically greatest in diameter in the head of the pancreas. The diameter of the pancreatic duct typically follows the '3-2-1 rule': the duct diameter measures approximately 3 mm in the head, 2 mm in the body, and 1 mm in the tail.
- The exocrine pancreas constitutes approximately 90% of the gland.
- The functional unit of the exocrine pancreas consists of the acinus and a corresponding ductule (Figure 17.2).
- Between the acinus and the ductule are the centroacinar cells.
- The ductules drain into larger interlobular ducts, which drain into the main pancreatic duct.

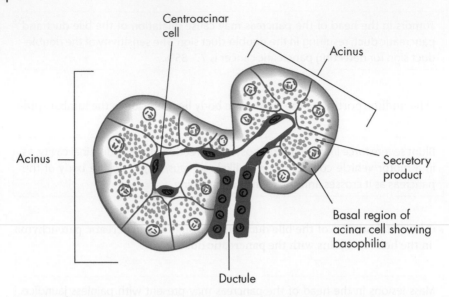

Figure 17.2 Diagram of a pancreatic acinus and ductule. Zymogen granules are stored at the apical aspect of the acinar cells. Enzymatic secretion is stimulated by small peptides, fat, and carbohydrate in the duodenum and is upregulated by cholecystokinin and acetylcholine. Adapted from Dr Thomas Caceci and Dr Samir El-Shafey; Virginia Tech, Blacksburg, VA, USA.

Embryology

- Pancreatic development begins around the fourth week of gestation.
- The pancreas develops from the endoderm and begins as dorsal and ventral buds.
- The dorsal bud grows more rapidly than the ventral bud, and forms the majority of the pancreas (the superior portion of the head, the body, and the tail).
- The ventral pancreas initially arises in the duodenum on the opposite side from the dorsal bud.
- The ventral bud rotates and fuses with the dorsal bud to become the inferior portion of the head and the uncinate process.
- The ventral and dorsal ducts anastomose to form the main pancreatic duct. The proximal portion of the dorsal duct becomes the duct of Santorini in most adults.

Developmental Anomalies

- **Pancreas divisum:**
  - Pancreas divisum is the most common pancreatic congenital anomaly.

- In pancreas divisum, the dorsal and ventral ducts do not fuse during development. The main dorsal pancreatic duct drains through the minor papilla, and the ventral duct drains separately through the major papilla.
- It is estimated that pancreas divisum may be present in up to 7% of the population.
- There may be a higher risk of pancreatitis in patients with pancreas divisum. This is thought to be due to reduced outflow of pancreatic secretions through a diminutive or stenotic minor papilla.
- Pancreas divisum may be found in 15% or more of patients with idiopathic pancreatitis undergoing endoscopic retrograde cholangiopancreatography (ERCP).
- Patients with recurrent pancreatitis due to pancreas divisum may be managed with sphincterotomy of the minor papilla and temporary placement of a pancreatic duct stent.
- **Annular pancreas:**
  - Annular pancreas describes a congenital anomaly in which a band of pancreatic tissue surrounds the second portion of the duodenum.
  - The condition results from abnormal fusion of the dorsal and ventral buds, which form a ring of pancreatic tissue around the duodenum.
  - There is a bimodal age distribution of the clinical presentation of annular pancreas, with a relatively increased frequency of presentation in the neonatal period and in adults in the fourth and fifth decades.

In infants, annular pancreas may present on imaging with the 'double-bubble sign.' The double-bubble sign reflects the regions of dilatation in the proximal duodenum and the distal stomach.

  - Annular pancreas is treated by performing a surgical bypass (duodeno-duodenostomy or gastrojejunostomy), because the pancreatic tissue may extend into the duodenal wall.
- **Ectopic pancreas:**
  - Ectopic pancreas refers to the presence of pancreatic tissue outside the pancreatic gland.
  - Ectopic pancreatic tissue may be found in many anatomic locations, but is most frequently observed in the stomach, duodenum, and distal small intestine.
  - Ectopic pancreas is usually an incidental finding.
  - A **pancreatic rest** is a focus of ectopic pancreas that has a classic appearance of a small nodule with a central umbilication, and is typically seen in the stomach as an incidental finding during esophagogastroduodenoscopy (Figure 17.3).

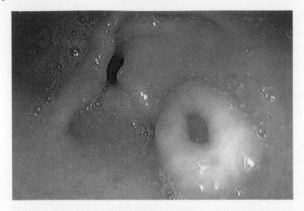

Figure 17.3 The classic appearance of a pancreatic rest in the gastric antrum adjacent to the pylorus on esophagogastroduodenoscopy. A pancreatic rest is a focus of ectopic pancreatic tissue with a characteristic central umbilication.

Physiology

Pancreatic Secretion

- Digestive enzymes are synthesized, stored, and secreted by the acinar cells. The enzymes are stored as inactive precursors (zymogens) in the zymogen granules located in the apical aspect of the acinar cells (see Figure 17.2).
- Activation of the zymogens is a multistage process which involves several proteolytic steps that occur sequentially during transport from the site of synthesis on ribosomes and endoplasmic reticulum to the final destination in the luminal space of the duodenum.
- The acinar cells are stimulated via basolateral membrane receptors, which trigger secretion of the zymogens into the lumen of the acinus.
- In the last stage, trypsinogen is converted into an active form, trypsin, by enteropeptidase (also called enterokinase), an enzyme produced by the crypts of Lieberkühn in the duodenum. Trypsin, in turn, converts the other pancreatic proenzymes into their active forms in the duodenum.

Inappropriate activation of pancreatic proenzymes within the pancreas leads to pancreatitis.

- The pancreas secretes 1–2.5 liters of fluid per day. As a consequence, dehydration can occur quickly in patients with a pancreatic fistula when secretions are not delivered to the intestinal lumen for subsequent reabsorption.

- There are two major types of pancreatic secretion: the aqueous fraction, and the enzymatic fraction:
  - The **aqueous fraction** is rich in bicarbonate and acts to neutralize the acidic chyme in the duodenum. The inorganic products of pancreatic secretion also include water, sodium, potassium, and chloride. The aqueous fraction is secreted by the centroacinar cells and ductal cells. Aqueous secretion is stimulated by the presence of H^+ ions in the duodenum and upregulated by secretin and acetylcholine.
  - The **enzymatic fraction** of pancreatic secretion acts on carbohydrates, proteins, and fat, and plays a key role in digestion and absorption.
- Pancreatic enzymes are secreted by the acinar cells:
  - The pancreatic enzymes amylase and lipase are secreted in the active form.
  - As mentioned earlier, proteases, trypsinogen and chymotrypsinogen, are secreted in an inactive form and require further steps for activation.
  - Enzymatic secretion is stimulated by small peptides, fat, and carbohydrates in the duodenum. Enzymatic secretion is upregulated by cholecystokinin and acetylcholine.
- As pancreatic flow increases, often due to secretin stimulation, the relative concentration of bicarbonate increases.
- Table 17.1 compares pancreatic enzymes and several gastrointestinal hormones.

Chronic diseases of the exocrine pancreas, such as cystic fibrosis and chronic pancreatitis, lead to a loss of pancreatic mass and deficiency of pancreatic enzymes, and may result in maldigestion. Maldigestion, in turn, leads to weight loss and nutritional deficiencies.

Endocrine Function

- The primary role of the endocrine pancreas is to secrete insulin and other hormones to control serum levels of glucose and triglycerides and amino acid balance.
- The endocrine portion of the pancreas constitutes approximately 10% of the gland and is made up of the islets of Langerhans.
- The majority of the cells in the islets are beta cells, which produce insulin.
- Other cell types within each islet are the alpha, delta, and PP cells.
- The alpha cells secrete glucagon; the delta cells secrete somatostatin; and the PP cells secrete pancreatic polypeptide.
- Autonomic nerves, metabolites such as glucose, circulating hormones, and local paracrine hormones regulate the function of the islets.

Table 17.1 Enzymes and gastrointestinal hormones involved in digestion.

Enzyme or hormone	Source	Function	Regulation	Comment
Amylase	Pancreas and salivary glands	Digests dietary starch and glycogen	Stimulated by the vagus nerve, acetylcholine, and CCK	Isolated hyperamylasemia may not be related to pancreatic disease
Lipase	Primarily pancreas	Hydrolyzes triglycerides and fatty acids	Stimulated by the vagus nerve, acetylcholine, and CCK	More specific to the pancreas than amylase
Gastrin	G-cells (in the antrum and duodenum)	Stimulates secretion of gastric acid, intrinsic factor, and pepsinogen Increases gastric motility	Stimulated by gastric distension, amino acids, peptides; and the vagus nerve Inhibited by secretin and very low gastric pH	Hypersecretion may be seen with gastrinoma (Zollinger–Ellison syndrome), leading to peptic ulceration and associated complications
CCK	I-cells (in the duodenum and jejunum)	Stimulates gallbladder contraction and pancreatic enzyme secretion. Inhibits gastric acid secretion	Stimulated by fat and acid	A HIDA scan uses a synthetic form of CCK to stimulate gallbladder contraction. Gallbladder dysfunction is defined as an ejection fraction less than 35%
Secretin	S-cells (in the duodenum)	Stimulates pancreatic secretion Inhibits gastric acid secretion	Stimulated by acid and fat in the duodenum	Secretin is involved in alkalinizing the duodenum; pancreatic enzymes are inactivated by an acidic pH
Somatostatin	D-cells (in the pancreatic islets and gastric and intestinal mucosa)	Inhibits gastric acid and pepsinogen secretion. Decreases gallbladder contraction. Inhibits release of insulin and glucagon	Stimulated by acid. Inhibited by the vagus nerve	An inhibitory hormone. Synthetic somatostatin, octreotide, is used to treat carcinoid syndrome, acute variceal bleeding, and acromegaly

CCK, cholecystokinin; HIDA, hydroxy iminodiacetic acid.

Pearls
• The splenic vein and artery course along the length of the pancreas. Splenic vein thrombosis may lead to isolated gastric varices (gastric varices in the absence of esophageal varices). Unlike cirrhosis, this presentation is not related to portal hypertension.
• It is estimated that symptoms of pancreatic insufficiency do not present until 85–90% of the pancreatic mass is compromised.

Questions

Questions 1 and 2 relate to the clinical vignette at the beginning of this chapter.

1 Which of the following is the most likely diagnosis?
   A Primary sclerosing cholangitis.
   B Acute cholecystitis.
   C Ascending cholangitis.
   D Acute pancreatitis.
   E Peptic ulcer disease.

2 Which of the following is the next best step in the evaluation of the patient's condition?
   A Esophagogastroduodenoscopy.
   B Cholecystectomy.
   C Endoscopic retrograde cholangiopancreatography (ERCP).
   D Magnetic resonance imaging (MRI)/magnetic resonance cholangio-pancreatography (MRCP).
   E Serum amylase isoforms.

3 A 26-year-old man is involved in a motor vehicle collision. He was the driver of the vehicle and was wearing his seat belt. The vehicle is 'totaled,' and the passengers are transported to the nearest trauma center. The driver complains of marked abdominal pain. Computed tomography shows fluid surrounding the pancreas. A traumatic injury would most likely be localized to which of the following regions?
   A Stomach.
   B Head of the pancreas.
   C Body of the pancreas.
   D Gallbladder.
   E Spleen.

4   An 84-year-old man is admitted to the hospital with lethargy and a change in mental status. Physical examination reveals a thin frail man. The blood pressure is 92/54 mmHg, pulse rate 115 per minute, and temperature 102 °F (38.9 °C). He is mildly jaundiced and oriented to person, but not to place or time. Abdominal examination reveals mild tenderness to palpation in the epigastrium. There is no rebound tenderness or guarding. Bowel sounds are present. Abdominal ultrasonography reveals dilatation of the bile duct to 12 mm, multiple gallstones in the gallbladder, but no gallbladder wall thickening or pericholecystic fluid. Laboratory tests show a normal complete blood count, total bilirubin level of 5 mg dl^{-1}, aspartate aminotransferase 145 U l^{-1}, alanine aminotransferase 79 U l^{-1}, amylase 196 U l^{-1}, and lipase 246 U l^{-1}. The patient is started on intravenous fluids and broad-spectrum antibiotics. Which of the following is most appropriate at this time?

A Laparoscopy.

B Cholecystectomy.

C Cholecystostomy tube placement.

D ERCP.

E MRCP.

5   A 55-year-old man presents to his primary care doctor with a complaint of abdominal discomfort, bloating, and early satiety. The primary care physician obtains an abdominal X-ray, which reveals air–fluid levels in the stomach and first portion of the duodenum. Esophagogastroduodenoscopy is performed and reveals narrowing in the second portion of the duodenum with normal-appearing duodenal mucosa. The patient's findings are consistent with which of the following diagnosis?

A Annular pancreas.

B Cystic fibrosis.

C Duodenal atresia.

D Pancreatic heterotopias.

E Pancreas divisum.

Answers

1 D

2 D

    This patient has mild acute pancreatitis as evidenced by epigastric pain and mildly elevated serum amylase and lipase levels. She may have pancreatitis secondary to pancreas divisum. Ultrasonography did not reveal features of cholecystitis such as gallbladder wall thickening, pericholecystic fluid, or gallstones. Ascending cholangitis is unlikely in the absence of fever, jaundice, or elevated liver enzyme levels. Peptic ulcer typically presents with epigastric pain and possibly with bleeding, but not typically with elevated serum amylase and lipase levels. Primary sclerosing cholangitis presents with elevated liver biochemical test levels in a cholestatic pattern (elevated serum bilirubin and alkaline phosphatase levels). ERCP could be considered if the bilirubin and alkaline phosphatase levels were elevated or there was other evidence of cholangitis or bile duct dilatation, but would not be the next test in this case. Amylase isoforms can be obtained to determine if the salivary amylase level is elevated in serum and can be helpful in a patient with isolated hyperamylasemia. This patient has elevation of both amylase and lipase levels (lipase is more specific for the pancreas) associated with abdominal pain and fluid around the pancreas, and the elevated amylase level is not likely to be from a salivary source. MRI/MRCP would be helpful to evaluate the pancreatic parenchyma, which is not seen well on abdominal ultrasonography. MRI/MRCP will also help visualize the pancreatic and biliary ductal systems. If MRI/MRCP shows pancreas divisum, ERCP could be considered as a therapeutic intervention for minor sphincterotomy and temporary stenting of the pancreatic duct via the minor papilla.

3 **C**

The patient sustained a pancreatic injury following a motor vehicle collision; this is a common occurrence following a 'seat-belt injury.' The most frequently injured segment of the pancreas is the body, which passes anterior to the spine. Traumatic pancreatic injuries frequently can be missed on abdominal imaging. The spleen can be injured in motor vehicle collisions; however, in this case ultrasonography revealed fluid around the pancreas and no damage to the spleen.

4 **D**

This patient has ascending cholangitis and gallstone pancreatitis. After fluid resuscitation and administration of antibiotics, ERCP is indicated for biliary decompression. The bile duct is dilated, and the serum aminotransferase and pancreatic enzyme levels are elevated. Together with the presence of gallstones, this pattern is most suggestive of bile duct obstruction secondary to choledocholithiasis. The patient has Charcot's triad with fever, jaundice, and abdominal pain, as well as Reynolds' pentad with the addition of hypotension and altered mental status. There is no evidence of cholecystitis on ultrasonography. Placement of a cholecystostomy tube may be considered for urgent decompression of the gallbladder in patients who are in the intensive care unit and in whom ERCP cannot be performed due to hemodynamic instability. MRCP would be unlikely to change the diagnosis, is not therapeutic, and could delay definitive management.

5 A

This patient has annular pancreas, a condition in which the pancreatic parenchyma encircles the second portion of the duodenum. A 'double-bubble sign' on an abdominal X-ray is characteristic of annular pancreas. A double-bubble sign may also be seen with duodenal atresia. Duodenal atresia typically presents in neonates and is rarely diagnosed in childhood or adulthood. Cystic fibrosis typically presents in neonates, infants, and children. Gastrointestinal manifestations of cystic fibrosis include pancreatic insufficiency, steatorrhea, failure to thrive, and abdominal pain. Pancreas divisum does not present with duodenal narrowing and obstruction. Pancreatic heterotopia is often an incidental finding on endoscopy and does not cause obstructive symptoms.

Further Reading

Costanzo, L.S. (1998) *Physiology*, 1st edition, W.B. Saunders, Pennsylvania, pp. 289–333.

Pandol, S.J. (2016) Pancreatic secretion, in *Sleisenger and Fordtran's Gastrointestinal and Liver Disease: Pathophysiology/Diagnosis/Management*, 10th edition (eds M. Feldman, L.S. Friedman, and L.J. Brandt), Saunders Elsevier, Philadelphia, pp. 934–943.

Weblink

http://www.pancreapedia.org/reviews/anatomy-and-histology-of-pancreas

18

Acute Pancreatitis

Steven Keilin

Clinical Vignette

A 52-year-old woman presents with a 3-day history of nausea and upper abdominal pain. The pain is sharp, radiates to the back, and is associated with a decrease in appetite. She reports that over the previous weekend she was at a wedding and drank six glasses of wine. Her past medical history is remarkable for hypertension and dyslipidemia. Her medications include hydrochlorothiazide, niacin, and naproxen one to two tablets per week for joint pain. She has never had surgery. Her family history is remarkable for hypertension and diabetes mellitus in her father. She is married and has two children, who are healthy. She used to smoke cigarettes but quit 3 years ago. She has consumed one to two glasses of red wine daily for many years, and admits to binge drinking on occasion. On physical examination, the blood pressure is 124/78 mmHg, pulse rate 110 per minutes, and respiratory rate 12 per minute. She is afebrile. There are no cutaneous stigmata of liver disease, tattoos, or needle tracks. There is no conjunctival icterus. The abdomen is tender to palpation in the epigastrium, but there is no guarding or rebound tenderness. There is no hepatosplenomegaly. Bowel sounds are normal. Laboratory tests are significant for a white blood cell count of 16 500 mm^{-3}, serum aspartate aminotransferase (AST) 112 U l^{-1}, alanine aminotransferase (ALT) 38 U l^{-1}, alkaline phosphatase 78 U l^{-1}, and total bilirubin 0.8 mg dl^{-1}.

General

- Acute pancreatitis is an acute inflammatory condition of the pancreas that may extend to local and distant extrapancreatic tissues.
- The clinical diagnosis of is based on the presence of two of the following three features: (1) serum amylase and lipase levels elevated at least three

Sitaraman and Friedman's Essentials of Gastroenterology, Second Edition.
Edited by Shanthi Srinivasan and Lawrence S. Friedman.
© 2018 John Wiley & Sons Ltd. Published 2018 by John Wiley & Sons Ltd.

times the upper limit of normal; (2) epigastric abdominal pain (often radiating to the back); and (3) typical imaging features on contrast-enhanced computed tomography (CT) or magnetic resonance imaging (MRI).

- Acute pancreatitis accounts for more than 200,000 hospital admissions each year in the US.

The majority (80%) of cases of acute pancreatitis are caused by gallstones or alcohol.

Etiology

Gallstones

- Gallstones account for 45% of cases of acute pancreatitis.
- Acute pancreatitis develops in only 3–7% of patients with gallstones.
- In addition, microlithiasis (small [<3 mm] stones) and sludge (biliary debris) cause acute pancreatitis.
- Gallstones cause acute pancreatitis by obstructing the pancreatic duct, or through reflux of bile or debris from the bile duct into the pancreatic duct.

Alcohol

- Alcohol accounts for 30–35% of cases of acute pancreatitis.
- Acute pancreatitis typically occurs after binge drinking. About 10% of heavy drinkers will develop acute pancreatitis.
- Persons with acute pancreatitis due to alcohol may have underlying chronic pancreatitis (see Chapter 19).

Other Causes

- These account for 10–15% of cases of acute pancreatitis:
  - Hypertriglyceridemia (serum triglyceride level >1000 mg dl^{-1}): the third most common cause, accounts for 3–5% of cases of acute pancreatitis.
  - Hyperparathyroidism/hypercalcemia.
  - Medications (e.g., asparaginase, azathioprine, 6-mercaptopurine, cytarabine, exatanide, didanosine, enalapril, estrogen and tamoxifen, liraglutide, mesalamine, methyldopa, metronidazole, nonsteroidal anti-inflammatory drugs including sulindac, pentamidine, procainamide, sitagliptin, sulfonamides, tetracyclines, thiazides, valproic acid).

- Infections (e.g., tuberculosis, *Mycobacterium avium* complex, cytomeg-alovirus, Coxsackie virus, ascariasis).
- Vascular diseases (e.g., polyarteritis nodosa, systemic lupus erythematosus, ischemic damage to the pancreas).

Anatomic Causes

- Pancreas divisum: affects up to 7% of the population, but pancreatitis occurs in 15–20% of persons with pancreas divisum.
- Annular pancreas.
- Anomalous pancreaticobiliary junction.
- Sphincter of Oddi dysfunction.

Genetic Causes

- These are associated with chronic pancreatitis that may present acutely:
  - Cystic fibrosis.
  - Hereditary pancreatitis:
    - Protease serine 1 (PRSS1) (also called cationic trypsinogen): a mutation in the *PRSS1* gene renders trypsinogen resistant to autolysis, thereby leading to the activation of trypsinogen within the pancreas. It is responsible for the majority of hereditary cases (60–80%).
    - Serine protease inhibitor Kazal type 1 (SPINK1): a mutation in the *SPINK1* gene, which codes for trypsin inhibitor, leads to trypsin activation within the pancreas.

Iatrogenic Causes

- Postsurgical.
- Post-endoscopic retrograde cholangiopancreatography (post-ERCP): acute pancreatitis occurs in an estimated 5% of diagnostic ERCPs and in up 25% of persons with sphincter of Oddi dysfunction who undergo ERCP;
- Post-double balloon enteroscopy: occurs in ~1% of procedures.

Autoimmune Pancreatitis

- Often associated with concomitant autoimmune disorders such as Sjögren's syndrome, autoimmune thyroiditis, and Raynaud's disease:
- Type I: Antinuclear antibodies (ANA) may be positive; immunoglobulin (Ig) G4 levels are increased; other organs (bile ducts, salivary glands, kidneys,

lymph nodes, orbits) are often involved. Imaging may show an irregular main pancreatic duct or 'sausage-shaped' pancreas or mimic pancreatic adenocarcinoma. A lymphoplasmacytic infiltrate is seen on biopsy of the pancreas. Usually responds to treatment with glucocorticoids only.

- Type II: IgG4-negative; tends to affect the pancreas, but some patients may also have inflammatory bowel disease. On pancreatic biopsy, granulocyte epithelial lesions that often cause destruction of the pancreatic ducts are seen. Usually responds to treatment with glucocorticoids.

Pancreatic Cancer

- Adenocarcinoma, intraductal papillary mucinous neoplasm.

Idiopathic Acute Pancreatitis

- The cause of pancreatitis is unknown in 5–10% of cases.

Differential Diagnosis

- Peptic ulcer disease.
- Gastritis/gastropathy.
- Intestinal perforation.
- Acute cholecystitis.
- Mesenteric ischemia.
- Small intestinal obstruction.
- Ruptured abdominal aortic aneurysm.
- Acute hepatitis.

Pathophysiology

- Normal mechanisms that protect the pancreas (see also Chapter 17):
  - Activation of pancreatic proenzymes occurs outside the pancreas within the duodenal lumen.
  - Enterokinase, the enzyme responsible for activating pancreatic proenzymes, is located only in the duodenum.
  - Trypsin inhibitor (SPINK1) partially blocks the activity of trypsin.
- Mechanisms of injury in acute pancreatitis (Figure 18.1):
  - Activation of pancreatic proenzymes into active forms occurs within the pancreatic acinar cells, thereby leading to autodigestion of pancreatic tissue.
  - Failure of normal protective mechanisms to inactivate trypsin such as SPINK1 dysfunction.

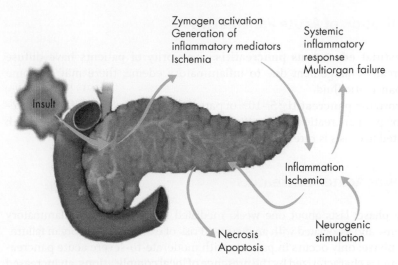

Figure 18.1 Mechanisms of injury in acute pancreatitis.

 - Microcirculatory injury and damage to the vascular endothelium in the pancreas lead to the activation of the complement system, release of proinflammatory mediators and cytokines and translocation of bacteria into the systemic circulation.

Clinical Features

Typical Symptoms

- Pain: 90–95% of patients with acute pancreatitis present with abdominal pain that is usually localized to the epigastrium and often radiates to the back. The pain may be worse after eating.
- Nausea and vomiting – in 80% of patients.
- Fever and chills may occur, but do not necessarily indicate infection.
- Anorexia and decreased appetite may also occur.

Physical Examination

- Common findings include tachycardia, fever, epigastric tenderness, localized guarding and rebound tenderness in the epigastrium, and decreased bowel sounds;
- Findings associated with severe pancreatitis include hypotension, jaundice, tachypnea, and a palpable mass (which may indicate a pseudocyst); pancreatic necrosis may track along the falciform ligament and into the retroperitoneum and can be seen as ecchymoses in the periumbilical region (Cullen's sign) and flanks (Grey–Turner's sign).

Classification of Acute Pancreatitis

- **Interstitial edematous pancreatitis**: a majority of patients have diffuse pancreatic enlargement due to inflammatory edema; there may be some peripancreatic fluid.
- **Necrotizing pancreatitis**: 5–10% of patients develop necrosis of the pancreatic or peripancreatic tissue, which can remain sterile or become infected; infected necrosis is rare during the first week of acute pancreatitis.

Phases of Acute Pancreatitis

- **Early phase**: lasts about one week, mediated by the systemic inflammatory response and associated with an increased risk of extrapancreatic organ failure.
- **Late phase**: only occurs in patients with moderate-to-severe acute pancreatitis, and is characterized by the presence of local complications, an increased risk of infection, and organ failure.

Complications

Local

- Pancreatic: ascites, fistula, peripancreatic fluid collection, pseudocyst, abscess, necrosis (sterile and infected).
- Nonpancreatic: bile duct obstruction, gastric outlet obstruction, duodenal ulcer, splenic and portal vein thrombosis.

Systemic

- Cardiovascular: hypotension, tachycardia, shock.
- Pulmonary: pleural effusion, pulmonary edema, acute respiratory distress syndrome (ARDS).
- Renal: decreased urine output, acute renal failure.
- Hematologic: vascular thrombosis, disseminated intravascular coagulation.
- Metabolic: metabolic acidosis, hyperglycemia, hypocalcemia.
- Infectious: sepsis, bacteremia, fungemia.
- Organ failure is best defined by the modified Marshall scoring system, which is based on pulmonary, cardiovascular, and renal dysfunction (Table 18.1).

Organisms most frequently seen in infected pancreatic necrosis include *Escherichia coli*, *Klebsiella* spp., *Pseudomonas* spp., *Enterococcus* spp., and rarely *Candida albicans*.

Table 18.1 Modified Marshall scoring system.

Organ system	Points				
	0	1	2	3	4
Respiratory (PaO_2/FiO_2)	>400	301–400	201–300	101–200	<101
Renal (serum Cr; mg dl^{-1})	<1.4	1.4–1.8	1.9–3.6	3.6–4.9	>4.9
Cardiovascular (systolic blood pressure; mmHg)	≥90	<90 fluid-responsive	<90 fluid-unresponsive	<90, pH <7.3	<90, pH <7.2

The score is the sum of the points for each organ system. A score of 2 or more in any system defines presence of organ failure.

Cr, creatinine; PaO_2, partial pressure of oxygen in arterial blood; FiO_2, fraction of inspired oxygen.

Prognosis

- The majority (75–80%) of cases of acute pancreatitis are mild and self-limiting.
- Some 20–25% of cases are severe, and despite aggressive efforts at initial resuscitation, up to 50% of these patients will develop multiorgan failure or pancreatic necrosis.
- The mortality rate in patients with severe acute pancreatitis is 10–30%.

Assessment of Severity

Several scoring systems have been developed to predict severity, in order to identify severe acute pancreatitis and predict pancreatic necrosis, mortality, and the need for prompt aggressive fluid resuscitation and intensive patient monitoring. The practical clinical application of these scoring systems has limitations.

- **Definition of severity**
  - Mild: absence of organ failure and absence of local/systemic complications.
  - Moderate severe: presence of transient (<48 hours) organ failure or local/systemic complications.
  - Severe: presence of persistent organ failure (>48 hours).
- **Ranson's criteria**: these are measured at admission and at 48 hours (Table 18.2). The presence of three or more criteria predicts a severe course and increased mortality.

Table 18.2 Ranson's criteria.

Admission	At 48 hours
Age >55 years	Hematocrit value decrease >10%
WBC >16 000 mm^{-3}	BUN increase >5 mg dl^{-1}
Serum glucose >200 mg dl^{-1}	Calcium <8 mg dl^{-1}
Serum LDH >350 U l^{-1}	Base deficit ≥4 mEq l^{-1}
Serum AST >250 U l^{-1}	Fluid sequestration >6 liters
	PaO$_2$ < 60 mmHg
No. of criteria	**Mortality (%)**
3–4	15
5–6	40
7–8	100

AST, aspartate aminotransferase; BUN, blood urea nitrogen; LDH, lactate dehydrogenase; PaO$_2$, partial pressure of oxygen in arterial blood; WBC, white blood cell count.

- **Acute Physiology and Chronic Health Evaluation (APACHE) III**
  - Used to predict mortality in critically ill patients admitted to the intensive care unit.
  - Can be measured at any time during the hospitalization.
  - Cumbersome method, some parameters may not be relevant to prognosis in acute pancreatitis.
- **CT severity index (Balthazar score):**
  - CT severity index utilizes the presence and degree of pancreatic necrosis and the presence or absence of peripancreatic fluid collections on CT to predict morbidity and mortality.
  - Limitations include variability in radiologists' interpretation of CT findings and lack of correlation of the score with the presence of organ failure, extrapancreatic complications, or peripancreatic vascular complications.
- **Atlanta classification:**
  - Original criteria (1992): developed to allow comparison among all aforementioned scoring systems (Ranson's, APACHE, and CT severity index); however, it only defines mild and severe acute pancreatitis.
  - Revised criteria (2012): defines criteria for diagnosis of acute pancreatitis, differentiates types of acute pancreatitis (interstitial edematous and necrotizing), classifies severity (mild, moderate, and severe), and defines morphology seen on imaging.

- **BISAP scoring system** (also called the Bedside Index of the Severity of Acute Pancreatitis):
  - Simple five-point scoring system: Blood urea nitrogen ($>25\,\text{mg}\,\text{dl}^{-1}$), Impaired mental status, Systemic inflammatory response (SIRS), Age ($>65\,\text{years}$), Pleural effusion.
  - BISAP is used to identify patients within the first 24 hours of admission at increased risk of in-hospital mortality.
- **HAPS** (Harmless Acute Pancreatitis Score):
  - Absence of rebound abdominal tenderness, a normal hematocrit value, and a normal serum creatinine level predict a nonsevere course with 98% accuracy.

Diagnosis

Pancreas-specific Laboratory Tests

- The diagnosis of acute pancreatitis relies on elevation of serum amylase and lipase levels greater than threefold the upper limit of normal. The tests are not specific for acute pancreatitis (Tables 18.3 and 18.4).
  - Amylase tends to rise earlier, within hours, and can remain elevated for 3–5 days.

Table 18.3 Causes of hyperamylasemia other than acute pancreatitis.

Ectopic pregnancy
Intestinal perforation
Macroamylasemia
Medications
Mesenteric ischemia
Parotitis/salivary gland disease
Peptic ulcer disease
Renal failure

Table 18.4 Causes of hyperlipasemia other than acute pancreatitis.

Gastritis/gastroenteritis
Intestinal obstruction
Intestinal perforation
Liver disease
Medications (e.g., chemotherapeutic agents)
Peptic ulcer disease

- Lipase is more specific for pancreatic disease and may remain elevated for longer periods than amylase.
- The degree of pancreatic enzyme elevation or trend over time does not correlate with the patient's prognosis.

Other Tests

- **Liver biochemical tests**:
  - Elevations of serum bilirubin and alkaline phosphatase levels are often seen with gallstone pancreatitis (see Chapter 21).
  - Greater than threefold elevation of the serum alanine aminotransferase (ALT) level is highly specific, but not sensitive for gallstone pancreatitis.
  - Elevation of the serum aspartate aminotransferase (AST) level greater than the serum ALT level may indicate acute pancreatitis due to alcohol consumption.
- The white blood cell (WBC) count is commonly elevated; however, an elevated WBC count does not necessarily indicate infection.
- Hyper/hypoglycemia, hypocalcemia, and renal insufficiency are of prognostic significance.
- Serum triglyceride levels should be checked; levels >1000 mg dl^{-1} may indicate hypertriglyceridemia as the cause of pancreatitis.

Imaging

Abdominal X-Ray

- Plain films of the abdomen are often normal in acute pancreatitis; however, they are used to exclude other causes of abdominal pain.
- May show ileus ('sentinel loop'), displacement or abnormal contour of other organs such as the stomach and colon ('colon cut-off sign'), gallstones, or pancreatic calcifications.

Ultrasonography

- Used to identify gallstones.
- May also show bile duct dilatation, ascites, or decreased echogenicity of the pancreas.
- Findings specific to acute pancreatitis may be seen and include pancreatic enlargement and inflammatory changes around the pancreas.
- Overlying bowel gas often obscures the pancreas, ultrasonography is a poor test to diagnose acute pancreatitis.

Computed Tomography (CT) (with Intravenous Contrast; Figure 18.2)

- CT is usually not necessary initially; however, it should be obtained if the patient is not improving clinically or to rule out other intra-abdominal disorders.
- CT may be used to:
  - Exclude other intra-abdominal disorders.
  - Assess the severity of pancreatitis.
  - Determine if complications are present: the presence of extraluminal gas in the pancreatic and/or peripancreatic tissues is indicative of infected necrosis.
- CT is useful for detecting:
  - Bile duct stones and bile duct dilatation.
  - Pancreatic pseudocysts.
  - Pancreatic necrosis and fluid collections (with administration of intravenous contrast).
- CT can be used to guide needle aspiration or biopsy to assess for infected pancreatic necrosis.

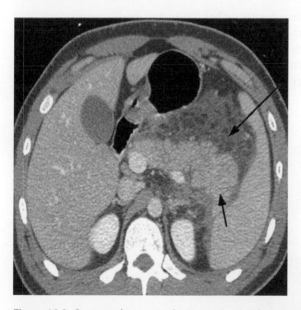

Figure 18.2 Computed tomography in a patient with acute pancreatitis. Findings include focal or diffuse pancreatic enlargement (short arrow), heterogeneous enhancement of the pancreas, obliteration of fat planes around the pancreas, and peripancreatic fluid collections (long arrow).

- Contraindications to performing CT include:
  - Contrast allergy.
  - Renal insufficiency.

Magnetic Resonance Imaging (MRI) and Magnetic Resonance Cholangiopancreatography (MRCP)

- MRI/MRCP uses gadolinium as a contrast agent; therefore, the test can be used in patients with an allergy to contrast dye.
- MRI/MRCP is useful for detecting:
  - Bile duct stones and bile duct dilatation.
  - Pancreas divisum.
  - Pancreatic duct disruption.
  - Pancreatic cysts and neoplasms.
  - Pancreatic necrosis.
- MRI/MRCP-guided needle biopsies are now utilized at some centers.

Endoscopic Retrograde Cholangiopancreatography (ERCP)

- ERCP is preferable as a therapeutic rather than a purely diagnostic tool.
- ERCP should be used with caution in patients with severe acute pancreatitis, because acute pancreatitis may worsen with the procedure.
- ERCP is useful for detecting and treating:
  - Bile duct stones (Figure 18.3) or microlithiasis.
  - Bile duct stricture.
  - Pancreas divisum.

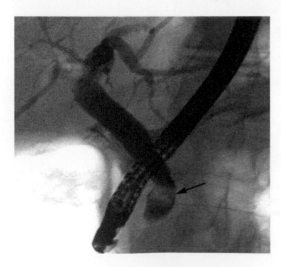

Figure 18.3 Endoscopic retrograde cholangiopancreatography showing a bile duct stone. A filling defect is seen in the distal bile duct (arrow) with dilatation of the bile duct proximal to the stone.

- Pancreatic duct disruption.
- Sphincter of Oddi dysfunction.
- Commonly performed interventions include:
  - Bile duct stone removal.
  - Stent placement to relieve bile duct obstruction or treat pancreatic duct disruption.

Treatment

Prevention

- Preventive strategies include cessation of alcohol and smoking and discontinuation of potentially causative medications.
- In high-risk patients undergoing ERCP, placement of a prophylactic pancreatic duct stent or administration of rectal indomethacin reduces the risk of pancreatitis.

Conservative and Supportive Care

- The majority (80%) of cases will resolve with supportive measures.
- Aggressive fluid resuscitation with Ringer's lactate or normal saline $250–300\,\text{ml}\,\text{h}^{-1}$ intravenously for the first 48 hours has been the mainstay of management of acute pancreatitis. Ringer's lactate may be preferable. However, >4 liters per day may have adverse outcomes, and a rate of $125–175\,\text{ml}\,\text{h}^{-1}$ may be appropriate.
- Patients should be given nothing by mouth.
- Nasogastric decompression should be considered in patients who have protracted vomiting.
- Electrolyte abnormalities should be corrected.
- Analgesics and anti-emetics should be given as needed.

Nutrition

- An oral diet may be initiated if the patient's pain is improved and appetite returns.
  - Start with clear liquids and advance to a low-fat diet.
- If the patient's symptoms do not improve within 72 hours, parenteral or enteral feeding should be initiated.
- Total parenteral nutrition (TPN):
  - Has been used widely in the past.
  - Does not stimulate pancreatic secretion.
  - Has been shown to decrease mortality.

- However, TPN is expensive and is associated with complications such as line infection, thrombophlebitis, electrolyte disturbances, and liver dysfunction (including cholestasis).
- Enteral nutrition through a nasogastric or nasojejunal feeding tube:
  - May stimulate pancreatic secretion.
  - Is less expensive than TPN.
  - Maintains intestinal integrity and prevents intestinal atrophy.
  - Reduces the rate of infections and shortens the length of hospitalization.
- Enteral nutrition is preferred to TPN. There appears to be no difference in efficacy between nasojejunal and nasogastric feeding.

Antibiotics

- Antibiotics are recommended in the following situations:
  - Persistent fever or leukocytosis while the source is being identified.
  - Acute necrotic pancreatic collection, both sterile (controversial) and infected.
  - Bacteremia.
  - Infected pancreatic pseudocyst.
  - Walled-off pancreatic necrosis.
- Antibiotics that have good pancreatic penetration include imipenem, meropenem, cefepime, and moxifloxacin.

> The routine use of prophylactic antibiotics is not recommended for mild acute pancreatitis, and is controversial in severe acute pancreatitis. Routine use of antibiotics does not affect the rate of infection or mortality. Use of antibiotics also increases the risk of fungal infections and infections with resistant bacteria.

Gallstones and Bile Duct Stones

- Indications for ERCP:
  - Severe acute gallstone pancreatitis in a hemodynamically stable patient.
  - Cholangitis.
  - Recurrent idiopathic pancreatitis: rule out microlithiasis, sphincter of Oddi dysfunction, or pancreas divisum.
  - If required during pregnancy, it is safest to do ERCP during the second trimester.
- Cholecystectomy for gallstone pancreatitis:
  - Recurrent pancreatitis occurs in about 30% of patients with gallstone pancreatitis; therefore, cholecystectomy is recommended.
  - Cholecystectomy should be performed during the hospitalization for acute pancreatitis, if possible, or within 2–4 weeks of discharge.

Pancreatic Ascites

- Patients should be placed on TPN.
- Octreotide administered intravenously has been shown to be beneficial.
- Antibiotics may be used, but the benefit is unclear.
- Diuretics are not helpful.
- Drainage options include:
  - Endoscopic stent placement into the pancreatic duct to bridge the leak or relieve duct obstruction.
  - Percutaneous drainage.
  - Surgical drainage.

Pancreatic Pseudocyst

- Pseudocysts usually take >4 weeks to mature. Immediate intervention is usually not necessary.
- Indications for drainage: worsening abdominal pain, infected pseudocyst, gastric outlet or bile duct obstruction, associated leak.
- Drainage may performed percutaneously, endoscopically (transgastric or transpapillary), or surgically.

Acute Necrotic Collection and Walled-off Necrosis

- Asymptomatic patients with a sterile necrotic fluid collection and walled-off necrosis do not require antibiotics.
- Antibiotics alone are indicated if the patient is minimally symptomatic.
- Antibiotics in conjunction with a drainage procedure with or without debridement (necrosectomy) are indicated for symptomatic or infected acute necrotic collection or walled-off necrosis or if the patient is not improving clinically.
- Drainage can be endoscopic or percutaneous.
- Endoscopic debridement is preferred over surgical debridement.

Pearls
<ul><li>Acute pancreatitis is a potentially fatal disease with a mortality rate of 5–10%.</li><li>Some 80% of all cases are caused by gallstones or alcohol.</li><li>The diagnosis of acute pancreatitis relies on elevations in serum amylase and lipase levels more than threefold times the upper limit of normal, in conjunction with epigastric pain and imaging evidence of pancreatitis.</li></ul>

- Patients with acute pancreatitis need hospitalization with close monitoring and frequent clinical assessment.
- Treatment of acute pancreatitis relies mainly on supportive care, which includes intravenous fluids, parenteral analgesia, anti-emetics, and attention to the patient's nutritional status.
- Antibiotics should be reserved for patients with a documented infection or symptomatic or infected acute necrotic collection or walled-off necrosis.

Questions

Question 1 relates to the clinical vignette at the beginning of the chapter.

1   The best next test to perform to make a diagnosis is which of the following:
   A Endoscopic retrograde cholangiopancreatography.
   B Serum amylase and lipase levels.
   C Abdominal ultrasonography.
   D Esophagogastroduodenoscopy.
   E Magnetic resonance imaging (MRI).

2   A 27-year-old obese woman with a history of diabetes mellitus, hypertension, dyslipidemia, and a prior cholecystectomy presents with her third episode of acute pancreatitis. There is no family history of pancreatitis or pancreatic cancer. Which of the following is the LEAST likely cause of acute pancreatitis in this patient?
   A Sitagliptin.
   B Hypertriglyceridemia.
   C Idiopathic pancreatitis.
   D Hereditary pancreatitis.
   E Sphincter of Oddi dysfunction.

3   A 53-year-old man has been hospitalized for 6 days with acute alcoholic pancreatitis. He is febrile (101.9 °F [38.7 °C]). The white blood cell count is 21 500 mm^{-3} and serum creatinine level 2.4 mg dl^{-1}. His abdominal pain is worsening. What of the following is not indicated at this time?
   A Nothing to eat by mouth.
   B Antibiotics.
   C Computed tomography (CT) of the abdomen.
   D Blood cultures.
   E MRI of the abdomen.

4 Enteral nutrition has been shown to be more beneficial than parenteral nutrition in severe or prolonged acute pancreatitis. The benefits of enteral nutrition compared with parenteral nutrition include all of the following EXCEPT that enteral nutrition:

A Does not stimulate pancreatic secretion.
B Shortens the length of hospitalization.
C Maintains intestinal integrity.
D Lowers the rate of infection.
E Is less expensive than parenteral nutrition.

5 In which of the following patients with acute pancreatitis should antibiotics be started?

A A patient with a fever of 100.5 °F (38 °C) on admission.
B A patient with a large asymptomatic pseudocyst.
C A patient with a white blood cell count of $22\,500\,mm^{-3}$ on admission.
D A patient with persistent abdominal pain on day 4 of hospitalization.
E A patient with continued abdominal pain and walled off necrosis on CT.

Answers

1 B

Elevated serum amylase or lipase levels in a patient with abdominal pain typical of acute pancreatitis will confirm the diagnosis of acute pancreatitis. Amylase and lipase are not included in a comprehensive metabolic panel and have to be ordered separately. Abdominal imaging is not necessary initially but should be obtained if the patient does not improve or requires evaluation for other causes of abdominal pain if the serum amylase and lipase are normal. Once a diagnosis of acute pancreatitis is made, abdominal ultrasonography is indicated to look for gallstones, and CT may be indicated in patients with severe acute pancreatitis.

2 D

All of the choices are likely causes of acute pancreatitis except hereditary pancreatitis. The patient does not have a family history of pancreatitis or pancreatic cancer.

3 C

The patient's elevated white blood cell count and persistent abdominal pain are concerning for complications of acute pancreatitis such as pancreatic necrosis, a fluid collection, or an abscess. Abdominal imaging should be performed. Intravenous contrast is contraindicated because of renal failure.

MRI (without gadolinium) is an alternative approach. The patient should have nothing to eat by mouth and have blood cultures drawn; antibiotics may be initiated.

4 A

Enteral nutrition, in contrast to parenteral nutrition, has the potential to stimulate pancreatic secretion. Nevertheless, enteral feeding has several advantages over parenteral nutrition and is the preferred method of nutrition in patients with severe acute pancreatitis.

5 E

Antibiotics are recommended for persistent fever or persistent leukocytosis, while the source is being identified; symptomatic or infected acute necrotic collection or walled-off necrosis; bacteremia; or an infected pancreatic pseudocyst.

Further Reading

Banks, P.A., Bollen, T.L., Dervenis, C., *et al.* (2013) Classification of acute pancreatitis-2012: revision of the Atlanta classification and definitions by international consensus. *Gut*, **62**, 102–111.

Loveday, B.P., Srinivasa, S., Vather, R., *et al.* (2010) High quantity and variable quality of guidelines for acute pancreatitis: a systematic review. *American Journal of Gastroenterology*, **105**, 1466–1476.

Singh, V.K., Bollen, T.L., Wu, B.U., *et al.* (2011) An assessment of the severity of interstitial pancreatitis. *Clinical Gastroenterology and Hepatology*, **9**, 1098–1103.

Tenner, S. and Steinberg, W.M. (2016) Acute pancreatitis, in *Sleisenger and Fordtran's Gastrointestinal and Liver Disease: Pathophysiology/Diagnosis/Management*, 10th edition (eds M. Feldman, L.S. Friedman, and L.J. Brandt), Saunders Elsevier, Philadelphia, pp. 969–993.

Weblinks

http://www.nlm.nih.gov/medlineplus/ency/article/000287.htm
http://emedicine.medscape.com/article/181364-overview
http://gi.org/guideline/acute-pancreatitis/

19

Chronic Pancreatitis

Anthony M. Gamboa and Qiang Cai

Clinical Vignette

A 47-year-old man is seen in the office for a 10-month history of abdominal pain. The pain is localized to the epigastrium and radiates to the back, is worse with eating, and is associated with nausea. Over the past 8 months he has had an unintentional weight loss of 15 lb (6.8 kg) and six episodes of oily-appearing diarrhea per day. He takes ibuprofen for the abdominal pain, with minimal relief. The past medical history includes hypertension, type 2 diabetes mellitus, and depression. For the past 25 years, he has consumed approximately six beers daily and has smoked one pack of cigarettes per day. On physical examination, the vital signs are within normal limits. There is mild abdominal tenderness in the epigastric area with no rebound tenderness or guarding. Bowel sounds are normal. There is no organomegaly. Laboratory tests reveal a normal complete blood count, glucose 206 mg dl^{-1}, aspartate aminotransferase 180 U l^{-1}, alanine aminotransferase 101 U l^{-1}, amylase 105 U l^{-1}, and lipase 210 U l^{-1}. A plain abdominal film reveals calcifications in the mid-upper abdomen. Computed tomography is remarkable for coarse calcifications of the pancreas and a dilated pancreatic duct with a diameter of 5 mm. A 2×2 cm fluid collection is noted adjacent to the pancreas.

General

- Chronic pancreatitis (CP) is defined as irreversible injury to the pancreas caused by chronic inflammation and fibrosis leading to impairment of the exocrine and endocrine functions of the pancreas (Figure 19.1).
- The incidence of CP in the US is 3–10 cases per 100 000 persons, with a prevalence of 27–35 per 100 000.

Sitaraman and Friedman's Essentials of Gastroenterology, Second Edition.
Edited by Shanthi Srinivasan and Lawrence S. Friedman.
© 2018 John Wiley & Sons Ltd. Published 2018 by John Wiley & Sons Ltd.

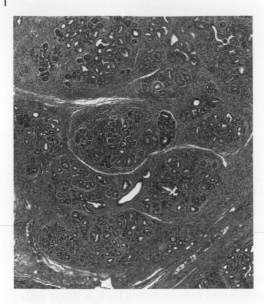

Figure 19.1 Histopathology of chronic pancreatitis, demonstrating atrophy and interstitial fibrosis. Hematoxylin and eosin staining, original magnification ×40.

Etiology and Pathogenesis

- **Alcohol**
  - The majority of cases of CP in Western countries are caused by chronic alcoholism. The median age of onset of CP is 36 years.
  - Most patients have a history of drinking 150 g per day for at least 5–10 years (a standard 12-ounce [350 ml] beer contains approximately 18 g of alcohol).
  - CP develops in only 5–10% of heavy drinkers. Proposed cofactors that contribute to the development of CP include genetic variations, including polymorphisms of proteins involved in cellular antioxidant defense or alcohol metabolism, consumption of high-protein and high-fat diets, hyperlipidemia, exposure to bacterial endotoxins, and smoking.
  - The pathogenesis may follow a necrosis–fibrosis pathway, in which repeated episodes of acute pancreatitis lead to irreversible fibrosis and atrophy. This is also referred to as the SAPE (sentinel acute pancreatitis event) hypothesis. Alcohol also causes zymogens to be activated prematurely, leading to autodigestion of the pancreas. Finally, alcohol use causes increased secretion of proteins and ionized calcium from acinar cells with a relative decrease in bicarbonate secretion; this leads to precipitation of proteins and obstruction of ductules.

- **Tobacco**
  - Smoking is also an independent risk factor for the development of CP and leads to the rapid development of pancreatic calcifications.
- **Idiopathic**
  - Some 10–30% of cases of CP are idiopathic. Contributing factors include genetic abnormalities (see later), modest alcohol consumption in susceptible patients, surreptitious alcohol use, trauma, and smoking.
- **Obstruction**
  - Chronic obstruction of the pancreatic duct can cause CP proximal to the obstruction, and relief of the obstruction occasionally reverses damage to the pancreas.
  - Causes of obstruction include pancreatic, ductal, or ampullary tumors, benign ductal strictures, and pancreatic divisum with stenosis of the minor papilla.
  - In Eastern countries, bile duct disorders, such as gallstone disease, are thought to be a major cause of CP.
- **Tropical pancreatitis**
  - Tropical pancreatitis is the most common form of CP in southwest India and other tropical areas including Africa, southeast Asia, and Brazil.
  - The etiology is unknown, but there is an association with mutations in the serine protease inhibitor Kazal type 1 (*SPINK1*) gene, which encodes a trypsin inhibitor and thereby leads to trypsin activation within the pancreas.
- **Hereditary pancreatitis**
  - Hereditary CP is associated with mutation of the protease serine 1 (*PRSS1*) gene, and is transmitted in an autosomal dominant manner with a penetrance of 80%.
  - The *PRSS1* gene encodes trypsinogen, and mutations lead to increased autoactivation of trypsin within the pancreas. This allows increased activation of various zymogens to their active proteolytic forms, leading in turn to autodigestion of the pancreas.
  - Other mutations may act as cofactors or increase susceptibility to or the severity of CP. These include mutations in *SPINK1* and the cystic fibrosis transmembrane conductance regulator (*CFTR*) genes.
- **Autoimmune pancreatitis**
  - Autoimmune pancreatitis is a chronic inflammatory and fibrosing disease of the pancreas.
  - The characteristic feature of autoimmune pancreatitis is a lymphoplasmacytic infiltration of the pancreas and other organs (bile duct, salivary glands, retroperitoneum). The inflammatory cells often express immunoglobulin (Ig)G4.
- **Metabolic disorders**
  - Hypertriglyceridemia and hypercalcemia are associated with CP.

Up to 70% of cases of CP in Western countries are caused by alcohol; however, only 5–10% of alcoholics develop chronic pancreatitis. A convenient mnemonic for the causes of CP is TIGAR-O: toxic–metabolic, idiopathic, genetic, autoimmune, recurrent and severe acute pancreatitis, or obstructive.

Clinical Features

- **Abdominal pain**
  - Abdominal pain is the most common symptom of CP and detracts significantly from the quality of life of patients with CP. The pain is typically epigastric and may radiate to the back and sometimes around to the flanks in a band-like manner. The pain is worse with eating, and may be associated with nausea and vomiting.
  - Pain may be absent in some patients who present with pancreatic insufficiency.
- **Malabsorption**
  - *Exocrine pancreatic insufficiency* typically occurs after acinar cell reserve is reduced by 90%. With inadequate lipase, fat maldigestion and steatorrhea occur. Patients may have loose, oily stools with a foul odor.
  - Osteopenia and osteoporosis are common due to malabsorption of vitamin D. Deficiencies in other fat-soluble vitamins – A, E, and K – and vitamin B_{12} may also occur.
  - Protein and carbohydrate deficiencies may occur at later stages and to a lesser degree than fat maldigestion.
- **Impaired glucose tolerance and diabetes mellitus**
  - Impaired glucose tolerance resulting in diabetes mellitus results from destruction of the islet cells and is similar to type I diabetes mellitus; however, alpha cells are also destroyed, so patients lose the ability to secrete glucagon, thereby making hypoglycemia more common and more severe.
- **Physical examination**
  - The only consistent finding on physical examination is epigastric tenderness.

Diagnosis

- **Imaging**
  - Imaging studies are frequently diagnostic in advanced disease. Diagnosing early CP is difficult.
  - **Plain abdominal films** show calcifications in about 30% of patients with CP. This finding, combined with loss of pancreatic function, can be diagnostic of CP. Calcifications develop over 5–25 years and are most common with alcoholic and tropical CP.

Figure 19.2 Magnetic resonance image (MRI) showing changes of chronic pancreatitis with a large pancreatic pseudocyst (arrow).

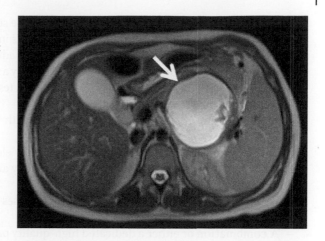

- **Transabdominal ultrasonography** is frequently limited by inadequate visualization of the pancreas due to body habitus or overlying bowel and is not routinely useful.
- **Computed tomography (CT)** findings include calcifications, ductal stones, abnormal size of the pancreas, a dilated pancreatic duct, and pseudocysts (Figure 19.2). Sensitivity and specificity are over 80%.
- **Endoscopic retrograde cholangiopancreatography (ERCP)** has a sensitivity and specificity of 70–90% and 80–100%, respectively, but use of ERCP purely for diagnostic purposes is limited by the potential for complications. Pancreatography reveals ductal abnormalities including stenoses, dilatation (normal diameter of the main pancreatic duct is up to 3 mm), and irregularities of the main pancreatic duct and its side branches. ERCP is typically used for therapeutic interventions, such as placement of stents through stenoses or removal of ductal stones from the pancreatic duct.
- **Magnetic resonance imaging (MRI) with magnetic resonance cholangiopancreatography (MRCP)** is noninvasive and has a sensitivity and specificity comparable to those of ERCP.
- **Endoscopic ultrasonography (EUS)** is highly sensitive and specific for detecting CP. Compared with ERCP, EUS has a lower risk of complications and can detect abnormalities suggestive of CP in the pancreatic parenchyma and ductal system that may not be visible with other imaging modalities.
- **Tests of pancreatic function**
  - Exocrine pancreatic insufficiency can be identified directly by sampling duodenal contents for pancreatic secretions after administration of secretin or cholecystokinin. Over a 1-hour intraduodenal collection, a bicarbonate concentration of $<80\,\mathrm{mEq\,l^{-1}}$ is diagnostic of CP. This method is sensitive and can be useful in early CP, but it is not widely available.

- Indirect measures of exocrine dysfunction include serum trypsinogen, fecal chymotrypsin, and fecal elastase levels. Low levels indicate exocrine insufficiency, but these tests are unreliable until CP is advanced. Of the indirect tests, fecal elastase is widely available, requires only a single stool sample, and may be the most sensitive and specific of the fecal tests for diagnosing CP.
- **Other laboratory studies**
  - A 72-hour stool fat quantitation in patients with CP is typically greater than 7 g per day.
  - Serum amylase and lipase levels may be slightly elevated in patients with symptomatic exacerbations of CP, but often they are normal.
- **Diagnostic approach** (Figure 19.3)
  - Fecal elastase is noninvasive and helpful in cases of suspected exocrine insufficiency.
  - A combination or either a dedicated high-quality pancreas protocol CT or MRI/MRCP and/or EUS is recommended.

> The diagnosis of CP depends largely on identifying characteristic clinical features by history, often in the setting of chronic alcohol abuse. Diagnostic tests for CP may be classified as those that detect abnormalities of pancreatic structure (imaging tests) and those that detect abnormalities of pancreatic function.

Treatment

- CP can cause a significant reduction in a patient's quality of life, and treatment should focus on alleviating symptoms (see Figure 19.3).
- Patients should undergo imaging evaluation for the presence of complicating or concurrent factors, including pseudocysts, biliary stricture, or pancreatic cancer.
- General treatment recommendations include abstaining from alcohol and smoking and eating small, frequent low-fat meals to limit pancreatic enzyme secretion and to reduce symptoms of malabsorption.
  - Medical treatment for pain includes:
    o Acetaminophen or nonsteroidal anti-inflammatory drugs (NSAIDs).
    o Uncoated pancreatic enzymes, which suppress the release of cholecystokinin, the hormone that stimulates pancreatic secretion.
    o Tricyclic antidepressant drugs, selective serotonin reuptake inhibitors, serotonin and norepinephrine reuptake inhibitors, gabapentin, or pregabalin.
    o Opioid analgesics; however, narcotic addiction is a major risk in patients with CP. Pain management clinics that emphasize non-narcotic approaches may be helpful.

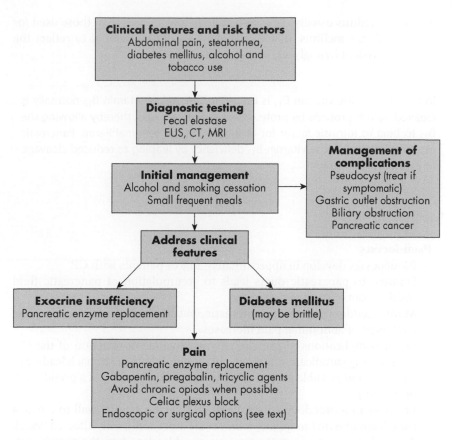

Figure 19.3 Algorithm for the diagnosis and treatment of chronic pancreatitis. CT, computed tomography; EUS, endoscopic ultrasonography; MRI, magnetic resonance imaging.

  - Surgical or endoscopic treatments include celiac plexus block, endoscopic stenting of the pancreatic duct, pancreatic duct stone removal, sphincter-otomy, and surgical resection or decompression of the pancreatic duct. Extracorporeal shock wave lithotripsy may also be helpful in cases of pancreatic duct stones.
- Maldigestion and steatorrhea:
  - Pancreatic enzyme replacement with enterically-coated formulations that contain at least 40 000 U of lipase with each meal is recommended.
  - Nonenteric-coated pancreatic enzymes may be inactivated in the acidic environment of the stomach; therefore, a proton pump inhibitor or histamine H_2 receptor antagonist is usually used in conjunction with such preparations.

- Diabetes mellitus usually requires insulin in lower doses than those used for type I diabetes mellitus. Insulin regimens should be tailored to reflect the increased risk of hypoglycemia in patients with CP.

> In the duodenum, vitamin B_{12} is bound to R-proteins. Vitamin B_{12} normally is cleaved from R-proteins by proteases from the pancreas, thereby allowing the B_{12} to bind to intrinsic factor for absorption in the terminal ileum. Pancreatic insufficiency may cause vitamin B_{12} deficiency by leading to reduced cleavage of B_{12} from R-proteins.

Complications

- **Pseudocysts**
  - Pseudocysts develop in approximately 25% of patients with CP.
  - Damage to pancreatic ducts leads to accumulation of pancreatic fluid inside or outside of the pancreas.
  - Many pseudocysts are asymptomatic, but as they increase in size, the likelihood of abdominal pain increases.
  - Other complications of pseudocysts may include obstruction of the bile duct causing jaundice, compression of the duodenum or stomach leading to vomiting and possible gastric outlet obstruction, infection of a pseudocyst, or bleeding.
  - Enzymes in a pseudocyst may digest an adjacent arterial wall to create a pseudoaneurysm; the splenic artery is the most commonly affected vessel. A pseudoaneurysm may rupture, causing bleeding into the pseudocyst, adjacent viscera, or the peritoneal cavity. They may also bleed into the pancreatic duct, causing hemosuccus pancreaticus, which may present as gastrointestinal bleeding.
  - Ultrasonography, CT, and MRI are used to diagnose pseudocysts.
  - The indications for draining a pseudocyst include rapid enlargement, persistent pain, compression of surrounding structures, marked early satiety, and infection. Transgastric or transduodenal endoscopic drainage with placement of conventional stents or lumen-apposing stents is often the preferred approach. Drainage may also be achieved by a percutaneous or surgical approach.
- **Pancreatic ascites and pleural effusion**
  - Disruption of the pancreatic duct or rupture of a pseudocyst can lead to accumulation of pancreatic fluid in the pleural or peritoneal space.
  - Diagnostic paracentesis or thoracentesis will reveal fluid with an elevated amylase level, usually higher than 1000 U l^{-1}.
  - Treatment includes withholding oral feeding to minimize pancreatic secretions. Diuretics, serial paracentesis or thoracentesis, and octreotide

are also used. Many patients benefit from endoscopic placement of a stent across a disrupted pancreatic duct. In some cases, surgical intervention is required.

- **Biliary or duodenal obstruction**
  - Obstruction of the bile duct or the duodenum occurs at rates of 10% and 5%, respectively. Obstruction may be caused by a pseudocyst or by fibrosis and inflammation in the pancreatic head.
  - Diagnostic studies include ERCP or MRCP for biliary obstruction and CT, upper endoscopy, or an upper gastrointestinal series for duodenal obstruction.
  - Treatment may include drainage of an obstructing pseudocyst, endoscopic stenting of a biliary obstruction, or surgery.
- **Splenic vein thrombosis**
  - Pancreatic inflammation can cause thrombosis of the splenic vein, which courses along the posterior aspect of the pancreas.
  - Splenic vein thrombosis may lead to isolated gastric varices.
  - Splenectomy is curative and is indicated for bleeding gastric varices.
- **Pancreatic cancer**
  - Patients with CP are at an increased risk for developing pancreatic cancer. The risk is about 4% after 20 years.

Prognosis

- The quality of life of patients with CP is significantly worse than that of the general population. Tobacco use and ongoing alcohol use predict a worse prognosis.
- Abdominal pain often abates after 10 years or more of CP; frequently this coincides with the development of pancreatic insufficiency. The mortality ratio is approximately 3.6 : 1 when compared with patients without CP. Continued alcohol use increases the mortality rate by another 60%.
- The survival rate is about 70% at 10 years, and 45% at 20 years. Most patients die from an associated condition, such as complications from continued alcohol use or smoking, or from pancreatic cancer or postoperative complications.

Pearls
• The diagnosis of chronic pancreatitis requires a high index of clinical suspicion in a patient presenting with chronic abdominal pain.
• Pain management is an important component of treatment of chronic pancreatitis.
• Tobacco use and ongoing alcohol use predict a worse prognosis, and patients should be encouraged to stop smoking and alcohol consumption.

Questions

Questions 1 and 2 relate to the clinical vignette at the beginning of this chapter.

1 The patient continues to drink beer and returns to clinic complaining of intractable vomiting and a 20-lb weight loss. Repeat CT scan shows a 10-cm pseudocyst adjacent to the pancreas compressing the stomach and duodenum. Which of the following is the best management approach to this patient?

  A Magnetic resonance cholangiopancreatography (MRCP).
  B Antibiotics.
  C Duodenal stent placement for gastric outlet obstruction.
  D Percutaneous aspiration of the pseudocyst to rule out infection.
  E Endoscopic ultrasonographic (EUS)- guided placement of a lumen-apposing stent from the stomach to the pseudocyst.

2 The patient presents to the ER with black tarry stools and syncope. EGD shows blood in the stomach and duodenum but no actively bleeding lesion. What is the best next step in diagnosis?

  A MRCP.
  B Endoscopic retrograde cholangiopancreatography (ERCP).
  C Tagged red blood cell scan.
  D Capsule endoscopy.
  E CT angiography.

3 A 55-year-old man with alcoholic chronic pancreatitis presents to the emergency department with hematemesis for the past hour. His blood pressure is 92/63 mmHg, pulse rate 115 per minute, and respiratory rate 18 per minute. He is afebrile. He has a history of chronic pancreatitis. Upper endoscopy reveals bleeding gastric varices. What is the appropriate treatment?

  A Endoscopic banding of gastric varices.
  B Splenectomy.
  C Endoscopic placement of hemoclips across gastric varices.
  D Blakemore tube placement.

4 A 58-year-old woman is referred for evaluation of a recent 30-lb weight loss and abnormal liver biochemical test results. She has a known history of chronic pancreatitis related to chronic tobacco use, and she takes pancreatic enzyme replacement for malabsorption and steatorrhea. On physical examination, she appears cachectic. There is mild tenderness in the epigastrium. Liver biochemical tests show a total bilirubin 1.1 mg dl^{-1}, alkaline phosphatase 203 U l^{-1}, aspartate aminotransferase 42 U l^{-1}, and alanine

aminotransferase 51 U l^{-1}. CT of the abdomen shows calcifications in the head and body of the pancreas. The bile duct is 7 mm in diameter compared with 5 mm on a previous imaging study 2 years earlier. Which of the following is the next best recommendation?

A EUS.

B ERCP.

C Percutaneous biopsy of the pancreatic head.

D Liver biopsy.

5 A 24-year-old woman presents with 3-month history of epigastric pain, nausea, and steatorrhea. Abdominal imaging shows pancreatic calcifications and a dilated pancreatic duct consistent with chronic pancreatitis. The patient moved to the US from southern India 2 months ago. She denies alcohol use. Which of the following is the most likely cause of her condition?

A Hereditary pancreatitis.

B Alcoholic chronic pancreatitis.

C Tropical pancreatitis.

D Gallstone disease.

E Autoimmune pancreatitis.

6 A 59-year-old man with alcoholic chronic pancreatitis presents with a complaint of oily stools seven or eight times per day. Which of the following is the most appropriate initial step in management?

A Loperamide.

B Psyllium fiber.

C Probiotics.

D Enteric-coated pancreatic enzyme replacement.

Answers

1 E

The patient is presenting with a gastric outlet obstruction caused by compression from the large pseudocyst. Appropriate therapy is endoscopic drainage of the symptomatic pseudocyst, which is commonly accomplished by stent placement under EUS guidance.

2 B

Patients with pseudocysts are at risk for having bleeding from either vessels within the pseudocyst or from pseudoaneurysm formation related to erosion of the pseudocyst into an adjacent vessel. The first step in diagnosis is EGD. If there is evidence of hemosuccus pancreaticus, or if no bleeding lesion is seen in the upper GI tract, the next diagnostic study should be CT angiography to look for pseudoaneurysm formation or blood in the pseudocyst. Appropriate treatment would involve embolization of a pseudoaneurysm by interventional radiology.

3 B

Pancreatic inflammation can cause thrombosis of the splenic vein, which courses along the posterior aspect of the pancreas. Splenic vein thrombosis may cause gastric varices. Splenectomy is the treatment of choice for bleeding gastric varices resulting from splenic vein thrombosis.

4 A

Patients with chronic pancreatitis are at increased risk of pancreatic cancer. The patient presents with weight loss and increasing dilatation of the bile duct, raising concern for possible malignancy in the head of the pancreas. If the patient had cholangitis, jaundice, or markedly dilated bile ducts, ERCP would be a reasonable step. In the absence of these factors, ERCP would not be indicated for diagnostic purposes. EUS is indicated to look for an occult pancreatic malignancy and for possible fine-needle aspiration of the pancreas.

5 C

The most common form of chronic pancreatitis in southern India and other tropical areas including Africa, southeast Asia and Brazil, is tropical pancreatitis. Hereditary pancreatitis and autoimmune pancreatitis are possible diagnoses in this case, but because the patient is from southern India, tropical pancreatitis is more likely. She does not drink alcohol, making alcoholic chronic pancreatitis unlikely. Gallstones commonly cause acute, not chronic, pancreatitis.

6 D

Patients with chronic pancreatitis may have exocrine pancreatic insufficiency, leading to malabsorption and steatorrhea. The most appropriate therapy is pancreatic enzyme replacement with coated pancreatic enzymes.

Further Reading

Braganza, J.M., Lee, S.H., McCloy, R.F., and McMahon, M.J. (2011) Chronic pancreatitis. *Lancet*, **377**, 1184–1197.

Forsmark, C.E. (2013) Management of chronic pancreatitis. *Gastroenterology*, **144**, 1282–1291.

Forsmark, C.E. (2016) Chronic pancreatitis, in *Sleisenger and Fordtran's Gastrointestinal and Liver Disease: Pathophysiology/Diagnosis/Management*, 10th edition (eds M. Feldman, L.S. Friedman, and L.J. Brandt), Saunders Elsevier, Philadelphia, pp. 994–1026.

Weblinks

http://emedicine.medscape.com/article/181554-overview
http://www.clevelandclinicmeded.com/medicalpubs/diseasemanagement/
gastroenterology/chronic-pancreatitis/

20

Bile Acid Metabolism

Nicole M. Griglione and Field F. Willingham

Clinical Vignette

A 34-year-old man with Crohn's disease presents with chronic diarrhea after undergoing resection of his terminal ileum 4 months ago. He describes his stools as watery and small in volume, but denies blood in the stool. He denies nausea, vomiting, fever, or abdominal pain. He does not take any prescription or over-the-counter medications, and denies recent antibiotic use. Physical examination is unremarkable. Rectal examination reveals brown stool without blood. Laboratory tests including a complete blood count, comprehensive metabolic panel, stool culture for bacteria, stool examination for ova and parasites, and stool *Clostridium difficile* toxin assay are negative. A capsule endoscopy shows normal small intestinal mucosa and a normal appearing ileocolonic anastomosis.

Bile

- Bile is an alkaline, lipid-rich micellar solution that is isosmotic with plasma and consists of water, electrolytes, and organic solutes such as bile acids, phospholipids (e.g., phosphatidylcholine), cholesterol, proteins, and bile pigments (e.g., bilirubin).
- The liver secretes 500–600 ml of bile per day, which is delivered to the duodenum via the bile duct.

Bile Acids and Bile Salts

- Hepatocytes synthesize the primary bile acids, cholic acid and chenodeoxycholic acid (Figure 20.1), from cholesterol.

Sitaraman and Friedman's Essentials of Gastroenterology, Second Edition.
Edited by Shanthi Srinivasan and Lawrence S. Friedman.
© 2018 John Wiley & Sons Ltd. Published 2018 by John Wiley & Sons Ltd.

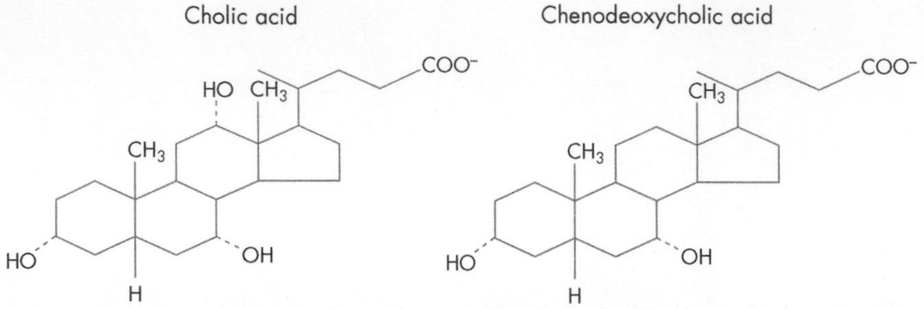

Figure 20.1 The primary bile acids, cholic acid and chenodeoxycholic acid.

- Prior to secretion into the bile canaliculi, primary bile acids are conjugated to glycine or taurine to form bile salts. Conjugation increases water solubility, preventing passive reabsorption from the small intestine.
  - Chenodeoxycholic acid is also epimerized to form the bile acid ursodeoxycholic acid, which is conjugated to taurine or glycine in hepatocytes.
  - Ursodeoxycholic acid represents less than 5% of the bile acid pool.
  - Ursodeoxycholic acid reduces cholesterol secretion into bile and improves biliary cholesterol solubility. Ursodeoxycholic acid has also been used as an oral therapy to dissolve small to medium-sized cholesterol gallstones.
- Primary bile acids and salts reach the small intestine, where they are converted by intestinal bacteria to secondary bile acids, deoxycholic acid and lithocholic acid, through dehydroxylation.
- The two major functions of bile acids and salts are:
  - Regulation of the total body pool of cholesterol:
    ○ Bile acids and bile salts serve as the major excretory form of cholesterol.
    ○ Factors that increase bile acid synthesis promote mobilization and excretion of cholesterol; factors that decrease bile acid synthesis increase the total body pool of cholesterol; factors that decrease intestinal reabsorption of bile acids increase synthesis of bile acids and therefore excretion of cholesterol.
  - Digestion and absorption of dietary lipid:
    ○ Bile acids and salts facilitate the formation of micelles, which aid in the digestion and absorption of dietary lipid and fat-soluble vitamins from the small intestine.

The Enterohepatic Circulation

- Enterohepatic circulation refers to the circulation of bile acids and salts from the liver to the small intestine and back to the liver via the portal vein after reabsorption from the small intestine (Figure 20.2). The enterohepatic

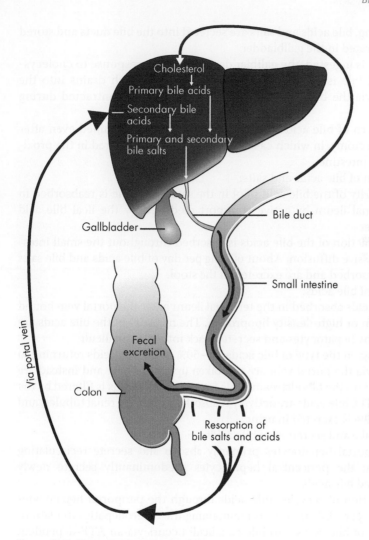

Figure 20.2 The enterohepatic circulation.

circulation helps to maintain an adequate bile acid pool for digestion and absorption and minimizes the need for production of bile acids by hepatocytes.

- Hepatocytes synthesize approximately 600 mg of primary bile acids and salts per day:
  - In normal healthy persons, the total bile acid pool is 2–4 g.
  - On average, the bile acid pool cycles through the enterohepatic circulation two to four times per meal.

- During fasting, bile acids and salts are secreted into the bile ducts and stored and concentrated in the gallbladder.
- After a meal is ingested, the gallbladder contracts in response to cholecystokinin, and bile is secreted into the cystic duct, which drains into the duodenum via the bile duct. The gallbladder remains contracted during the meal.
  - This pattern of bile acid secretion and storage is maintained even after cholecystectomy, in which case the bile acids may be stored in the proximal small intestine.
- Reabsorption of bile acids and salts:
  - The majority of the bile acid pool in the small intestine is reabsorbed in the terminal ileum by active transport mediated by the ileal bile acid transporter.
  - A small fraction of the bile acids is absorbed throughout the small intestine by passive diffusion. About 600 mg per day of bile acids and bile salts are not absorbed and are excreted in the stool.
- Circulation of bile acids:
  - The bile acids absorbed in the terminal ileum enter the portal vein bound to albumin or high-density lipoprotein. The majority of the bile acids are taken up by hepatocytes and secreted back into bile canaliculi.
  - Depending on the type of bile acids, 10–50% of the bile acids returning to the liver via the portal vein are not taken up by the liver and instead are absorbed into the bloodstream. This fraction of bile acids is filtered by the kidneys. The bile acids are actively reabsorbed from the renal tubules, and less than 2% is excreted in urine.
- Hepatic uptake and secretion of bile acids:
  - The periportal hepatocytes primarily absorb and secrete recirculating bile acids; the pericentral hepatocytes predominantly secrete newly synthesized bile acids.
  - The secretion of recycled bile acids through the periportal hepatocytes induces hepatic bile flow, thus maintaining the enterohepatic circulation.
  - Secretion of bile acids into bile canaliculi occurs via an ATP-dependent bile acid efflux pump and is the rate-limiting step in the transport of bile acids from the portal system to the bile duct.

Disorders of Bile Acid Metabolism

Cholesterol Gallstones (see also Chapter 21)

- Up to 20% of women and 8% of men over age 40 develop cholesterol gallstones.

- These stones are comprised mostly of cholesterol monohydrate. Bile pigments, proteins, calcium salts, and fatty acids make up the remainder of the stone.
- Three main factors contribute to gallstone formation:
  - Increased biliary secretion of cholesterol:
    o When excess cholesterol is secreted into bile, adequate micelle formation with phospholipids and bile acids cannot occur. This results in the precipitation of cholesterol crystals.
    o Increased biliary excretion of cholesterol is associated with obesity, high-fat diets, certain medications, increased 3-hydroxy-3-methylglutaryl-coenzyme A (HMG-CoA) reductase activity, and increased hepatic uptake of cholesterol from the bloodstream.
  - Nucleation, the formation of crystal nuclei in supersaturated bile:
    o Certain glycoproteins and mucin promote the nucleation of cholesterol monohydrate crystals.
  - Gallbladder hypomotility:
    o Incomplete emptying of supersaturated and crystal-rich bile from the gallbladder allows stones to increase in size.
- Pregnancy predisposes to gallstone formation because of increased cholesterol saturation during the third trimester and sluggish postprandial gallbladder contraction.
- Women taking oral contraceptive pills have increased hepatic uptake of dietary cholesterol, stimulation of hepatic lipoprotein receptors, and biliary cholesterol secretion, which predispose to gallstone formation.
- Patients who experience rapid weight loss, as occurs after gastric bypass surgery, often develop cholesterol stones secondary to increased mobilization of tissue cholesterol and increased biliary secretion of cholesterol, as well as decreased enterohepatic circulation of bile acids.
- Biliary sludge can also lead to gallstone formation and can be seen in conditions that cause gallbladder hypomotility such as prolonged fasting, burns, surgery, pregnancy, total parenteral nutrition, and oral contraceptive use.

Pigment Gallstones (see also Chapter 21)

- **Black pigment stones** may be seen with hemolytic anemia as in sickle cell anemia, in which elevated levels of bilirubin result from an increased breakdown of red blood cells. By contrast, cholesterol stones are yellow.
- **Brown pigment stones** contain calcium bilirubinate, calcium phosphate, cholesterol, and organic material and may form in the setting of biliary stasis, as occurs with a bile duct stricture.

Table 20.1 Characteristic features of the two different mechanisms of bile salt diarrhea.

	Bile acid excess	Bile acid deficiency
Length of resection	<100 cm	≥100 cm
Compensatory hepatic synthesis of bile acid	Yes	No
Steatorrhea	No	Yes
Response to low-fat diet	No	Yes
Response to oral cholestyramine	Yes	No

Bile Salt Diarrhea

- Impaired bile acid reabsorption due to surgical resection of the terminal ileum, loss of terminal ileal surface area (e.g., after radiation therapy or in Crohn's disease), or congenital defects in the ileal bile acid transporter may lead to diarrhea.
- The nature of bile salt diarrhea and its management depend on the length of terminal ileum that is compromised (Table 20.1):
  - **Secretory diarrhea** results when excessive amounts of bile acids are delivered to the colon, thereby stimulating fluid and electrolyte secretion. Bile acid exposure may also increase colonic mucosal permeability and cause direct mucosal damage.
  - **Steatorrhea** occurs when more than 100 cm of ileum is lost or diseased and the liver is unable to keep up with bile salt losses, thereby resulting in a lack of micelle formation and impaired dietary lipid digestion.

Cholecystectomy

- Cholecystectomy has little effect on bile acid secretion. However, patients may experience post-cholecystectomy diarrhea if the bile acid pool size exceeds the amount of bile acid absorbed by the ileal transport system. This state is usually only transient, and patients often respond to treatment with an oral bile acid sequestrant such as cholestyramine, colestipol, or colesevelam.

Small Intestinal Bacterial Overgrowth

- Small intestinal bacterial overgrowth can lead to deconjugation of bile acids in the proximal small intestine, thereby reducing intraluminal bile acid distribution, impairing formation of micelles, and in some cases leading to steatorrhea.

Pearls

- Bile acids and salts serve as the major excretory pathway for cholesterol.
- The enterohepatic circulation plays a vital role in dietary lipid and fat-soluble vitamin digestion, as well as in the excretion of cholesterol and certain medications.
- Interruption or impairment of the enterohepatic circulation occurs in certain conditions, such as liver disease, terminal ileal resection, Crohn's disease, and small intestinal bacterial overgrowth, and may lead to diarrhea, drug toxicity, or gallstone formation.

Questions

Question 1 relates to the clinical vignette at the beginning of this chapter.

1   Which of the following is the most likely cause of diarrhea in this patient?
   A Active Crohn's disease.
   B Bile acid-induced diarrhea.
   C Fat malabsorption.
   D Viral enteritis.

2   Which of the following are the primary bile acids?
   A Deoxycholic acid and lithocholic acid.
   B Glycocholic acid and taurocholic acid.
   C Hydrochloric acid and ursodeoxycholic acid.
   D Cholic acid and chenodeoxycholic acid.
   E Taurocholic acid and lithocholic acid.

3   The secondary bile acids are produced in the:
   A Liver.
   B Bile ducts.
   C Portal vein.
   D Small intestine.
   E Stomach.

4   Absorption of bile acids occurs predominantly in which of the following segments of the gastrointestinal tract, and by which mechanism?
   A Duodenum via an active carrier-mediated process.
   B Jejunum via passive diffusion.
   C Terminal ileum via an active carrier-mediated process.
   D Ascending colon via passive diffusion.

5 Which of the following is TRUE regarding the enterohepatic circulation?
  A During fasting, bile acids are stored and concentrated in the gallbladder.
  B A fraction of bile salts is absorbed throughout the small intestine by passive diffusion.
  C Less than 10% of bile acids is excreted in the feces.
  D All of the above.

6 Which of the following persons are predisposed to developing cholesterol gallstones?
  A Pregnant women.
  B Persons with a history of gastric bypass surgery.
  C Thin white men.
  D A and B.
  E All of the above.

Answers

1 B
The patient likely has bile acid-induced diarrhea. He has undergone resection of the terminal ileum, which likely resulted in interruption of the enterohepatic circulation. The liver compensates by increasing the synthesis of bile acids and bile salts, which overwhelm the already compromised reabsorption of bile acids and salts in the terminal ileum and leads to increased exposure of the colon to bile acids and salts, thereby resulting in the stimulation of fluid and electrolyte secretion. A trial of a bile acid-sequestrant, such as cholestyramine, before meals may be helpful in this patient. Some patients with a greater portion of affected ileum may experience substantial bile acid losses in the feces. If the liver is unable to compensate by increasing production, intestinal fat malabsorption and steatorrhea can result. Diarrhea in these patients is less responsive to bile acid-sequestrant medications and is best treated with a low-fat diet supplemented with medium-chain triglycerides.

2 D
Primary bile acids are cholic acid and chenodeoxycholic acid. They are synthesized in hepatocytes from cholesterol.

3 D
Primary bile acids and salts are converted by bacteria in the small intestine to secondary bile acids, deoxycholic acid and lithocholic acid, through dehydroxylation.

4 C

The majority of the bile acids are reabsorbed in the terminal ileum by active transport mediated by the ileal bile acid transporter.

5 D

All of the statements are true. During fasting, bile acids are stored and concentrated in the gallbladder. A fraction of bile salts is absorbed throughout the small intestine by passive diffusion and less than 10% of the bile acids are excreted in the feces.

6 D

Pregnancy and rapid weight loss (especially the significant weight loss seen after gastric bypass surgery) are both risk factors for gallstone formation. Hemolytic disorders such as sickle cell anemia also predispose to stone formation, albeit of a different type (pigment gallstones). A thin body habitus and male gender do not increase the risk of gallstone formation.

Further Reading

Chiang, J.Y. (2013) Bile acid metabolism and signaling. *Comprehensive Physiology*, 3, 1191–1212.

Dawson, P.A. (2016) Bile secretion and the enterohepatic circulation, in *Sleisenger and Fordtran's Gastrointestinal and Liver Disease: Pathophysiology/Diagnosis/Management*, 10th edition (eds M. Feldman, L.S. Friedman, and L.J. Brandt), Saunders Elsevier, Philadelphia, pp. 1085–1099.

Ferrebeea, C.B. and Dawson, P.A. (2015) Metabolic effects of intestinal absorption and enterohepatic cycling of bile acids. *Acta Pharmaceutica Sinica B*, 5, 129–134.

Weblinks

http://themedicalbiochemistrypage.org/bileacids.php
http://www.meddean.luc.edu/lumen/meded/orfpath/bileacids.htm

21
Gallstones and Complications
Julia Massaad

Clinical Vignette

A 46-year-old woman is seen in the office for a 4-month history of intermittent right upper quadrant pain. She reports a dull pain that usually begins shortly after a meal and radiates to the right shoulder. The pain lasts 1–2 hours and resolves spontaneously. These episodes have occurred three times in the past year. She denies any change in bowel habits, nausea, vomiting, jaundice, or fever. She has tried over-the-counter ranitidine for the pain, with no improvement. Her past medical history is unremarkable. Her father has hypertension, and her mother has diabetes mellitus. She has four children who are healthy. She does not smoke cigarettes, drink alcohol, or use illicit drugs. On examination she is moderately obese (BMI 32). The physical examination is otherwise unremarkable. Laboratory tests, including a complete blood count and comprehensive metabolic panel, are unremarkable.

Gallstones (Cholelithiasis)

Pathogenesis

- Gallstones and their complications are among the most common gastrointestinal disorders with a prevalence of 10–15% in Western countries.
- Types of gallstones (see also Chapter 20):
  - Cholesterol stones: in Western countries, cholesterol is the principal constituent of 80% of gallstones. Cholesterol gallstones are composed mainly of cholesterol (70%), mixed with calcium salts, bile pigment, and glycoproteins.

Sitaraman and Friedman's Essentials of Gastroenterology, Second Edition.
Edited by Shanthi Srinivasan and Lawrence S. Friedman.

– Non-cholesterol stones:
  ○ Black pigment stones, composed predominantly of calcium bilirubi-nate, are found in patients with cirrhosis or chronic hemolytic states.
  ○ Brown pigment stones, composed of varying amounts of calcium biliru-binate, calcium phosphate, cholesterol, and organic material, are usually formed in the setting of biliary stasis, secondary to biliary stricture, or small-bowel diverticula.
- Three principal defects are involved in the pathogenesis of gallstone forma-tion: (1) supersaturation of bile with cholesterol; (2) accelerated nucleation; and (3) gallbladder hypomotility. The extent of cholesterol saturation in the bile stored in the gallbladder is the most important determinant of gallstone formation.

Risk Factors

- Age: approximately 50% of women will have gallstones by age 70.
- Female sex: two- to threefold increased risk compared with males.
- Multiparity.
- Diabetes mellitus.
- Hypertriglyceridemia.
- Total parenteral nutrition.
- Ethnicity: 70% of Pima Indian women have gallstones by age 25, and 50% of Scandinavian women have gallstones by age 50.
- Medications: ceftriaxone, octreotide, oral contraceptives.
- Diseases involving the terminal ileum (such as Crohn's disease).
- Rapid weight loss.

Natural History

- Some 80% of persons with gallstones are asymptomatic. Of those, 20% will develop symptoms over 15 years of follow-up.
- Complications of gallstones include biliary pain, cholecystitis, choledocho-lithiasis, cholangitis, acute pancreatitis, gallstone ileus, and Mirizzi syn-drome (see later). Gallbladder carcinoma is a rare complication of chronic cholelithiasis.
- The cumulative rate of complications in persons with asymptomatic chole-lithiasis is estimated to be 1–4% at 10 years. Therefore, treatment of asymp-tomatic gallstones is not recommended except for persons who are at high risk for gallbladder cancer, such as Native Americans and persons with a porcelain gallbladder (see later).
- In contrast, up to 50% of patients with gallstones and biliary pain will have recurrent pain, and the risk of biliary complications is estimated to be 1–2% per year. Therefore, cholecystectomy should be recommended for persons who have symptoms.

Clinical Features

- The typical symptom of gallstones is biliary pain, conventionally referred to as 'biliary colic.' Biliary pain is characterized by severe, steady, epigastric or right upper quadrant pain that usually begins abruptly and peaks within 1 hour of onset. The pain may radiate to the right shoulder or scapula in approximately 50% of patients. Although termed 'colic,' the pain is steady and not intermittent.
  - Biliary pain is caused by intermittent obstruction of the cystic duct by a gallstone.
  - Biliary pain usually resolves gradually within 3 hours. Prolonged pain (>3 hours) should raise suspicion of a complication such as cholecystitis, cholangitis, or pancreatitis.

Diagnosis

- Laboratory tests (complete blood count, liver biochemical tests) are often normal in the setting of biliary pain, and a high index of suspicion is needed to confirm the diagnosis.
- The diagnosis of cholelithiasis is made by right upper quadrant ultrasonography, which has >95% sensitivity and specificity for the detection of gallstones that are larger than 2mm (see Chapter 27).

Treatment

- Symptomatic gallstone disease is treated surgically with laparoscopic cholecystectomy.
- Medical treatment of gallstone disease with oral ursodeoxycholic acid, with or without extracorporeal shock wave lithotripsy, is considered a treatment option in persons with small cholesterol stones who are not surgical candidates.

> Asymptomatic gallstones do not require treatment except in persons who are at high risk for gallbladder cancer such as Native Americans or persons with a porcelain gallbladder.

Common Gallstone Complications

Acute Cholecystitis

- Acute cholecystitis is the most common complication of gallstones. It occurs in up to 11% of patients followed over 7–11 years. It is usually caused by prolonged obstruction of the cystic duct by an impacted stone (Table 21.1).

Table 21.1 Clinical manifestations, pathophysiology, diagnosis, and treatment of gallstones and their complications.

	Biliary pain	Acute cholecystitis	Choledocholithiasis	Acute cholangitis
Pathophysiology	Intermittent obstruction of the cystic duct	Continuing obstruction of the cystic duct	Intermittent obstruction of the BD	Continuing obstruction of the BD and infection
Symptoms	Infrequent epigastric/right upper quadrant pain <3 hours	Epigastric/right upper quadrant pain >3 hours, associated nausea and vomiting	Asymptomatic or similar to biliary pain (more frequent episodes)	Fever, jaundice, right upper quadrant pain (Charcot's triad)
Physical examination	Normal	Murphy's sign, fever, mild jaundice	Normal, possibly jaundice	Charcot's triad, + hypotension, altered mental status (Reynolds' pentad)
Laboratory tests (CBC, AST, ALT, ALP, bilirubin)	Normal	Leukocytosis, elevated bilirubin (<4 mg dl^{-1}), mildly elevated AST, ALT, ALP	Elevated bilirubin, elevated AST, ALT, ALP	Leukocytosis, elevated AST, ALT, ALP
Imaging test(s)	Abdominal ultrasonography	Abdominal ultrasonography, HIDA scan	MRCP, EUS, ERCP, PTC	MRCP, EUS, ERCP, PTC
Treatment	Cholecystectomy	Antibiotics, cholecystectomy	ERCP followed by cholecystectomy; PTC if ERCP unsuccessful or unavailable	Antibiotics, ERCP, followed by cholecystectomy; PTC if ERCP unsuccessful or unavailable

ALP, alkaline phosphatase; ALT, alanine aminotransferase; AST, aspartate aminotransferase; BD, bile duct; CBC, complete blood count; ERCP, endoscopic retrograde cholangiopancreatography; EUS, endoscopic ultrasonography; HIDA, hydroxy iminodiacetic acid; MRCP, magnetic resonance cholangiopancreatography; PTC, percutaneous transhepatic cholangiography.

- Acalculous cholecystitis: in 10% of patients, cholecystitis occurs in the absence of gallstones. Acalculous cholecystitis typically occurs in critically ill patients in the setting of major surgery, prolonged total parenteral nutrition, or extensive trauma. It is usually associated with a high morbidity and mortality.

Clinical Features

- Typical symptoms include a prolonged (>3 hours) episode of biliary pain that may be associated with nausea, vomiting, and fever.
- The physical finding that is nearly pathognomonic of acute cholecystitis is a positive Murphy's sign, which is the abrupt arrest of breathing during inspiration when the right costal margin is palpated and the inflamed gallbladder touches the examiner's hands.

Diagnosis

- Laboratory tests: leukocytosis as well as a mild elevation of the serum aminotransferases, alkaline phosphatase, and bilirubin (usually $<4\,\mathrm{mg\,dl^{-1}}$) levels may be seen.
- Imaging studies:
  - Right upper quadrant ultrasonography is the single best test to confirm acute cholecystitis. Findings on ultrasonography include gallbladder wall thickening, pericholecystic fluid, and a sonographic Murphy's sign (see Chapter 27).
  - Hepatobiliary scintigraphy (hydroxy iminodiacetic acid, or HIDA, scan) can be used to confirm or exclude acute cholecystitis with a high degree of sensitivity and specificity:
    - A HIDA scan is performed after the intravenous administration of ^{99m}Tc-labeled HIDA.
    - A positive scan is defined by the lack of visualization of the gallbladder and normal excretion into the bile duct and small bowel within 30–60 minutes of the administration of ^{99m}Tc-labeled HIDA. False-positive HIDA scan results can be seen in patients with severe liver disease or prior biliary sphincterotomy, and in fasting patients receiving total parenteral nutrition
  - Computed tomography (CT) is indicated if there is a concern for other complications of cholecystitis such as fistula or abscess.

Treatment

- Patients suspected of having acute cholecystitis should be admitted to the hospital, and intravascular volume and electrolytes should be repleted.

- Broad-spectrum antibiotics should be initiated. A cephalosporin such as cefuroxime or ceftriaxone is effective in mild acute cholecystitis. In severely ill patients, piperacillin-tazobactam, a carbapenem, or a third-generation cephalosporin, each in combination with metronidazole, is recommended.
- Cholecystectomy, preferably laparoscopic, is definitive treatment.

> A prolonged (>3 hours) episode of biliary pain associated with nausea, vomiting, and fever should raise suspicion for acute cholecystitis.

Choledocholithiasis

- Choledocholithiasis is defined as the presence of gallstones in the bile duct (BD). BD stones usually have migrated from the gallbladder, but they can also form *de novo*.

Clinical Features

- Typically, symptoms of choledocholithiasis include right upper quadrant pain with associated nausea and vomiting; however, the majority of persons with BD stones are asymptomatic.
- Physical examination is usually normal. If there is biliary obstruction, jaundice may be noted.

Diagnosis

- Laboratory tests: elevated serum alkaline phosphatase level and mild jaundice (serum bilirubin $<5\,\mathrm{mg\,dl^{-1}}$) are the most common laboratory findings.
- Imaging studies:
  - 50% of BD stones can be missed on ultrasonography; however, ultrasonography can suggest the presence of BD stones with the finding of a dilated bile duct.
  - Endoscopic ultrasonography has >98% sensitivity and specificity for the detection of choledocholithiasis, but requires an invasive endoscopic procedure.
  - Magnetic resonance cholangiopancreatography (MRCP) detects BD stones with >95% sensitivity and specificity.
  - Endoscopic retrograde cholangiopancreatography (ERCP) is the 'gold standard' for the diagnosis of choledocholithiasis. Importantly, therapeutic interventions, including biliary decompression, stone extraction, and stent placement, can be performed with ERCP.
  - ERCP is the diagnostic test of choice when the suspicion for choledocholithiasis is high and an intervention is likely to be required, as in patients with jaundice secondary to BD stones. MRCP is generally the test of choice when the suspicion for choledocholithiasis is low or intermediate.

Treatment

- Treatment of asymptomatic choledocholithiasis is recommended due to the risk of life-threatening complications, including acute pancreatitis and cholangitis.
- Treatment includes ERCP with stone extraction, as well as a cholecystectomy to prevent further stone formation and migration into the BD.
- Treatment with ERCP alone is sufficient in patients who are considered to be at high surgical risk for cholecystectomy.

Choledocholithiasis is the most common cause of acute pancreatitis. Cholangitis is a life-threatening complication of choledocholithiasis. Therefore, choledocholithiasis should be treated even in asymptomatic persons.

Acute Cholangitis

- Acute cholangitis is a life-threatening complication of gallstones usually caused by an impacted stone in the BD.
- The impacted stone predisposes to bacterial infection and septicemia.
  - The most common organisms include *Escherichia coli*, *Klebsiella* spp., *Pseudomonas*, and *Enterococcus*.

Clinical Features

- Typical symptoms, which comprise Charcot's triad, include fever, jaundice, and right upper quadrant pain.
  - A smaller proportion of patients (10–20%) also have altered mental status and hypotension (Reynolds' pentad), which is associated with a higher morbidity and mortality than Charcot's triad alone.

Diagnosis

- Laboratory tests: leukocytosis with a left shift, hyperbilirubinemia, and elevated serum alkaline phosphatase and aminotransferase levels are the typical laboratory findings.
- Imaging studies:
  - CT is more accurate than ultrasonography for the diagnosis of acute cholangitis; however, neither CT nor ultrasonography is good for excluding a BD stone.
  - ERCP is recommended as a diagnostic test and therapeutic modality.
  - As in choledocholithiasis, MRCP may be used for diagnosis.

Treatment

- A single intravenous broad-spectrum antibiotic, such as cefoxitin, is sufficient in mild cases. In severely ill patients, broad-spectrum antibiotics similar to those used in acute cholecystitis are indicated. The antibiotic regimen should be adjusted if blood cultures grow the offending organism.

- Urgent biliary decompression: the urgency of decompression depends on the patient's initial response to supportive therapy with fluid resuscitation and antibiotics. In patients who remain symptomatic, urgent ERCP is recommended.
  - In patients who are hemodynamically unstable, such as those with hypotension, ERCP cannot be performed; instead, a percutaneous cholecystostomy tube insertion is recommended to decompress the biliary system.
  - Cholecystectomy is recommended to prevent further gallstone formation or migration of a stone into the BD.

> Acute cholangitis is a life-threatening complication of gallstones that should be identified early and treated promptly.

Uncommon Gallstone Complications

Gallstone Ileus

- Gallstone ileus is defined as small-bowel obstruction caused by a gallstone.
- The gallstone passes into the intestine through a cholecystoenteric fistula that forms after an episode of cholecystitis. Cholecystoenteric fistulas are typically seen in persons 65–75 years of age.
- The most common location of a cholecystoenteric fistula is the duodenum (an impacted gallstone within the fistula that results in gastric outlet obstruction is termed Bouveret's syndrome), followed by the colon, stomach, and jejunum. The most common site of gallstone impaction is the terminal ileum or ileocecal valve.
- Many patients with gallstone ileus may have serious concomitant medical illnesses such as coronary artery disease, diabetes mellitus, or pulmonary disease. Delayed diagnosis due to the intermittency of symptoms is not uncommon and leads to a high mortality rate (50%).

Diagnosis

- Gallstone ileus is diagnosed with a plain film of the abdomen: radiographic findings include pneumobilia (air in the biliary tract), dilated small-bowel loops suggestive of partial or complete small-bowel obstruction, and a stone impacted in the bowel (see Chapter 27). The treatment is surgical.

Mirizzi Syndrome

- Mirizzi syndrome is a rare complication of prolonged cholelithiasis. It is defined as jaundice caused by obstruction of the extrahepatic duct secondary to a gallstone impacted in the cystic duct.

- A stone impacted in the cystic duct can lead to pressure necrosis and obstruction of, or even a fistula to, the common hepatic duct (type I and type II Mirizzi syndrome, respectively).
- The diagnosis can be made by CT, ERCP, or MRCP. The characteristic extrinsic compression of the common hepatic duct is usually evident on ERCP or MRCP.
- Open cholecystectomy is the treatment of choice, in addition to repair of the fistula or creation of a bilio-enteric anastomosis depending on the degree of injury; however, ERCP with endoscopic stenting is being used increasingly as a primary therapeutic modality.

Porcelain Gallbladder

- Porcelain gallbladder is defined as intramural calcification of the gallbladder wall, and is associated with gallstones in more than 95% of cases. It is also associated with an increased risk of gallbladder carcinoma, which can occur in up to 5% of individuals.
- The incidence of gallbladder cancer depends on the pattern of gallbladder wall calcification, with selective mucosal calcification causing a significant cancer risk compared with diffuse intramural calcification, which does not seem to increase the risk of gallbladder cancer.
- Patients are usually asymptomatic, and laboratory tests are normal. The diagnosis is made with a plain abdominal X-ray or CT that shows calcifications in the gallbladder wall.
- Prophylactic cholecystectomy is indicated to prevent gallbladder carcinoma.

Emphysematous Cholecystitis

- Persons with emphysematous cholecystitis have a clinical presentation similar to those with acute cholecystitis.
- The etiology of emphysematous cholecystitis is related to cystic duct ischemia secondary to atherosclerosis. Therefore, elderly persons (without gallstones) and persons with diabetes mellitus are at increased risk of developing emphysematous cholecystitis.
- Gas-forming organisms infect the gallbladder wall and lead to gas pockets that are evident on abdominal imaging.
- The risk of gallbladder perforation is high. Therefore, emergent treatment with broad-spectrum antibiotics that include anaerobic coverage and early cholecystectomy is recommended.

Gangrenous Cholecystitis

- Gangrenous cholecystitis is a severe form of acute cholecystitis that results in gallbladder wall necrosis and perforation. It is associated with high mortality and morbidity.

- Persons who are at high risk of gangrenous cholecystitis are elderly men with multiple comorbidities.
- The clinical presentation is similar to that of acute nongangrenous cholecystitis; gangrene is often not suspected preoperatively.
- Treatment is with broad-spectrum antibiotic coverage and emergent, usually open, cholecystectomy.

Pearls

- The most common type of gallstones are cholesterol stones; women are affected much more commonly than men.
- Asymptomatic gallstones generally do not require treatment except in persons at high risk of gallbladder cancer.
- Prolonged biliary pain (>3 hours) suggests acute cholecystitis.
- Even asymptomatic choledocholithiasis should be treated. Acute cholangitis requires immediate antibiotic therapy and urgent bile duct decompression.

Questions

Question 1 relates to the clinical vignette at the beginning of this chapter.

1 Which of the following is the best test to confirm the diagnosis?
   A Right upper quadrant ultrasonography.
   B Computed tomography.
   C Magnetic resonance cholangiopancreatography.
   D Endoscopic retrograde cholangiopancreatography.

2 A 92-year-old woman with a history of dementia, coronary artery disease, critical aortic stenosis, and atrial fibrillation presents to the office for evaluation of a 6-month history of occasional right upper quadrant pain. The pain is infrequent (every few months) and is often precipitated by a fatty meal. She denies nausea, vomiting, fevers, chills, or jaundice. Laboratory tests, including a complete blood count and comprehensive metabolic panel, are normal except for a mildly elevated serum alkaline phosphatase level. Right upper quadrant ultrasonography shows cholelithiasis. Which of the following is the best next step in the management of this patient?
   A Upper endoscopy.
   B Laparoscopic cholecystectomy.
   C Magnetic resonance cholangiopancreatography (MRCP).
   D Oral ursodeoxycholic acid.

3   A 24-year-old African American man with sickle cell disease is admitted to the hospital for fevers, chills, right upper quadrant pain, and jaundice of 2 days' duration. Laboratory tests show a white blood cell count of 24 000 mm^{-3} with 89% neutrophils, serum aspartate aminotransferase level 125 U l^{-1}, alanine aminotransferase 214 U l^{-1}, and bilirubin 5 mg dl^{-1}. Right upper quadrant ultrasonography shows cholelithiasis, with no evidence of cholecystitis, and a dilated bile duct with intraductal stones. The best next step in the management of this patient is which of the following?

   A Emergent cholecystectomy.
   B Broad-spectrum antibiotics and endoscopic retrograde cholangio-pancreatography (ERCP).
   C Broad-spectrum antibiotics and percutaneous transhepatic cholangiography (PTC).
   D Broad-spectrum antibiotics only.

4   A false-positive HIDA scan can result from each of the following EXCEPT:
   A Severe hyperbilirubinemia.
   B Incomplete cystic duct obstruction.
   C Total parenteral nutrition (TPN).
   D Prior biliary sphincterotomy.

5   A 79-year-old man is admitted to the hospital with fever, abdominal pain, jaundice, and altered mental status of 1 day's duration. Laboratory tests show a white blood cell count of 18 000 mm^{-3}, serum alkaline phosphatase level 400 U l^{-1}, aspartate aminotransferase 200 U l^{-1}, alanine aminotransferase 216 U l^{-1}, and bilirubin 4 mg dl^{-1}. Right upper quadrant ultrasonography is unremarkable. Blood cultures are positive for *E. coli*. He continues to be febrile despite treatment with broad-spectrum antibiotics for 24 hours. Which of the following is the next best step in the management of this patient?

   A Computed tomography (CT) of abdomen and pelvis.
   B Urgent endoscopic retrograde cholangiopancreatography (ERCP).
   C Magnetic resonance imaging and magnetic resonance cholangiopancreatography (MRI/MRCP).
   D An intravenous antifungal agent.

6   A 73-year-old woman with history of hypertension and diabetes mellitus is admitted to the hospital with a 2-day history of right upper quadrant pain and fever. Laboratory tests show a white blood cell count of 27 000 mm^{-3} and elevated serum alkaline phosphatase and bilirubin levels. Ultrasonography shows gallbladder wall thickening, and air in the

gallbladder wall. A Murphy's sign is positive. Which of the following is the most appropriate next step in the management of this patient?

A Antibiotics for 2 weeks followed by cholecystectomy.

B HIDA scan.

C Antibiotics and urgent cholecystectomy.

D Endoscopic retrograde cholangiopancreatography (ERCP).

7 All of the following are indications for cholecystectomy EXCEPT:

A Calcifications in the gallbladder wall detected incidentally on a CT.

B Prolonged TPN.

C Asymptomatic gallstones in a Native American.

D A patient with an asymptomatic 8-mm stone in the bile duct.

8 A 32-year-old woman is seen for follow up of right upper quadrant ultrasonography that was ordered to evaluate hepatomegaly noted on a routine annual physical examination. The patient is asymptomatic. Ultrasonography shows evidence of gallstones but no other abnormality; the liver size is normal. Laboratory tests including serum aminotransferase, alkaline phosphatase, and bilirubin levels are normal. Which of the following is the best next step in the management of this patient?

A Reassurance.

B Repeat ultrasonography in 1 year.

C Cholecystectomy.

D Treatment with ursodeoxycholic acid.

Answers

1 A

The patient describes symptoms consistent with biliary pain, likely from cholelithiasis. Her age, sex, and parity are risk factors for cholelithiasis. The differential diagnosis includes choledocholithiasis, cholecystitis, pancreatitis, gastroesophageal reflux disease, and peptic ulcer disease. Ultrasonography is the best test to confirm cholelithiasis.

2 D

The clinical presentation is suggestive of biliary pain. The differential diagnosis includes choledocholithiasis, cholecystitis, pancreatitis, gastroesophageal reflux disease, and peptic ulcer disease. Ultrasonography has >95% sensitivity and specificity for the detection of gallstones or cholecystitis, and is a cost-effective test compared with MRCP. The treatment of choice for symptomatic cholelithiasis is cholecystectomy. However, the patient's age and comorbidities make her a high surgical risk. In patients who are not surgical candidates, oral ursodeoxycholic acid can be considered for the treatment of symptomatic gallstones. Upper endoscopy is not indicated at this time.

3 **B**

This patient has classic symptoms of acute cholangitis (Charcot's triad – right upper quadrant pain, fever, and jaundice). Acute cholangitis is caused by a stone impacted in the bile duct, with secondary bacterial proliferation. It is likely that this patient has black pigment stones, given his history of sickle cell disease. Irrespective of the type of gallstone, the treatment of choice for acute cholangitis is broad-spectrum antibiotics followed by biliary decompression. The preferred method of biliary decompression is ERCP. PTC is reserved for cases in which ERCP is not available or not possible, given the lower risk of complications with an ERCP. A cholecystectomy is not required urgently but should be considered once the acute cholangitis resolves.

4 **B**

Incomplete cystic duct obstruction can give a false-negative, not a false-positive, HIDA scan result. Severe hyperbilirubinemia or liver disease, prior biliary sphincterotomy, and prolonged fasting and TPN can give a false-positive HIDA scan result.

5 **B**

The patient has acute cholangitis as evidenced by fever, abdominal pain, jaundice, and altered mental status. He has bacteremia and is not responding to intravenous antibiotic treatment. Cholangitis is a life-threatening condition and requires urgent biliary decompression. The next best step in the management of this patient is biliary decompression and removal of the bile duct (BD) stone by ERCP. If the patient is hemodynamically unstable, percutaneous cholecystostomy should be performed. Ultrasonography that is negative for gallstones does not alter the management of cholangitis. CT and MRI are better diagnostic modalities than ultrasonography for visualizing BD stones, but they do not have any therapeutic potential and will only delay treatment.

6 **C**

Air in the gallbladder wall is indicative of emphysematous cholecystitis, which has a high mortality and morbidity – hence the need for urgent treatment. Antibiotic coverage should be initiated and followed immediately by a cholecystectomy. Delaying surgery increases the risk of gallbladder perforation, which can lead to serious complications. The clinical presentation and ultrasonographic findings confirm the diagnosis of emphysematous cholecystitis; a HIDA scan or ERCP is not indicated in this situation.

7   B

Prolonged TPN can lead to a false-positive HIDA scan result, but is not an indication for cholecystectomy. Stones in the bile duct, even if asymptomatic, should be removed because of an increased risk of complications. Stone removal alone is not sufficient, however; cholecystectomy should be considered to prevent additional migration of gallbladder stones to the bile duct. The risk of gallbladder malignancy is markedly increased in Native Americans with gallstones; therefore, in this case, as well as in patients with calcifications in the gallbladder wall (porcelain gallbladder), cholecystectomy is indicated.

8   A

Treatment of asymptomatic gallstone disease is not recommended, given the low risk of complications. The patient is asymptomatic and does not need further therapy or follow up of the stones unless symptoms of biliary disease develop.

Further Reading

Chen, Y., Kong, J. and Wu, S. (2015) Cholesterol gallstone disease: focusing on the role of the gallbladder. *Laboratory Investigation*, **95**, 124–131.

Glasgow, R.E. and Mulvihill, S.J. (2016) Treatment of Gallstone Disease, in *Sleisenger and Fordtran's Gastrointestinal and Liver Disease: Pathophysiology/ Diagnosis/Management*, 10th edition (eds M. Feldman, L.S. Friedman, and L.J. Brandt), Saunders Elsevier, Philadelphia, pp. 1134–1151.

Khan, Z.S., Livingston, E.H. and Huerta, S. (2011) Reassessing the need for prophylactic surgery in patients with porcelain gallbladder: case series and systematic review of the literature. *Archives of Surgery*, **146**, 1143–1147.

Wang, D. and Afdhal, N. (2016) Gallstone disease, in *Sleisenger and Fordtran's Gastrointestinal and Liver Disease: Pathophysiology/Diagnosis/Management*, 10th edition (eds M. Feldman, L.S. Friedman, and L.J. Brandt), Saunders Elsevier, Philadelphia, pp. 1100–1133.

Weblink

http://www.aafp.org/afp/20000315/1673.html

Common Problems in Gastroenterology

Emad Qayed and Meena A. Prasad

22

Acute Gastrointestinal Bleeding

Tanvi Dhere

Clinical Vignette

A 63-year-old man presents to the emergency department (ED) with hematemesis that started 2 hours ago. He was working at his computer, began to feel nauseated, and vomited two cups of bright red blood. He vomited once more in the ED. He also noted passage of black, tarry stool. He takes ibuprofen 1 g daily for osteoarthritis of his knees. He drinks up to six to eight beers a day, does not smoke cigarettes, and has no history of illicit drug use. Vital signs show a blood pressure of 145/86 mmHg supine and 100/65 mmHg upright; pulse rate 112 per minute supine and 130 per minute upright; respiratory rate 14 per minute; and oxygen saturation 94% on room air. The abdomen is soft and nontender, and bowel sounds are normal. The liver edge cannot be palpated. The spleen tip is palpable in the left upper quadrant. There is fluid wave and shifting dullness suggesting the presence of ascites. A few spider telangiectasias are noted on the chest. Rectal examination shows maroon stools. Laboratory tests show a white blood cell count of 7200 mm^{-3}, hemoglobin level 10 g dl^{-1}, platelet count 100 000 mm^{-3}, and mean corpuscular volume 99 fl. A comprehensive metabolic panel shows a sodium of 128 mEq l^{-1}, potassium 4.2 mEq l^{-1}, blood urea nitrogen 45 mg dl^{-1}, creatinine 1.3 mg dl^{-1}, alanine aminotransferase 32 U l^{-1}, aspartate aminotransferase 92 U l^{-1}, alkaline phosphatase 90 U l^{-1}, and total bilirubin 1.5 mg dl^{-1}. The prothrombin time is 13.4 seconds and international normalized ratio (INR) 1.4.

Sitaraman and Friedman's Essentials of Gastroenterology, Second Edition.
Edited by Shanthi Srinivasan and Lawrence S. Friedman.
© 2018 John Wiley & Sons Ltd. Published 2018 by John Wiley & Sons Ltd.

General

- Acute gastrointestinal (GI) bleeding accounts for >350 000 hospital admissions in the US each year.
- The overall mortality rate for upper GI bleeding is 5–10% and for lower GI bleeding 2–3%.

Definitions

- The ligament of Treitz, a suspensory ligament located between the duodenum and jejunum and connecting to the diaphragm, is the key landmark separating **upper GI bleeding** (UGIB) from **lower GI bleeding** (LGIB). UGIB refers to hemorrhage proximal to, whereas LGIB refers to hemorrhage distal to, the ligament of Treitz.
- Hematemesis, coffee ground emesis, or melena typically indicates UGIB (Table 22.1).
- **Melena** is black, tarry, malodorous stool that usually indicates hemorrhage proximal to the ligament of Treitz. Occasionally, bleeding from a source in the small bowel or right colon may also cause melena. The black color is caused by oxidation of the iron in hemoglobin by gastric acid or by bacteria. A volume of approximately 100–200 ml of blood in the upper GI tract is needed to cause melena. Melena may persist for several days after bleeding has ceased.
- Black stool that does not contain occult blood may result from ingestion of iron, bismuth, or various foods and should not be mistaken for melena.

Table 22.1 GI bleeding nomenclature.

Presentation	Definition	Association with UGIB	Association with LGIB
Coffee ground emesis	Dark gastric contents; usually signifies prolonged exposure to gastric acid	+	−
Hematemesis	Emesis of bright red color	+	−
Melena	Black, tarry stool with a characteristic smell	+	+
Hematochezia	Passage of bright blood per rectum; may be admixed with stool	+	+

LGIB, lower gastrointestinal bleeding; UGIB, upper gastrointestinal bleeding.

Etiology

UGIB

- UGIB constitutes 75% of all cases of acute GI bleeding. Causes of UGIB (Table 22.2) include:
  - **Peptic ulcer disease**: Duodenal and gastric ulcers, gastropathy, and duodenitis (see Chapter 3) are the most common causes of UGIB, and account for 70% of all cases. Less common causes of peptic ulcer include Cushing ulcer (gastric and duodenal ulcers associated with increased intracranial pressure) and Curling ulcer (acute ulcer of the duodenum associated with severe burns).
  - **Erosive esophagitis** accounts for 10–15% of cases of UGIB.
    - Common causes of erosive esophagitis in immunocompetent patients include gastroesophageal reflux disease and radiation therapy.
    - In immunosuppressed persons, erosive esophagitis is typically caused by infections, such as *Candida* spp., cytomegalovirus, herpes simplex virus, or human immunodeficiency virus, or may be idiopathic.
  - **Esophageal and gastric varices** account for 10% of cases of UGIB.
  - **Mallory–Weiss tears** account for 5% of cases of UGIB; they are tears at the gastroesophageal junction in the mucosa due to retching, repeated vomiting, or coughing.
  - **Vascular lesions** account for less than 5% of cases of UGIB. Examples of vascular lesions include Dieulafoy's lesion (a superficial ectatic submucosal arteriole), arteriovenous malformations, telangiectasias (as in hereditary hemorrhagic telangiectasia, or Osler–Weber–Rendu disease), and gastric vascular antral ectasia (GAVE, or 'watermelon' stomach), which may be associated with chronic renal failure, portal hypertension, or collagen vascular disease.
  - **Neoplasms** of the esophagus, stomach, or duodenum may cause UGIB.
  - Uncommon causes:
    - **Hemobilia** (bleeding into the biliary tract) may occur in patients who have undergone liver biopsy or experienced trauma or hepatobiliary manipulation.
    - **Hemosuccus pancreaticus** (bleeding into the pancreatic duct) may occur with acute or chronic pancreatitis, pancreatic cancer, or pancreatic duct manipulation.
    - **Aortoenteric fistula** (communication between the abdominal aorta, usually an aneurysm or graft, and the third portion of the duodenum). Bleeding from an aortoenteric fistula often presents as a brief 'herald' bleed followed by an acute massive bleed and is associated with a high mortality rate.

Table 22.2 Differential diagnosis of upper gastrointestinal bleeding (UGIB).

Cause (% of all cases of UGIB)	Pathogenic factors	Presentation	Course	Treatment
PUD (70%)	NSAIDs *H. pylori* infection, Curling ulcer, Cushing ulcer	Melena Hematemesis Coffee ground emesis Hematochezia	Self-limited in 80% of cases Endoscopic therapy needed in 20% of cases	Intravenous PPI Endoscopic hemostasis
Erosive esophagitis (10–15%)	GERD Alcohol NSAIDs Infection Radiation	Hematemesis Coffee ground emesis Melena	<5% risk of rebleeding	PPI Sucralfate Treatment of infection
Esophageal/gastric varices (10%)	Chronic liver disease Splenic vein thrombosis (gastric varices)	Severe hypovolemia Melena Hematemesis Hematochezia	In 80–90% of cases, bleeding ceases following urgent endoscopic intervention performed within 12 hours Mortality rate 15–40%	Octreotide Antibiotics Endoscopic hemostasis Sengstaken–Blakemore tube TIPS Splenectomy for splenic vein thrombosis
Mallory–Weiss tear (5%)	Retching Heavy alcohol ingestion Coughing	Hematemesis Coffee ground emesis	Resolves spontaneously in >95% of cases <10% have continued bleeding	Supportive Endoscopic hemostasis if ongoing bleeding

Vascular malformation (<5%)	Angiodysplasias associated with CKD Anticoagulation Osler–Weber–Rendu disease Dieulafoy's lesion GAVE Portal hypertensive gastropathy	Hematemesis Coffee ground emesis Melena Iron-deficiency anemia	Dieulafoy's lesion may result in significant blood loss Recurrent GI bleeding can occur in one third of patients with Osler–Weber–Rendu disease, most commonly above age 40 Patients with bleeding diatheses have worse outcomes than those without diatheses Bleeding from angiodysplasias in the setting of aortic stenosis may improve with aortic valve replacement	Endoscopic ablation
Neoplasms (1%)	Family history Smoking Age >65 H. pylori infection	Iron deficiency + FOBT Weight loss Dyspepsia	Majority present with advanced disease	Chemotherapy, radiation, surgery

CKD, chronic kidney disease; FOBT, fecal occult blood test; GAVE, gastric antral vascular ectasia; GERD, gastroesophageal reflux disease; *H. pylori*, *Helicobacter pylori*; NSAIDs, nonsteroidal anti-inflammatory drugs; PPI, proton pump inhibitor; PUD, peptic ulcer disease; TIPS, transjugular intrahepatic portosystemic shunt.

> Hematochezia in the setting of UGIB is an ominous sign because it signifies that the patient is bleeding at a rapid rate.

LGIB

- Causes of LGIB (Table 22.3) include:
  - **Diverticulosis** accounts for 25–40% of cases of LGIB. Right-sided diverticula bleed more frequently than left-sided diverticula. They are more common in persons >65 years of age and in those with chronic constipation.
  - **Angiodysplasia** accounts for 3–37% of cases of LGIB.
    - Angiodysplasias (or angioectasias) are ecstatic thin-walled venules or capillaries in the mucosa or submucosa. Their development is age-related.
    - They are typically seen in the cecum or ascending colon, but may occur anywhere in the GI tract, including the small bowel. Although angiodysplasias can bleed spontaneously, bleeding is associated with the use of anticoagulants and aspirin or other nonsteroidal anti-inflammatory drugs (NSAIDs). They may also bleed in the setting of uremia due to platelet dysfunction from uremia.
    - Bleeding from angiodysplasia may be associated with aortic stenosis (Heyde's syndrome).
  - **Neoplastic disease** accounts for 15% of cases of LGIB. Most present as chronic occult blood loss and iron-deficiency anemia rather than acute blood loss.
  - **Colitis** accounts for 10% of cases of LGIB. Causes of colitis include ischemia, infection, radiation therapy, and inflammatory bowel disease.
  - **UGIB** may present as LGIB. Approximately 10% of patients suspected initially of having a LGIB are found to have a UGI source of bleeding.
  - **Internal hemorrhoids**. Bleeding from internal hemorrhoids is typically intermittent, small in quantity, and self-limited but can be massive, resulting in hemodynamic compromise.
  - Uncommon causes of LGIB include intestinal intussusception, colonic varices, solitary rectal ulcer syndrome, and aortoenteric fistula.

> A clue to esophageal or gastric malignancy as a cause of UGIB is the presence of iron-deficiency anemia in the setting of acute GI bleeding.

Table 22.3 Differential diagnosis of lower gastrointestinal bleeding (LGIB).

Cause (% of all cases of LGIB)	Pathogenic factors	Presentation	Course	Treatment
Diverticulosis (25–40%)	Constipation Older age Low fiber intake	Abrupt onset of painless maroon stools or bright red blood per rectum	>60% cease spontaneously within 12 hours of onset Rebleeding in 25–35% of cases	Colonoscopy Angiography with embolization Surgery
Angiodysplasia (3–37%)	CKD Anticoagulation Aortic stenosis	Intermittent melena Iron-deficiency anemia Painless hematochezia	>80% success rate of endoscopic treatment	Endoscopic hemostasis Estrogen Octreotide
Internal hemorrhoids (10%)	Constipation	Painless intermittent bloody stools	Majority present with small-volume bleeding	Suppositories Band ligation Hemorrhoidectomy
Neoplasms (15%)	Family history Older age Polyposis syndromes Lynch syndrome (HNPCC) IBD	Iron deficiency	40% mortality rate	Chemotherapy, radiation, surgery
Colitis (10%)	Ischemia IBD Infection (e.g., *Shigella*, *Salmonella*, CMV) Radiation therapy	Bloody stools Bright red blood per rectum	Most cases of ischemic colitis resolve with no complications 20% of patients with extensive colitis due to IBD require surgery	Supportive treatment for ischemic colitis Glucocorticoids, biologic agents, cyclosporine, surgery for IBD Antibiotics/antiviral agents for infections Argon plasma coagulation for radiation proctitis
UGIB (10%)	NSAIDs *H. pylori* infection	Brisk hematochezia	Mortality rate can be up to 30%	Endoscopic hemostasis Angiography Surgery

CKD, chronic kidney disease; CMV, cytomegalovirus; IBD, inflammatory bowel disease; HNPCC, hereditary nonpolyposis colorectal cancer; NSAIDs, nonsteroidal anti-inflammatory drugs; UGIB, upper gastrointestinal bleed.

General Risk Factors for GI Bleeding

- Older age.
- Prior history of GI bleed.
- Chronic liver disease.
- Coagulation disorders.
- Use of medications such as anticoagulants, aspirin and other NSAIDs, and antiplatelet agents such as clopidogrel.

Clinical Features

History

- The onset, duration, severity, and character of emesis (bright red blood, coffee ground), quantity of emesis, and presence of melena or hematochezia and associated nausea, retching, and abdominal pain should be determined.
- Associated symptoms including long-standing heartburn, chronic constipation, diarrhea, and nosebleeds should be ascertained.
- A history of chronic liver disease should be elicited. The history should also include an assessment of risk factors for liver disease such as a history of illicit drug use, alcohol abuse, blood transfusions and unprotected sex, as well as a family history of liver disease.
- Key features of the past medical history include previous GI bleeding, abdominal surgery, and concomitant medical conditions.
- A thorough medication history should be obtained. Use of NSAIDs, anticoagulants, and antiplatelet agents such as clopidrogrel should be determined. Gingko biloba (a herbal supplement) and selective serotonin reuptake inhibitors may also increase the risk of bleeding. Prior ingestion of a caustic agent should be determined.
- The social history should include alcohol, tobacco, and illicit drug use.
- The family history should include liver disease, bleeding disorders, cancer, and inflammatory bowel disease.

Physical Examination

- The assessment of hemodynamic stability is of utmost importance in patients with acute GI bleeding. Patients should be evaluated immediately for symptoms and signs of shock, and those without overt tachycardia or hypotension should be examined for orthostatic hemodynamic changes.
- Orthostatic changes in pulse rate and blood pressure are indicative of hypovolemia in the setting of GI bleeding. An increase in the pulse rate of 20 per minute and a drop in blood pressure of 20 mmHg systolic or 10 mmHg

diastolic from the supine to standing position indicate roughly 700 ml of blood loss. Lightheadedness or dizziness when standing from a sitting position is a sensitive marker for the presence of orthostasis.

- Patients should be examined for stigmata of chronic liver disease (e.g., spider telangiectasias, ascites, palmar erythema, splenomegaly, caput medusae). Peritoneal signs (abdominal rebound tenderness, guarding, or rigidity) may indicate a perforated ulcer, perforated colon (from ischemic colitis, inflammatory bowel disease), or toxic megacolon (due to inflammatory bowel disease).

Treatment

General

- Regardless of the source of bleeding, fluid resuscitation is the first and most important step in the management of GI bleeding, especially in patients with hemodynamic compromise. Measures include the following:
  - Placement of two large-bore (16- or 18-gauge) intravenous (IV) lines or a central venous line.
  - Immediate volume expansion with IV fluids.
  - Transfusion of packed red blood cells to a hemoglobin level goal of $7\,g\,dl^{-1}$ (up to $8\,g\,dl^{-1}$ in patients with coronary artery disease).
  - Treatment of coagulopathy. Transfuse platelets to maintain the platelet count $>50\,000\,mm^{-3}$. Endoscopy may be performed safely at an INR <2.5. The use of fresh-frozen plasma (FFP) or prothrombin complex should be individualized.
  - Vasopressors may be indicated in some patients if volume expansion alone does not stabilize the blood pressure.
- Hemodynamic instability or evidence of significant ongoing blood loss (active hematemesis, melena, or at least moderately severe hematochezia) is an indication for admission to an intensive care unit for close monitoring. Intubation may be required for protection of the airway in patients with massive hematemesis.
- Laboratory tests including a complete blood count, comprehensive metabolic panel, prothrombin time, and partial prothrombin time should be obtained in all patients. Blood should be typed and cross-matched.
- All anticoagulants should be withheld. Antihypertensive medications should be used with caution.

UGIB

- If UGIB is suspected, an urgent consultation with a gastroenterologist should be obtained.

- The hemoglobin level at the time of presentation of acute GI bleeding may be higher than the patient's actual hemoglobin level due to hemoconcentration.
- A 2–3% decrease in the hematocrit value reflects blood loss of ~500 ml.
- A blood urea nitrogen-to-creatinine ratio >36 may be found in patients with UGIB (without underlying renal insufficiency) due to prerenal azotemia and absorption of digested blood during intestinal transit.
- In addition to a low hemoglobin level, patients with cirrhosis may have low white blood cell and platelet counts and an increased INR.

> Use of a nasogastric (NG) tube is controversial. NG lavage may be negative in 10% of patients with UGIB, and a clear aspirate does not necessarily rule out UGIB. NG lavage may be useful, however, in the setting of hematochezia that results in hemodynamic compromise when an UGIB may be the source. If the NG lavage shows bilious return (indicating no blood in stomach and duodenum), then an upper source is unlikely, and management for LGIB can proceed (see later). If the aspirate is clear and not bilious, bleeding from the duodenum cannot be ruled out definitively, and esophagoduodenoscopy (EGD) should be performed.

- Variceal UGIB (see Chapter 16):
  - In patients with suspected variceal bleeding, octreotide should be administered intravenously in a dose of 50 μg bolus followed by 50 μg h^{-1}. Octreotide is preferred to IV vasopression plus nitroglycerin.
  - Antibiotics should be administered in all cases of suspected variceal bleeding. Antibiotics reduce the incidence of spontaneous bacterial peritonitis associated with acute variceal bleeding. Ceftriaxone 1 g IV or norfloxacin 400 mg orally twice daily for 7 days is recommended.
  - EGD can be diagnostic as well as therapeutic, and should be performed once a patient is hemodynamically stable:
    o For active bleeding from esophageal varices, upper-endoscopic band ligation or sclerotherapy can be used to stop bleeding; where available, band ligation is preferred.
    o Gastric varices are not amenable to these endoscopic treatments in most cases; where available, injection of cyanoacrylate may be an option.
    o Insertion of a Sengstaken–Blakemore or Minnesota tube may be necessary for massive variceal hemorrhage. These tubes have gastric and esophageal balloons that can be inflated to tamponade varices.
    o A transjugular intrahepatic portosystemic shunt (TIPS) may be placed to manage patients with variceal bleeding that does not respond to medical or endoscopic treatment. TIPS reduces elevated portal

Table 22.4 Endoscopic predictors of peptic ulcer rebleeding.

Endoscopic finding	Frequency (%)	Risk of rebleeding without endoscopic hemostasis (%)	Treatment
Arterial spurting	10	90	PPI + endoscopic hemostasis
Nonbleeding visible vessel	25	50	PPI + endoscopic hemostasis
Adherent clot	10	25–30	PPI ± endoscopic hemostasis
Oozing without visible vessel	10	10–20	PPI ± endoscopic hemostasis
Pigmented spot	10	7–10	PPI Consider discharge from ED
Clean-based ulcer	35	3–5	PPI Consider discharge from ED

ED, emergency department; PPI, proton pump inhibitor.

pressure by creating a communication between the hepatic vein and an intrahepatic branch of the portal vein.

- Nonvariceal UGIB:
  - If peptic ulcer disease is suspected, a proton pump inhibitor (PPI) should be given either intravenously (e.g., esomeprazole or pantoprazole 40 mg twice daily) or orally (40 mg twice daily). Once endoscopic treatment is performed or if there is no rebleeding within 72 hours, the patient can be transitioned to an oral PPI once daily.
  - EGD can be diagnostic as well as therapeutic and should be performed once the patient is hemodynamically stable (Table 22.4).
  - For active bleeding from a gastric or duodenal ulcer, endoscopic hemostatic modalities such as injection of epinephrine plus electrocautery or placement of hemoclips may be used.
  - Angiography may be used when endoscopic control of bleeding cannot be achieved.
  - Surgery is indicated in patients with ongoing bleeding despite medical and endoscopic treatment (see Chapter 4).

LGIB

- UGIB should be ruled out before attempting to localize the source of presumed LGIB that results in hemodynamic compromise. NG lavage may be useful but may be negative in 10% of cases. EGD may be necessary to rule out an UGIB.

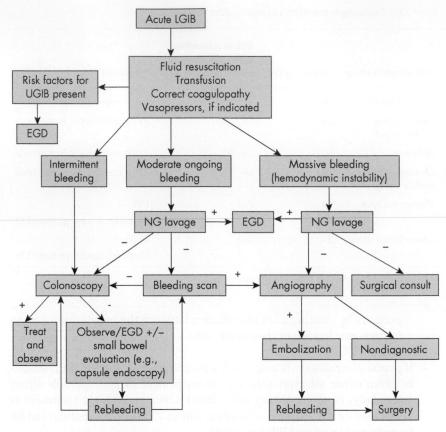

Figure 22.1 Algorithm for the management of lower gastrointestinal bleeding (LGIB). EGD, esophagogastroduodenoscopy; NG, nasogastric; UGIB, upper GI bleeding.

- Colonoscopy is generally considered the test of choice for diagnosis and potential therapy (Figure 22.1).
  - If bleeding stops spontaneously, subsequent colonoscopy is recommended. Colonoscopy identifies the source of bleeding in >70% of patients.
  - In patients who are hemodynamically stable but continue to bleed, colonoscopy can be performed after a rapid purge with polyethylene glycol solution administered through a NG tube. If the source is not found, a bleeding scan can be considered.
- A bleeding (tagged red blood cell) scan utilizes technetium sulfur colloid-labeled autologous red blood cells, which are infused back into the patient to detect the site of bleeding.

- The study detects GI bleeding that occurs at a rate of >0.1 ml min^{-1}, and is more sensitive than angiography.
  - A bleeding scan does not localize the site of bleed precisely and is not therapeutic.
- In patients who continue to bleed and are hemodynamically unstable, multidetector computed tomography angiography may be diagnostic, and angiography may be diagnostic and therapeutic (with embolization or intra-arterial infusion of vasopressin).
  - The study detects GI bleeding that occurs at a rate of 0.5–1.5 ml min^{-1}.
  - The diagnostic yield is variable and depends on the timing of the procedure, patient selection, and experience and skill of the radiologist.
  - Complications of angiography include acute kidney injury, cholesterol emboli, and bowel infarction.
- Surgery may be required for uncontrolled bleeding or in some cases of recurrent diverticular bleeding, which can occur in up to 35% of cases.
- Although colonoscopy is the diagnostic test of choice for LGIB, a plain abdominal X-ray and/or computed tomography (CT) may be used to diagnose ischemic colitis.
  - Irregular thickening of the mucosal folds may lead to classic 'thumbprinting' on plain film.
  - The presence of pneumatosis cystoides intestinalis (air in the wall of the colon) or portomesenteric venous gas may be an ominous sign indicating transmural infarction.
  - CT may show a thickened colonic wall.
- Capsule endoscopy, a noninvasive modality to image the small bowel, and/or deep enteroscopy can be used to identify the source of bleeding when EGD, colonoscopy, and other modalities fail to reveal a source.

Pearls

- Regardless of the source of bleeding, fluid resuscitation is the first and most important step in the management of GI bleeding.
- Upper endoscopy is the diagnostic test of choice for UGIB.
- Bleeding from esophageal or gastric varices carries a mortality rate of 50% if untreated.
- An UGI source of bleeding should be ruled out in patients with hemodynamically significant LGIB.
- The diagnostic test of choice for LGIB depends on the rapidity of bleeding; colonoscopy is often the preferred initial test.

Questions

Questions 1 and 2 relate to the clinical vignette at the beginning of this chapter.

1 Which of the following should be the first step in the management of this patient?
   A A proton pump inhibitor.
   B Angiography.
   C Fluid resuscitation.
   D Intravenous octreotide.
   E Consultation with a gastroenterologist or surgeon.

2 Which of the following medications is preferred in the treatment of this patient's acute GI bleeding?
   A A proton pump inhibitor and octreotide.
   B Octreotide alone.
   C Vasopressin and nitroglycerin.
   D Vasopressin alone.

3 A 27-year-old man presents to the emergency department with three episodes of bright red blood per rectum the day after completing a marathon. The bleeding has resolved. He notes cramping lower abdominal discomfort prior to bowel movements. His vital signs include a blood pressure of 95/50 mmHg and pulse rate 112 per minute. The hemoglobin level is 14 g dl^{-1}. The remainder of the laboratory tests are normal. Which of the following is the next best step in the management of this patient?
   A Perform a rapid purge with polyethylene glycol for immediate colonoscopy.
   B Provide supportive care with intravenous fluids and perform an elective colonoscopy.
   C Perform a bleeding scan.
   D Consult a surgeon for possible colectomy.

4 A 23-year-old woman presents to the emergency department with an episode of vomiting bright red blood. She has had flu-like symptoms and nausea for the past week and has been retching and vomiting straw-colored fluid. She denies rectal bleeding or melena. She denies use of nonsteroidal anti-inflammatory drugs (NSAIDs) or anticoagulants. The past medical history is unremarkable. Vitals signs include a blood pressure of 123/76 mmHg and pulse rate 95 per minute. Rectal examination shows brown stool that is negative for occult blood. The hemoglobin value is 15.2 g dl^{-1}. Which of the following would you recommend?

A Reassure the patient and provide anti-emetics for nausea.
B Computed tomography (CT) scan.
C Nasogastric (NG) lavage.
D Angiography.

5 A 25-year-old man presents with a moderate amount of bright red blood in his bowel movements. He reports diarrhea (four to six loose stools per day) over the past 6 months, and notes that many bowel movements have been mixed with blood in the past month. He has urgency and tenesmus. He also reports cramping lower abdominal pain that is relieved by a bowel movement but has no nausea, vomiting, or melena. He reports an unintentional weight loss of 18 lb (8 kg) over the past 6 months. Physical examination reveals a blood pressure of 120/80 mmHg, pulse rate 80 per minute, and temperature 100.3 °F (38 °C). The remainder of the examination is unremarkable except for maroon stool on rectal examination. Laboratory tests show a hemoglobin level of 7.8 g dl^{-1} with a mean corpuscular volume of 68 fl. The white blood cell count is 14 200 mm^{-3} and platelet count 556 000 mm^{-3}. The remainder of the blood tests are normal. Which of the following is the most likely diagnosis?
A Ulcerative colitis.
B Diverticulosis.
C Portal hypertensive gastropathy.
D Colonic arteriovenous malformation.
E Hemorrhoids.

6 A 68-year-old man presents to the emergency department with bright red blood per rectum that started 4 hours ago. He denies abdominal pain, nausea, vomiting, hematemesis, or melena. He has no prior history of gastrointestinal bleeding. He is otherwise healthy. He takes no prescription or over-the-counter medications. He does not drink alcohol or smoke cigarettes. Vital signs include a blood pressure of 82/46 mmHg and pulse rate 124 per minute. Physical examination is unremarkable. There are no stigmata of chronic liver disease. Rectal examination shows clots. The patient refuses an NG tube. Laboratory tests, including a complete blood count and comprehensive metabolic panel, are normal except for a hemoglobin level of 6.8 g dl^{-1}. Colonoscopy is performed after a rapid purge, and is normal. Which of the following tests should be considered next?
A Capsule endoscopy.
B Bleeding scan.
C Esophagogastroduodenoscopy (EGD).
D Repeat colonoscopy.
E Angiography.

Answers

1 C

2 A

This patient has an acute UGIB and is hemodynamically unstable, as suggested by tachycardia and orthostasis. Fluid resuscitation with two large-bore IV lines should be the first step in the management of this patient. Although the patient appears to have signs of liver disease, a bleeding peptic ulcer cannot be excluded. Therefore, continuous infusion of a proton pump inhibitor (in case of an ulcer) and octreotide (in case of varices) is warranted. Once the patient is hemodynamically stable, esophagogastroduodenoscopy (EGD) should be performed to determine the source of bleeding. Angiography has no role in the initial management of an UGIB. Vasopressin and nitrates may be used in variceal bleeding as an alternative to octreotide.

3 B

This patient has LGIB, likely due to intestinal ischemia, a not uncommon occurrence in marathon runners. The bleeding has ceased, and the patient does not require a rapid purge for immediate colonoscopy or a bleeding scan. Hypotension and tachycardia indicate hypovolemia, which requires fluid resuscitation. A colonoscopy can be performed electively during the same hospital admission after adequate fluid resuscitation and blood transfusion.

4 A

This patient presents with classic symptoms of a Mallory–Weiss tear, as indicated by several episodes of retching and nonbloody emesis prior to hematemesis. The diagnosis of a Mallory–Weiss tear can often be suspected by history alone. Bleeding is self-limited in 90% of patients with a Mallory–Weiss tear. Endoscopic therapy in indicated if there is evidence of ongoing bleeding. Reassuring the patient and providing anti-emetics to help relieve nausea related to an acute viral illness would be the most appropriate management.

5 A

The patient is young and is presenting with chronic diarrhea that has become bloody. The presentation is suggestive of ulcerative colitis. He has significant weight loss and elevated white blood cell and platelets counts, as well as anemia. He has no stigmata of liver disease, and therefore portal hypertensive gastropathy is unlikely. Diverticulosis and colonic arteriovenous malformation are unlikely given the patient's age. Hemorrhoids present with bright red blood per rectum without weight loss, microcytic anemia, or other systemic features.

6 C

Approximately 10% of cases of LGIB are due to an upper GI source; therefore, an EGD should be performed. A bleeding scan and angiography may be considered if the EGD is negative and the patient has ongoing bleeding. Repeat colonoscopy is not indicated at this time. Capsule endoscopy may be considered if the EGD is negative and the patient is hemodynamically stable.

Further Reading

Garcia-Tsao, G., Sanyal, A.J., Grace, N.D., *et al.* (2007) Practice Guidelines Committee of the American Association for the Study of Liver Diseases; Practice Parameters Committee of the American College of Gastroenterology: Prevention and management of gastroesophageal varices and variceal hemorrhage in cirrhosis. *Hepatology*, **46**, 922–938.

Hwang, J.H., Fisher, D.A., Ben-Menachem, T., *et al.* (2012) Standards of Practice Committee ASGE Guideline: the role of endoscopy in acute non-variceal hemorrhage. *Gastrointestinal Endoscopy*, **75**, 1132–1138.

Jensen, D. and Savides, T. (2016) Gastrointestinal bleeding, in *Sleisenger and Fordtran's Gastrointestinal and Liver Disease: Pathophysiology, Diagnosis, and Management*, 10th edition (eds M. Feldman, L.S. Friedman, and L.J. Brandt), Saunders Elsevier, Philadelphia, pp. 297–335.

Pasha, S.F., Shergill, A., Acosta, R.D., *et al.* (2014) Standards of Practice Committee ASGE Guideline: the role of endoscopy in the patient with lower GI bleeding. *Gastrointestinal Endoscopy*, **79**, 875–885.

Weblinks

http://www.merckmanuals.com/professional/gastrointestinal-disorders/gi-bleeding/overview-of-gi-bleeding
http://www.aafp.org/afp/2005/0401/p1339.html

23

Abdominal Pain

Kamil Obideen

Clinical Vignette 1

A 65-year-old man presents with a 2-month history of progressive dull constant epigastric abdominal pain. The pain is associated with early satiety and a 5 lb (2.2 kg) weight loss. His past medical history is significant for hypertension. His medications include amlodipine and low-dose aspirin. He does not drink alcohol and quit smoking cigarettes 3 years ago. On physical examination, he is afebrile with a blood pressure of 140/85 mmHg, pulse rate 93 per minute, and respiratory rate 15 per minute. Abdominal examination reveals epigastric tenderness on deep palpation. Laboratory tests were normal except for an elevated serum alkaline phosphatase of 370 IU l^{-1} and total bilirubin of 1.7 mg dl^{-1}.

Clinical Vignette 2

A 31-year-old woman is seeking a second opinion for abdominal pain of 10 years' duration. Her symptoms began at age 20. The abdominal pain occurs daily, is usually diffuse, constant, dull, or cramping in nature, and is unrelated to eating, bowel movements, physical activity, or her menstrual cycle. The pain has increased in intensity and duration over the past 5 years. She denies blood in the stool, diarrhea, constipation, anemia, weight loss or nocturnal pain, but occasionally sees mucus in the stool. She has missed a substantial number of days at work because of abdominal pain and has had several visits to the emergency department. She is usually treated with morphine and phenargan and discharged with a prescription for narcotics. A review of her medical records indicates extensive diagnostic testing that has been negative for major medical disorders. Tests performed include two colonoscopies, three esophagogastroduodenoscopies, multiple computed tomographies of the abdomen and

---

Sitaraman and Friedman's Essentials of Gastroenterology, Second Edition.
Edited by Shanthi Srinivasan and Lawrence S. Friedman.
© 2018 John Wiley & Sons Ltd. Published 2018 by John Wiley & Sons Ltd.

pelvis, and magnetic resonance imaging of the abdomen. All the test results were normal. She underwent cholecystectomy 6 years ago. A laparoscopy done 3 years ago showed some adhesions but was otherwise normal. She is currently under the care of a psychiatrist who diagnosed posttraumatic stress disorder resulting from a childhood history of physical abuse and family deprivation. She takes paroxetine 20 mg daily. She is single and has one daughter from a previous marriage. She lives with her mother. On examination, she appears to be in moderate pain and 'wincing' while holding her abdomen. She is afebrile with a blood pressure of 110/60 mmHg and pulse rate 80 per minute. Abdominal examination is unremarkable when she is distracted.

General

- Abdominal pain is a complex sensation, the manifestations of which depend on an interplay between pathophysiologic and psychosocial factors.
- Abdominal pain is one of the most common causes of visits to a primary care provider, accounting for 2.5 million visits to office-based physicians per year. It is the most frequent reason for a gastroenterology consultation.

Classification

Abdominal pain can be classified based on neurologic origin or clinical presentation.

- Based on **neurologic** origin, abdominal pain can be divided into three types:
  - **Visceral pain**: stimulation of visceral nerves produces dull, poorly localized pain felt in the midline. Pain is perceived in the abdominal region corresponding to the affected organ's embryonic origin (Table 23.1). Ischemia, inflammation, distention of a hollow organ, or capsular stretching of a solid organ produces visceral pain.
  - **Somatoparietal pain** arises from stimulation of the parietal peritoneum. It is generally more intense and more precisely localized than visceral pain.
  - **Referred pain** is felt in areas remote from the affected organ (e.g., gallbladder disease may be experienced as pain in the right subscapular area). Referred pain is the result of convergence of visceral afferent neurons and somatic afferent neurons from different anatomic regions on second-order neurons in the spinal cord at the same spinal segment.
- Based on **clinical** presentation, abdominal pain can be divided into acute, subacute, or chronic:
  - **Acute**: pain of less than a few days' duration that has worsened progressively until the time of presentation (see Chapter 25).

Table 23.1 Localization of visceral pain based on embryonic origin.

Embryonic origin	Location of pain	Organ	Nerves stimulated
Foregut	Epigastrium	Stomach First two portions of the duodenum Liver Gallbladder Pancreas	Vagus nerve (parasympathetic) Greater thoracic splanchnic nerve (sympathetic)
Midgut	Periumbilical	Third and fourth portions of the duodenum Jejunum Ileum Cecum Appendix Ascending and proximal two thirds of the transverse colon	Vagus nerve (parasympathetic) Greater thoracic splanchnic nerve (sympathetic)
Hindgut	Hypogastrium	Distal one third of the transverse colon, descending colon, sigmoid colon, and rectum Upper portion of the anal canal Ovaries, fallopian tubes, and uterus Seminal vesicles and prostate gland Ureters and urinary bladder	Pelvic splanchnic nerve (parasympathetic) Lesser thoracic splanchnic nerve (sympathetic)

- **Subacute**: pain that lasts a few days to <6 months.
- **Chronic**: pain that has remained unchanged for months to years.

Etiology

- Chronic abdominal pain may be 'functional' (no identifiable structural disease) or 'organic' (identifiable structural disease) (Table 23.2). Neuro-musculoskeletal disorders such as anterior cutaneous nerve entrapment, myofascial pain syndromes, and thoracic nerve radiculopathy may present as abdominal pain.

Table 23.2 Some causes of chronic abdominal pain.

	Structural disorders	Functional gastrointestinal disorders
Chronic intermittent pain	**Inflammatory** Chronic appendicitis Chronic or relapsing pancreatitis Fibrosing mesenteritis Inflammatory bowel disease **Vascular** Mesenteric ischemia **Metabolic** Diabetic neuropathy Familial Mediterranean fever Porphyria Uremia **Musculoskeletal** Anterior cutaneous nerve entrapment syndrome Myofascial pain syndrome **Others** Gallstones Intermittent bowel obstruction (hernia, intussuception, adhesion, volvulus) Peptic ulcer disease	Biliary pain (sphincter of Oddi dysfunction) Centrally mediated abdominal pain syndrome (CAPS)* Functional dyspepsia Irritable bowel syndrome Levator ani syndrome Narcotic bowel syndrome Pelvic floor dysfunction Severe gastroparesis
Chronic constant pain	Abscess Chronic pancreatitis Inflammatory bowel disease Malignancy Pelvic inflammatory disease	CAPS Functional dyspepsia

* Rome IV criteria for the diagnosis of CAPS: all the following must be present for the previous 3 months with symptom onset at least 6 months before diagnosis:
1) continuous or nearly continuous abdominal pain;
2) no or only occasional relationship of pain with physiological events (e.g., eating, defecation, menses);
3) pain limits some aspect of daily functioning;
4) the pain is not feigned;
5) pain is not explained by another structural or functional gastrointestinal disorder or other medical condition.

- The most common cause of chronic abdominal pain is a functional disorder such as irritable bowel syndrome (see Chapter 7) or centrally mediated abdominal pain syndrome (CAPS; formerly functional abdominal pain syndrome [FAPS]).

Approach to Diagnosis

History and Physical Examination

- The initial work-up of a patient with chronic abdominal pain should focus on differentiating functional from organic causes. The history is critical.

Clinical features that suggest an organic etiology include weight loss, fever, change in appetite, nocturnal awakening with pain, association of pain with bowel movements, dehydration, electrolyte abnormalities, symptoms or signs of gastrointestinal blood loss, anemia, and signs of malnutrition.

- On the basis of the history there often is no need for an extensive diagnostic work-up, if the characteristics of the abdominal pain fit the so-called Rome IV criteria for irritable bowel syndrome (Chapter 7), functional dyspepsia, or CAPS.
- CAPS is considered a biopsychosocial disorder in which symptoms can be attributed to brain–gut dysfunction or abnormal perception of normal gut function. The cognitive and emotional centers of the central nervous system are the primary modulator of pain in CAPS. Psychosocial factors including major depression, anxiety disorder, somatoform disorder, and life stresses such as physical, sexual, or emotional abuse are common in patients with CAPS. CAPS is usually associated with loss of daily functioning including work or school absenteeism and limitations in social activities.
- A thorough physical examination should be performed. The abdominal examination should include inspection, auscultation (for bruits), percussion, and palpation (for organomegaly, masses, and ascites). The patient should be evaluated for signs of malnutrition (e.g., muscle wasting).

Diagnostic Tests

The following tests are recommended in most patients with suspected organic chronic abdominal pain. Judicious use of laboratory and imaging tests is recommended in patients suspected of having functional abdominal pain.

- Complete blood count with differential cell count
- Comprehensive metabolic profile

- Serum amylase and lipase levels
- Urinalysis
- Imaging and endoscopic studies should be guided by symptoms and signs:
  - Ultrasonography is recommended for patients presenting with right upper quadrant pain; ultrasonography is sensitive and specific for the detection of gallstones and their complications.
  - Computed tomography of the abdomen and pelvis.
  - Endoscopy (esophagogastroduodenoscopy, colonoscopy, capsule endoscopy).
- Other specialized tests include magnetic resonance imaging, magnetic resonance cholangiopancreatography, endoscopic ultrasonography, gastric emptying scan, and mesenteric angiography in selected cases.
- If the diagnosis is not clear after initial assessment and testing, watchful waiting with close monitoring is appropriate.

Pearls

- Chronic abdominal pain in patients over 50 years of age or in immunocompromised persons always requires work-up for an organic illness.
- Laboratory and diagnostic imaging evaluation must be tailored to answer specific questions arising from a carefully derived differential diagnosis based on a detailed history and physical examination. Unnecessary laboratory testing is costly, and often clouds the diagnostic picture.

Questions

Questions 1 and 2 relate to the clinical vignettes at the beginning of this chapter.

1 What is the most appropriate next step in the management of the patient presented in clinical vignette 1?
   A Esophagogastroduodenoscopy (EGD).
   B Trial of a proton pump inhibitor.
   C Abdominal ultrasonography.
   D Computed tomography (CT) of the abdomen and pelvis.

2 What is the most appropriate next step in the management of the patient presented in clinical vignette 2?
   A Abdominal ultrasonography.
   B CT of the abdomen and pelvis.
   C Colonoscopy.
   D No further testing.

3   A 23-year-old woman presents with a 6-week history of periumbilical abdomi-
    nal pain associated with diarrhea. She reports a 5 lb (2.3 kg) weight loss during
    this time. On physical examination she appears thin and pale; she has mild
    diffuse tenderness on palpation but has no rebound tenderness or guarding.
    Laboratory tests are remarkable for a hemoglobin level of 11 g dl^{-1}. Stool
    cultures and tests for ova and parasites, and *Clostridium difficile* toxin are
    negative. Which of the following tests is most likely to establish the diagnosis?
    A Small-bowel capsule endoscopy.
    B Ultrasonography.
    C CT of the abdomen and pelvis.
    D Colonoscopy.

4   A 21-year-old woman is seeking a second opinion for 1-year history of pro-
    gressive dull intermittent left lower quadrant and suprapubic abdominal
    pain; she reports that the pain has increased in intensity and duration over
    the past 6 months. The pain is not related to eating or bowel movements,
    but increases in intensity around her menstrual cycle. She awakens at night
    because of the pain. She has had multiple visits to the emergency depart-
    ment for severe abdominal pain. A review of her medical records reveals an
    extensive diagnostic work-up, including colonoscopy, EGD, multiple CTs of
    the abdomen and pelvis, and ultrasonography of the abdomen and pelvis.
    All the tests have been normal. She had normal laboratory results except for
    a hemoglobin level of 11.2 g dl^{-1}. Physical examination reveals a thin woman
    with mild tenderness in the left lower quadrant. The remainder of the exam-
    ination is unremarkable. Which of the following is the most appropriate
    next step in the management of this patient?
    A Capsule endoscopy.
    B CT enterography.
    C Laparoscopy.
    D No further testing.

Answers

1   D
    The patient is over 50 years of age and has a history of cigarette smoking
    with 'alarm' symptoms, including weight loss, early satiety, and an elevated
    serum bilirubin level. A CT of the abdomen and pelvis is the best initial
    test to evaluate the patient for suspected biliary or upper gastrointestinal
    disease. Abdominal ultrasonography would be an appropriate test in the
    absence of alarm symptoms; however, in a patient with alarm symptoms, it
    is best to proceed with a CT of the abdomen and pelvis.

2 **D**

The patient is young and presents with symptoms typical of chronic functional abdominal pain with no alarm symptoms (e.g., weight loss, anemia, fever, nocturnal pain). She has already had extensive diagnostic testing and meets the Rome IV criteria for centrally mediated abdominal pain syndrome (CAPS). Therefore, no further testing is indicated.

3 **D**

The patient has chronic abdominal pain associated with diarrhea, weight loss, and anemia. Her clinical presentation is suspicious for inflammatory bowel disease, and colonoscopy is the best initial test to confirm the diagnosis.

4 **C**

The patient presents with symptoms suggestive of endometriosis. Laparoscopy will confirm the diagnosis. All the other tests listed are not indicated.

Further Reading

Millham, F.H. (2016) Acute abdominal pain, in *Sleisenger and Fordtran's Gastrointestinal and Liver Disease: Pathophysiology/Diagnosis/Management*, 10th edition (eds M. Feldman, L.S. Friedman, and L.J. Brandt), Saunders Elsevier, Philadelphia, pp. 161–174.

Penner, R., Fishman, M.B., and Majumdar, S. (2016) Evaluation of the adult with abdominal pain. http://www.uptodate.com/contents/evaluation-of-the-adult-with-abdominal-pain. (Updated 26 February, 2016).

Yarze, J.C. and Friedman, L.S. (2016) Chronic abdominal pain, in *Sleisenger and Fordtran's Gastrointestinal and Liver Disease: Pathophysiology/Diagnosis/Management*, 10th edition (eds M. Feldman, L.S. Friedman, and L.J. Brandt), Saunders Elsevier, Philadelphia, pp. 175–184.

Weblinks

http://www.webmd.com/digestive-disorders/abdominal-pain
http://www.merckmanuals.com/professional/sec02/ch011/ch011b.html
http://www.nature.com/ajg/journal/v105/n4/full/ajg201068a.html

24

Jaundice

Nader Dbouk and Preeti A. Reshamwala

Clinical Vignette

A healthy neonate delivered 3 days ago is scheduled for discharge. During feeding, the mother notices that the baby's eyes are yellow and notifies the nurse. The mother and baby are otherwise well, and the pregnancy had been uneventful. The pediatrician notes no abnormalities on physical examination except for jaundice; he orders several laboratory studies. Results reveal a serum total bilirubin level of 18 mg dl^{-1}, direct bilirubin 1.0 mg dl^{-1}, and indirect bilirubin 17 mg dl^{-1}. A complete blood count is normal, and there is no evidence of hemolysis on the peripheral blood smear. On further questioning, the infant's father recalls that he had an older brother who died at age 3 years. The infant remains in the hospital for phototherapy due to frank jaundice, while the pediatrician obtains a genetic counselor to consult on the case.

Definition

- **Jaundice** (also known as **icterus**) is the clinical manifestation of hyperbilirubinemia, and is characterized by yellow discoloration of the skin, mucous membranes, and conjunctivae.

Bilirubin Metabolism

- Bilirubin, a hydrophobic and potentially toxic compound, is the end-product of heme degradation (Figure 24.1). In healthy adults, 70–80% of bilirubin is derived from the breakdown of senescent erythrocytes. Most of the

Sitaraman and Friedman's Essentials of Gastroenterology, Second Edition.
Edited by Shanthi Srinivasan and Lawrence S. Friedman.
© 2018 John Wiley & Sons Ltd. Published 2018 by John Wiley & Sons Ltd.

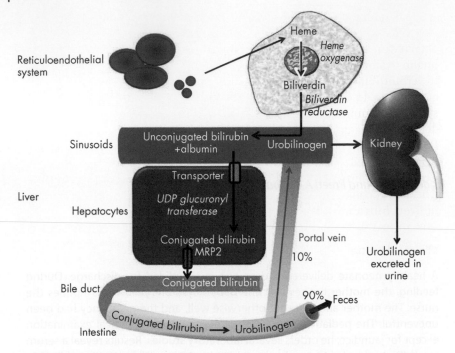

Figure 24.1 Bilirubin metabolism. MRP2, multidrug associated protein 2; UDP, uridine diphosphate.

remaining 20–30% is derived from the breakdown of hemoproteins such as catalase and cytochrome oxidases in the liver, and a minor component arises from the premature destruction of erythrocytes in the bone marrow or circulation.

- Bilirubin is the breakdown product of red blood cells. Heme is metabolized to biliverdin by the enzyme heme oxygenase; biliverdin is then converted to unconjugated bilirubin by the enzyme biliverdin reductase, mainly in the reticuloendothelial system.
- Unconjugated bilirubin is a hydrophobic molecule that circulates in the plasma noncovalently bound to albumin.
- Unconjugated bilirubin passes through the sinusoids into the space of Disse, where the bilirubin dissociates from albumin and is taken up by the hepatocytes by a transporter (an organic anion transporter that has not been fully characterized). Unconjugated bilirubin is converted to a water-soluble form through conjugation to glucuronic acid, which is mediated by the enzyme uridine diphosphate (UDP) glucuronyl transferase.
- The majority (up to 98%) of conjugated bilirubin is then secreted into the bile through an apically located active transport process mediated by the multidrug resistance-associated protein 2 (MRP2).

- A small amount of conjugated bilirubin is secreted into the hepatic sinusoids, enters the circulation, and is filtered by renal glomeruli and detected in the urine. (A small amount of conjugated bilirubin may be bound to albumin ['delta bilirubin'] and not filtered by the glomeruli.) With hyperbilirubinemia, filtered bilirubin gives the urine a classic tea-colored appearance. In contrast, unconjugated bilirubin is hydrophobic, bound to serum albumin, and not filtered by the glomeruli; therefore, it is not detected in the urine.
- Bilirubin is detected by the **van den Bergh reaction**. Bilirubin is cleaved to form a colored compound that can be assayed by spectrophotometry. Conjugated bilirubin is cleaved rapidly and is referred to as **direct bilirubin**, whereas unconjugated bilirubin is cleaved slowly and is referred to as **indirect bilirubin**.
- The normal serum bilirubin level is $1-1.5\,mg\,dl^{-1}$. The conjugated fraction constitutes <15% of the total bilirubin (normal value $<0.3\,mg\,dl^{-1}$).
- Jaundice develops at bilirubin concentrations $\geq 3\,mg\,dl^{-1}$. Other symptoms such as pruritus, diarrhea, and fatigue also may develop when the serum bilirubin level is $\geq 3\,mg\,dl^{-1}$.

In general, total serum bilirubin correlates with poor outcomes in patients with alcoholic hepatitis and chronic liver disease. Serum bilirubin is a critical component of the Model for End-Stage Liver Disease (MELD) score, which is used to assess survival of patients with end-stage liver disease (see Chapter 16).

Differential Diagnosis

- Clinically, causes of jaundice may be classified as: (1) isolated disorders of bilirubin metabolism; (2) liver disease; and (3) obstruction to bile flow.

Isolated Disorders of Bilirubin Metabolism

- Isolated unconjugated hyperbilirubinemia can be due to increased bilirubin production, decreased hepatocellular uptake, or decreased conjugation.
- Increased bilirubin production can be seen in patients with the following conditions:
  - Hemolytic anemias, which can be hereditary (e.g., hereditary spherocytosis, sickle cell disease) or acquired (e.g., autoimmune hemolytic anemia).
  - Large hematomas: the increase in bilirubin occurs during the resorption phase of the hematoma.
  - Repeated blood transfusions.
  - Ineffective erythropoeisis (e.g., thalassemia).

- Decreased hepatocellular uptake can be seen in patients taking certain drugs such as rifampin or cyclosporine.
- Impaired conjugation of bilirubin can be seen in Gilbert's syndrome, Crigler–Najjar syndrome, and physiologic jaundice of the newborn (see later).
  - Gilbert's syndrome:
    - Most common inherited cause of hyperbilirubinemia.
    - Autosomal recessive disorder, with a prevalence of 10% among Caucasians.
    - A mutation in the TATAA region in the 5′ promoter region of UDP glucuronyl transferase results in reduced levels of UDP glucuronyl transferase.
    - Serum bilirubin levels may increase two- to threefold with fasting, dehydration, alcohol ingestion, or acute illness.
    - Gilbert's syndrome has a benign course, and affected persons are asymptomatic. Elevated levels of unconjugated bilirubin generally are detected as an incidental finding on routine laboratory testing.
  - Crigler–Najjar syndrome type I:
    - Autosomal recessive disorder.
    - UDP glucuronyl transferase activity is absent, and patients often die in the neonatal period due to kernicterus.
    - Phototherapy can prevent kernicterus, and liver transplantation is curative.
  - Crigler–Najjar syndrome type II:
    - Autosomal recessive disorder.
    - Intermediate UDP glucuronyl transferase activity.
    - Patients are usually asymptomatic in the neonatal period, but present with jaundice in early childhood.
    - Phenobarbital increases UDP glucuronyl transferase activity, reduces bilirubin levels, and should be administered to help prevent neurologic complications.
- Isolated conjugated hyperbilirubinemia is seen in two other disorders associated with reduced excretion of bilirubin into the bile canaliculi and inherited in an autosomal recessive pattern, Dubin–Johnson syndrome and Rotor's syndrome.
  - Patients with Dubin–Johnson syndrome have mutations in the *ABCC2* (MRP2) gene, which encodes MRP2, and characteristic black pigmentation in the liver that is not present in Rotor's syndrome.
  - The genetic defect in Rotor's syndrome is in the OATP1B1/1B3 genes, which encode another hepatic transporter involved in bilirubin uptake by hepatocytes.
  - Both syndromes have a benign course and do not cause impairment in liver function.

Liver Disease

- Jaundice associated with liver disease is characterized by an increase in the serum bilirubin level that usually occurs in association with elevated liver biochemical test (serum aminotransferase, alkaline phosphatase) levels and prolongation of the prothrombin time. Bilirubin is predominantly conjugated in liver disease. Hyperbilirubinemia can occur with acute liver injury, chronic liver disease, or liver disease associated with cholestasis. Jaundice is typically an initial presentation of acute liver disease. In contrast, jaundice develops in late stages of chronic liver disease (e.g., cirrhosis).

Acute Liver Disease

- Jaundice is typically a part of the initial clinical presentation in patients with acute or subacute liver injury. These conditions are associated with markedly elevated serum aminotransferase levels out of proportion to the bilirubin and alkaline phosphatase levels (see Chapter 12). Examples of acute liver injury include:
  - Viral hepatitis (e.g., hepatitis A, B, C, D, and E and Epstein–Barr virus infection).
  - Drugs and hepatotoxins (e.g., alcohol, acetaminophen).
  - Ischemic hepatitis.
  - Reye's syndrome.
  - Acute fatty liver of pregnancy.
  - Pre-eclampsia associated with the hemolysis, elevated liver enzymes, and low platelets (HELLP) syndrome.

Chronic Liver Disease

- In chronic liver disease, jaundice is seen late in the course when cirrhosis is present, and is an ominous sign of hepatic decompensation (see Chapters 13, 14, and 15). Examples of chronic liver disease include the following:
  - Chronic viral hepatitis (hepatitis B, C, and D).
  - Chronic exposure to toxins, particularly alcohol.
  - Alpha-1 antitrypsin deficiency.
  - Autoimmune hepatitis.
  - Nonalcoholic fatty liver disease.
  - Hereditary hemochromatosis.
  - Wilson disease.

Liver Disease with Prominent Cholestasis

- Cholestasis signifies an impairment of bile flow from the liver. This can be due either to hepatocyte dysfunction and impaired transport of bilirubin to the bile canaliculi (intrahepatic cholestasis), or to obstruction of the extrahepatic bile ducts (extrahepatic cholestasis, discussed later). Cholestatic disorders are typically associated with predominant elevation of serum bilirubin and alkaline phosphatase levels relative to aminotransferase levels (see Chapter 12). Major causes of intrahepatic cholestasis include the following:

- Infiltrative diseases:
  o Granulomatous disorders of the liver: these can be caused by infections (tuberculosis, syphilis, parasites, fungal diseases, leprosy, *Mycobacterium avium* complex infection, and brucellosis), drugs (allopurinol, sulfonamides, and quinidine), and systemic disorders (sarcoidosis, Wegner's granulomatosis, and Hodgkin's lymphoma).
  o Systemic amyloidosis, which can present with hepatomegaly and jaundice: other findings may include macroglossia, heart failure, renal failure, and intestinal malabsorption.
- Disorders involving the biliary ductules:
  o Primary biliary cholangitis is characterized by inflammation of the small intrahepatic bile ducts and occurs primarily in middle-aged women (see Chapter 15).
  o Graft-versus-host disease occurs in up to 10% of bone marrow transplant recipients.
  o Drug-induced cholestasis: either 'bland' cholestasis or, in some cases, accompanied by features of immunoallergy, including arthralgias, fever, and rash, in addition to peripheral eosinophilia (drug reaction with eosinophilia and systemic symptoms [DRESS] syndrome). Medications that can cause cholestasis includes estrogen, anabolic steroids, erythromycin, mirtazapine, trimethoprim–sulfamethoxazole, terbinafine, amoxicillin–clavulinic acid, oral contraceptives, clopidogrel, and tricyclic antidepressants, as well as total parenteral nutrition.

Obstruction to Bile Flow

- Obstruction of the bile ducts can be due to intrinsic disorders of the bile ducts, extrinsic compression, or occlusion of the bile duct lumen.
- Diseases of the bile ducts:
  - Congenital disorders such as choledochal cysts and biliary atresia.
  - Inflammatory disorders such as primary sclerosing cholangitis (see Chapters 8 and 15).
  - Infectious disorders such as acquired immunodeficiency syndrome (AIDS) cholangiopathy.
  - Cholangiocarcinoma.
- Extrinsic compression of the bile ducts (e.g., by neoplasms such as pancreatic carcinoma, hepatocellular carcinoma, ampullary adenoma, and lymphoma or by pancreatitis or an aneurysm).

- Choledocholithiasis (see Chapter 21).
  - The most common of cause of bile duct obstruction is gallstones.

Chronic cholestasis may lead to various complications including hypercholesterolemia, fat-soluble vitamin deficiencies, osteopenia, pruritus, and steatorrhea. Patients should be screened routinely with bone densitometry, and supplementation with calcium and vitamin D should be recommended. Serum levels of fat-soluble vitamins (A, D, E, and K) should be measured and supplemented in case of deficiency.

Clinical Features

- The history should include the onset and duration of jaundice. Important associated symptoms may include fatigue, abdominal pain, nausea, vomiting, pruritus, fever or chills, weight loss, and arthralgias or arthritis.
- Conjugated hyperbilirubinemia can cause darkening of the urine, which may precede the onset of jaundice. Tea-colored urine, therefore, may be a more accurate indicator of the onset of hyperbilirubinemia than skin yellowing.
- Potential risk factors for liver disease or other systemic disorders that may be associated with jaundice should be identified. Assessment for risk factors for liver disease should include a history of illicit drug use, alcohol abuse, blood transfusions, unprotected sex, and a family history of liver or pancreatic disease.
- A meticulous medication history, including prescription, over-the-counter, and herbal agents, should be obtained (see Chapter 12).
- The past medical and surgical history should identify disorders associated with jaundice such as hepatobiliary disease, hemolytic anemia (e.g., sickle cell disease), AIDS, inflammatory bowel disease, and previous biliary surgery.
- The physical examination should focus on signs of systemic infection (fever, tachycardia, tachypnea), chronic liver disease (ascites, spider telangiectasias, palmar erythema, gynecomastia and testicular atrophy in men, hepatosplenomegaly, and encephalopathy), and heart failure.

The characteristic symptom of hyperbilirubinemia is jaundice (yellowing of the skin, conjunctivae, and mucous membranes). Jaundice develops at bilirubin concentrations $\geq 3\,\mathrm{mg\,dl^{-1}}$. Both conjugated and unconjugated hyperbilirubinemia result in jaundice.

Diagnosis

- Simple laboratory tests provide clues to the etiology of jaundice. These tests include a complete blood count and liver biochemical tests, including serum total bilirubin, alkaline phosphatase, alanine aminotransferase (ALT), and aspartate aminotransferase (AST) levels and the prothrombin time (Figure 24.2).
- Patients with an elevated serum bilirubin level but otherwise normal liver enzyme levels and liver function should be evaluated for evidence of hemolysis and genetic disorders associated with hyperbilirubinemia. In these disorders, most often, the majority of the elevated bilirubin is unconjugated.
- Patients with abnormal liver enzymes should undergo abdominal imaging (ultrasonography or computed tomography) to look for evidence of liver disease or biliary obstruction.
- Patients suspected of having liver disease should undergo a work-up to identify the specific cause of liver disease (see Chapters 12, 13, and 15). Screening laboratory studies may include viral serologies (including those for hepatitis B and C), serum levels of iron, transferrin, and ferritin

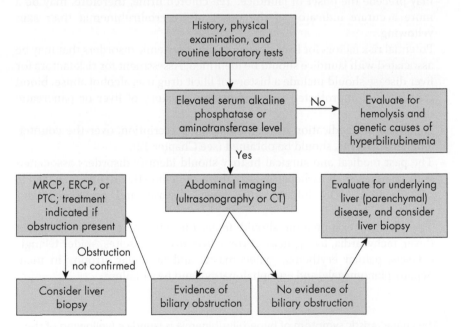

Figure 24.2 Algorithm for the approach to the patient with jaundice. CT, computed tomography; ERCP, endoscopic retrograde cholangiopancreatography; MRCP, magnetic resonance cholangiopancreatography; PTC, percutaneous transhepatic cholangiography.

(for hemochromatosis), serum ceruloplasmin (for Wilson disease), antimitochondrial antibodies (for primary biliary cholangitis), and antinuclear antibodies, smooth muscle antibodies, and serum protein electrophoresis or serum immunoglobulins (for autoimmune hepatitis).

- Patients with biliary obstruction should undergo further evaluation with magnetic resonance cholangiopancreatography (MRCP), endoscopic retrograde cholangiopancreatography (ERCP), or percutaneous transhepatic cholangiography (PTC) to visualize the bile ducts. ERCP and PTC also offer the potential for therapeutic intervention to relieve the obstruction when the index of suspicion for obstruction is high (see Chapter 21).
- A liver biopsy may be necessary in patients with abnormal liver enzymes without evidence of biliary obstruction on imaging when the laboratory evaluation is otherwise unrevealing.

Treatment

- The management of the patient with jaundice depends on the cause. When jaundice is caused by liver disease, management should be directed toward the underlying cause.
- Elevation of unconjugated bilirubin in neonates and infants has the potential to cause kernicterus, with irreversible brain injury, and should be treated promptly. Phototherapy reduces the risk of neurotoxicity by rendering bilirubin more water-soluble.
- If drug-induced cholestasis is suspected, all potential culprits should be discontinued and the patient observed for resolution of symptoms.
- Patients with biliary tract obstruction due to choledocholithiasis or malignancy often require endoscopic or surgical intervention to restore adequate biliary drainage (see Chapter 21).
- **Pruritus** can be treated with antihistamines, cholestyramine or other bile acid-binding resins, and rifampin.
- **Steatorrhea** is common in patients with advanced cholestatic liver disease and can be managed by a reduction in oral fat intake and substitution of dietary fat with medium-chain triglycerides (see Chapter 6).

Special Patient Populations

- Jaundice in the **postoperative patient** is often multifactorial. Predisposing factors include drug-induced liver toxicity from inhalational anesthetics, intraoperative or perioperative hypotension with ischemic liver injury, blood transfusions, total parenteral nutrition, antimicrobials/antifungals, and sepsis.

- Jaundice in the **critically ill patient** is often a manifestation of liver dysfunction occurring in a patient with sepsis and multiorgan dysfunction syndrome. Other potential etiologies include drug-induced hepatocellular injury or cholestasis, blood transfusions, and hypotension causing ischemic injury (ischemic hepatitis or ischemic cholangiopathy).
- Jaundice in **pregnancy** can be due to intrahepatic cholestasis of pregnancy, which usually presents in the third trimester and resolves within 2 weeks of delivery. Other less common conditions include acute fatty liver of pregnancy, which also occurs in the third trimester and is a life-threatening condition that necessitates urgent delivery. HELLP syndrome, a complication of pre-eclampsia, is characterized by hemolysis and elevated liver enzymes and is also treated by urgent delivery.
- **Neonatal jaundice** occurs in 60% of term and 80% of pre-term infants. Physiologic jaundice occurs due to increased hemolysis of fetal erythrocytes coupled with reduced hepatic conjugation of bilirubin due to a developmental delay in the expression of UDP glucuronyl transferase, thus leading to unconjugated hyperbilirubinemia. Bilirubin levels usually peak at around 72 hours, and 5–10% of infants develop serum bilirubin levels >10 mg dl^{-1}. In such cases, phototherapy can be used to reduce the risk of neurologic damage. Pathologic jaundice usually presents within the first 24 hours and can be due to infections, inherited enzyme deficiencies such as glucose-6-phosphate dehydrogenase (G6PD) deficiency, congenital deficiencies of bilirubin-conjugating enzymes and bile acid transporters, fetal–maternal ABO incompatibility, breast-milk jaundice, and dehydration.

Pearls

- Jaundice is a clinical manifestation of both unconjugated and conjugated hyperbilirubinemia, and usually indicates a total bilirubin level ≥3 mg dl^{-1}.
- A thorough history, physical examination, and simple laboratory tests should provide clues to the etiology of jaundice.
- Isolated hyperbilirubinemia is unlikely to be due to liver disease or biliary obstruction, and generally indicates increased bilirubin production (e.g., hemolysis), impaired hepatic uptake (e.g., rifampin), or impaired conjugation (e.g., Gilbert's syndrome).
- Liver disease and biliary obstruction are associated with predominantly conjugated hyperbilirubinemia.
- Imaging studies are helpful in evaluating a jaundiced patient for extrahepatic biliary obstruction and the presence of chronic liver disease.
- A liver biopsy is the final step in the evaluation of intrahepatic causes of jaundice.

Questions

Question 1 relates to the clinical vignette at the beginning of this chapter.

1 Which of the following is the most likely diagnosis?
 A Gilbert's syndrome.
 B Dubin–Johnson syndrome.
 C Crigler–Najjar syndrome type I.
 D Crigler–Najjar syndrome type II.
 E Rotor syndrome.

2 Cholestasis may be a consequence of which of the following conditions?
 A Biliverdin reductase deficiency.
 B Hemolysis.
 C Organic anion transporter deficiency.
 D Bile duct obstruction by gallstones.
 E All of the above.

3 A 20-year-old male college student is referred to you for evaluation of hyperbilirubinemia noted on routine laboratory testing. He has no complaints and feels well. His total bilirubin level is $3\,mg\,dl^{-1}$ (unconjugated bilirubin $2.7\,mg\,dl^{-1}$). Liver biochemical tests are otherwise normal, and the hematocrit value is normal. He does not drink alcohol and is on no medications. There is no family history of liver disease. He states that he recalls being told in the past that he had a slightly elevated bilirubin level, but the elevation resolved spontaneously on follow up. Which of the following should be done next?
 A Percutaneous liver biopsy.
 B Magnetic resonance image.
 C Endoscopic retrograde cholangiopancreatography.
 D Check a urine drug screen for barbiturates and a serum blood-alcohol level.
 E Reassurance.

4 A 15-year-old African American boy presents with jaundice. He has no other symptoms. His past medical history is unremarkable. He does not take any prescription or over-the-counter medications. Physical examination is unremarkable. Laboratory tests including a complete blood count and serum electrolyte, creatinine, aminotransferase, and alkaline phosphate levels are normal except for a hemoglobin of $5.8\,g\,dl^{-1}$, mean corpuscular volume $78\,fl$, total bilirubin $16\,mg\,dl^{-1}$, and direct bilirubin $2\,mg\,dl^{-1}$.

Which of the following is most likely to be found on further laboratory investigation?

A Immunoglobulin (Ig)M antibody to hepatitis A virus.

B Low serum ceruloplasmin level.

C Crescent shaped erythrocytes on peripheral blood smear.

D Elevated serum level of angiotensin-converting enzyme.

E None of the above.

Answers

1 C

Crigler–Najjar syndrome types I and II are autosomal recessive disorders associated with absent and reduced levels of UDP glucuronyl transferase, respectively. Patients with Crigler–Najjar syndrome present with marked unconjugated hyperbilirubinemia and little, if any, direct, or conjugated, bilirubin. Crigler–Najjar syndrome type I is a lethal disease; patients present in the neonatal period with jaundice, and mortality is due to kernicterus (the accumulation of unconjugated bilirubin in the brain). Liver transplantation is curative because it replaces the UDP glucuronyl transferase that has been deleted by the autosomal recessive mutation that causes the disease. Phototherapy is life-saving and serves as a bridge to liver transplantation. Crigler–Najjar syndrome type II presents in childhood. Because some activity of UDP glucuronyl transferase is present, the disease is not lethal and can be treated with phenobarbital. Gilbert's syndrome is a benign condition that is usually not detected until childhood or adolescence. Dubin–Johnson and Rotor syndromes are associated with direct hyperbilirubinemia and are not lethal.

2 D

Cholestasis is a condition in which the flow of bile from the liver is impaired. This can occur because of hepatocyte dysfunction and impaired transport of bilirubin to the bile canaliculi (intrahepatic cholestasis) or obstruction of the extrahepatic bile ducts (extrahepatic cholestasis). Cholestatic disorders are typically associated with a serum elevation of direct bilirubin (conjugated fraction) and alkaline phosphatase levels relative to the aminotransferase levels. Choices B and C are associated with isolated hyperbilirubinemia. Biliverdin reductase deficiency results in a decreased production of bilirubin.

3 E

The patient has Gilbert's syndrome, a benign condition characterized by elevation of unconjugated bilirubin levels, often triggered by physiologic stress or fasting, in an otherwise healthy person. No testing is indicated.

4 C

The patient is an African American who has isolated unconjugated hyper-bilirubinemia and microcytic anemia; therefore, the most likely cause of his marked hyperbilirubinemia is hemolytic anemia due to sickle cell disease. Hemolytic anemia is a common cause of indirect, or unconjugated, hyperbilirubinemia, and sickle cell disease is a leading cause of hemolysis. Note that patients with sickle cell disease may also present with cholestasis due to pigmented gallstones (see Chapter 21), in which case elevated con-jugated bilirubin levels along with elevated alkaline phosphatase levels may be seen. Acute hepatitis A, diagnosed by an antibody to hepatitis A virus in serum, presents with elevated aminotransferase levels and, in some cases, jaundice (see Chapter 13). A low serum ceruloplasmin level may be indicative of Wilson disease, a disorder in which copper accumu-lates in the liver and hemolytic anemia and indirect hyperbilirubinemia may occur. This disease is found primarily in Caucasians, and the red blood cells do not display the typical crescent, or sickle, shape seen in sickle cell disease (see Chapter 15). The angiotensin-converting enzyme level is a test used to aid in the diagnosis of granulomatous hepatitis, which typically is associated with jaundice and cholestasis, as may occur in patients with sarcoidosis. Because the alkaline phosphatase level is normal and the patient has hemolytic anemia, this diagnosis is unlikely.

Further Reading

Lidofsky, S.D. (2016) Jaundice, in *Sleisenger and Fordtran's Gastrointestinal and Liver Disease: Pathophysiology/Diagnosis/Management*, 10th edition (eds M. Feldman, L.S. Friedman, and L.J. Brandt), Saunders Elsevier, Philadelphia, pp. 336–348.

Wolkoff, A.W. and Berk, P.D. (2012) Bilirubin metabolism and jaundice, in *Shiff's Diseases of the Liver*, 11th edition (eds E. Shiff, W. Maddrey, and M. Sorrell), John Wiley & Sons, West Sussex, UK, Part II.

Weblinks

http://www.merckmanuals.com/professional/sec03/ch022/ch022d.html
http://www.uptodate.com/contents/diagnostic-approach-to-adult-with-jaundice-or-asymptomatic-hyperbilirubinemia

25

Abdominal Emergencies

Stephan Goebel

Clinical Vignette 1

A 55-year-old woman presents to the emergency department with severe, constant, periumbilical pain that began 5 hours earlier. Her past medical history is significant for coronary artery disease and a laparoscopic appendectomy 10 years ago, complicated by postoperative right lower extremity deep venous thrombosis. On physical examination, the blood pressure is 120/95 mmHg, pulse rate 120 per minute, and respiratory rate 12 per minute. She is afebrile but in moderate distress. Abdominal examination shows mild diffuse abdominal tenderness to palpation without guarding or rebound tenderness. Bowel sounds are normal. A plain radiograph, complete blood count, comprehensive metabolic panel, and erythrocyte sedimentation rate are normal.

Clinical Vignette 2

A 60-year-old man presents to the emergency department with the abrupt onset of severe diffuse abdominal pain a few hours earlier. He has a history of long-standing rheumatoid arthritis, and has been using a combination of aspirin and other non-steroidal anti-inflammatory drugs to control his pain. For the past 3 weeks he has had intermittent dyspepsia that is relieved by food or the ingestion of milk products. He denies rectal bleeding, melena, or nausea and vomiting. His past medical history is otherwise unremarkable, and his family history is noncontributory. He does not drink alcohol, smoke cigarettes, or use illicit drugs. On physical examination, he is in moderate distress and lying still on the examining table, refusing to move. The temperature is 101.4°F (38.6°C). The blood pressure is 90/55 mmHg,

Sitaraman and Friedman's Essentials of Gastroenterology, Second Edition.
Edited by Shanthi Srinivasan and Lawrence S. Friedman.

and pulse rate 130 per minutes. There is rigidity, guarding, and rebound tenderness on abdominal examination. Bowel sounds are absent. The patient refuses a rectal examination. Laboratory investigations reveal a white blood cell count of 16 500 mm^{-3}, hemoglobin 15 g dl^{-1}, and platelet count of 460 000 mm^{-3}.

General

- Most abdominal emergencies have acute abdominal pain (also referred to as 'an acute abdomen') as the initial presenting symptom. The pain is usually severe and of recent onset (<2 days).
- Acute abdominal pain is the reason for 5–10% of all visits to the emergency department. Up to 10% of patients are estimated to have a life-threatening cause or require surgery.
- A brief algorithm for the expedited evaluation of a patient with acute abdominal pain is shown in Figure 25.1.

Etiology

- The causes of acute abdominal pain can be diverse, from benign self-limited disorders to surgical emergencies.
- Common causes of acute abdominal pain and their locations are outlined in Table 25.1.

Clinical Features

- Patients with hemodynamic instability or peritoneal signs should be identified promptly, and tests to confirm the etiology and a surgical consultation should be obtained expeditiously.
- Focused history taking and physical examination are the cornerstones of identifying the cause of acute abdominal pain and guiding diagnostic testing and treatment.

History

- Elucidation of the rapidity of onset of pain may be helpful in identifying the cause and directing emergent diagnostic and therapeutic intervention.
  - **Sudden or abrupt onset** (maximal pain within minutes): perforated viscus, mesenteric infarction, ruptured aneurysm, ovarian/testicular torsion, acute myocardial infarction, pulmonary embolism.

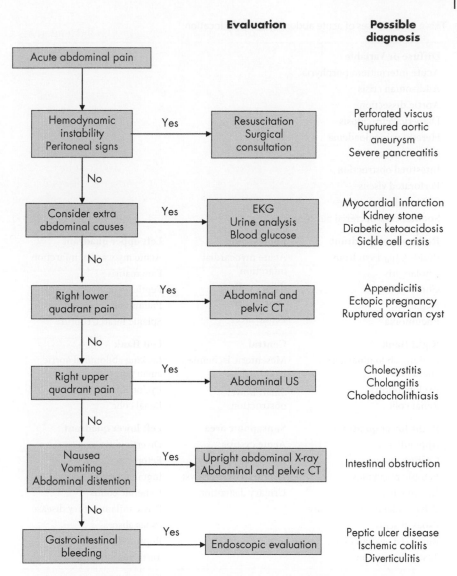

Figure 25.1 Algorithm for the evaluation and management of a patient with acute abdominal pain. CT, computed tomography; EKG, electrocardiogram; US, ultrasonography.

- **Rapid onset** (maximal pain reached in minutes to hours): strangulated hernia, volvulus, intussusception, biliary colic, renal colic, acute pancreatitis.
- **Gradual onset** (maximal pain reached in hours): acute appendicitis, peptic ulcer disease, pyelonephritis, acute cystitis, diverticulitis, ischemic colitis.

Table 25.1 Causes of acute abdominal pain by location.

Diffuse or Variable

Acute intermittent porphyria

Addisonian crisis

Aortic dissection

Diabetic ketoacidosis

Hereditary angioedema

Herpes zoster

Intestinal obstruction

Perforated viscus

Sickle cell crisis

Spontaneous bacterial peritonitis

Right upper quadrant	Epigastrium	Left upper quadrant
Budd–Chiari syndrome	Acute myocardial infarction	Acute myocardial infarction
Cholangitis		Pancreatitis
Cholecystitis	Biliary colic	Peptic ulcer
Hepatitis	Pancreatitis	Pneumonia
Pneumonia	Peptic ulcer	Splenic infarct/rupture
Right flank	**Central**	**Left flank**
Leaking abdominal aortic aneurysm	Mesenteric ischemia	Leaking abdominal aortic aneurysm
Pyelonephritis	Pancreatitis	Pyelonephritis
Renal colic	Small-bowel obstruction	Renal colic
Right lower quadrant	**Suprapubic area**	**Left lower quadrant**
Appendicitis	Acute cystitis	Diverticulitis
Crohn's disease	Ectopic pregnancy	Ectopic pregnancy
Ectopic pregnancy	Ruptured ovarian cyst	Inguinal hernia
Inguinal hernia	Urinary distention	Ischemic colitis
Pelvic inflammatory disease		Pelvic inflammatory disease
Psoas abscess		Psoas abscess
Ruptured ovarian cyst		Ruptured ovarian cyst
Testicular torsion		Testicular torsion

- The history should also include details of the duration, location, radiation, severity, and quality or character of the pain as well as any exacerbating or alleviating factors.

Persons at the extremes of age, those who are immunocompromised, pregnant women, and patients in an intensive care unit with an acute abdominal process often have nonspecific symptoms and may deteriorate rapidly.

- Associated symptoms such as fever, chills, nausea, vomiting, diarrhea or constipation, hematemesis, hematochezia or melena, jaundice, and a change in color of urine or stool should be elicited.
- The past medical and surgical history, a complete medication history, alcohol and illicit drug consumption, and a family history should be obtained.
- The review of systems should include changes in diet, bowel habits, and urination. An expeditious evaluation for cough, chest pain, and shortness of breath is necessary. In a female patient, the obstetric and gynecologic history, including menstrual history, is of utmost importance.

Physical Examination

- Changes in vital signs that indicate a potentially life-threatening condition include fever, tachycardia, and hypotension.
- The patient's demeanor may help to focus the differential diagnosis: patients with peritonitis tend to lie still, whereas those with colicky pain cannot find a comfortable position.
- The physical examination, particularly the abdominal examination, should be repeated serially in a patient with acute abdominal pain.
- The physical examination should be guided by the location of the pain. Examination of the structures surrounding the abdomen, i.e., heart, lungs, extremities, and peripheral pulses, should always be performed. Rectal and/ or pelvic examinations are mandatory in patients with lower abdominal or pelvic pain.
- Certain signs are highly predictive of some diseases (Table 25.2).

Laboratory Studies

- The laboratory evaluation for most patients should include the following: complete blood count; serum electrolytes, liver biochemical tests; renal function tests; serum amylase/lipase; urinalysis; troponin.
- Up to 25% of patients with acute abdominal pain may have a normal white blood cell count; this should not deter further investigations.
- A pregnancy test (urine or serum) should be obtained in all female patients of childbearing age.

Imaging

- Initial imaging studies should include a chest X-ray to assess for pneumonia and free air under the diaphragm, and abdominal X-rays to assess for intestinal obstruction, free air, pneumatosis cystoides intestinalis, or 'thumbprinting.'

Table 25.2 Signs on examination of the abdomen associated with specific conditions.

Sign	Location	Description	Associated condition
Carnett	Epigastric	Pain elicited when supine patient tenses the abdominal wall by lifting the head and shoulders off the examination table	Abdominal wall conditions (hematoma, myositis)
Chandelier	Suprapubic	Manipulation of the cervix causes the patient to lift buttocks off the table	Pelvic inflammatory disease
Cullen	Central	Bluish discoloration in the periumbilical region	Hemorrhage from pancreatitis, ruptured AAA
Grey-Turner	Right or left flank	Bluish discoloration of the flanks	Retroperitoneal hemorrhage from pancreatitis, ruptured AAA
Iliopsoas	RLQ	Abdominal pain with hyperextension of the hip	Appendicitis, abscess from Crohn's disease
Kehr		Severe left shoulder pain	Splenic rupture
McBurney	RLQ	Tenderness in the RLQ, 2/3 between iliac crest and umbilicus	Appendicitis
Murphy	RUQ	Abrupt inspiratory arrest on palpation of RUQ	Acute cholecystitis
Obturator	RLQ	Abdominal pain with internal rotation of the hip	Appendicitis, abscess from Crohn's disease
Rovsing	RLQ	RLQ pain on palpation of the LLQ	Appendicitis

AAA, abdominal aortic aneurysm; LLQ, left lower quadrant; RLQ, right lower quadrant; RUQ, right upper quadrant.

- If no diagnosis has been made, secondary imaging studies are needed:
  - Ultrasonography is sensitive for detecting gallstones in patients with RUQ pain.
  - Transvaginal ultrasonography should be considered in patients suspected of having an ectopic pregnancy.
  - In all other patients, computed tomography (CT) with intravenous contrast is recommended.
  - Magnetic resonance imaging may be employed in patients in whom CT is contraindicated (e.g., contrast dye allergy, pregnancy).

Approach to Treatment

- The patient should undergo aggressive fluid resuscitation, electrolyte repletion, and, if necessary, transfusion of blood products. Broad-spectrum antibiotic therapy should be initiated, if indicated.
- Surgical emergencies should be promptly identified and a surgical consultation obtained.
- Specific treatment is guided by the etiology (see later).
- Small, repeated doses of intravenous narcotics may be used for symptomatic pain management until a final diagnosis is made.
- Many causes of acute abdominal pain such as pancreatitis, peptic ulcer disease, and cholecystitis are discussed in other chapters of this book. In the following discussion, the most common diseases presenting with acute abdominal pain to an emergency department are reviewed.

Acute Appendicitis

General

- Acute appendicitis is the most common cause of acute abdominal pain requiring surgical intervention in the US.
- The incidence of appendicitis in the US is 90–110 per 100 000 inhabitants, with an estimated 250 000 cases annually.
- The overall lifetime risk for men is 8.7% and for women 6.7%.

Pathophysiology

- Direct luminal obstruction (by a fecolith, lymphoid hyperplasia, impacted stool, or tumor) as the cause of acute appendicitis is actually the exception. Recent theories focus on genetic factors, environmental influences, and infections.

Clinical and Laboratory Features

- Steady severe epigastric or periumbilical pain with rebound tenderness:
    - Pain frequently shifts to the right lower quadrant.
    - Aggravation of pain with walking or moving indicates perforation.
    - McBurney sign, obturator sign, Rovsing sign, or iliopsoas sign (see Table 25.2) are highly specific for acute appendicitis; however, these signs are present in <50% of patients.
- Nausea, vomiting, anorexia, and fever are common.

- Symptoms can be mild or nonspecific in pregnant women, young children, and the elderly.
- Leukocytosis is frequent.
- Treatment decisions are rarely based on clinical risk scores (e.g., the Alvarado score based on a combination of symptoms, signs, and laboratory findings).

Imaging

- CT with intravenous and oral (with or without rectal) contrast is the most commonly used modality:
  - Sensitivity 92%, diagnostic accuracy 95–98%.
  - Findings:
    o Dilated appendix with wall thickening and adjacent inflammatory reaction.
    o Possibly abscess formation.
    o Underlying malignancy in the elderly.
- Transabdominal ultrasonography is generally reserved for children and pregnant women in order to avoid radiation exposure.
  - Sensitivity 86%, specificity 81%, diagnostic accuracy 76–96%, operator-dependent.
  - Findings:
    o Appendiceal diameter >6 mm.
    o Muscular wall thickening >3 mm.
    o Presence of a complex mass.

Treatment

- Urgent initiation of broad-spectrum antibiotic therapy.
- In clinically mild cases, continued conservative management may be considered (25–30% will require surgery within a year).
- Appendiceal abscess should be treated with drainage and antibiotics.
- Operative appendectomy:
  - Laparoscopic versus open depending on local expertise and clinical situation.
  - Open appendectomy in the presence of perforation.

Acute Diverticulitis

General

- Acute diverticulitis accounts for 4% of all patients who present with acute abdominal pain to an emergency department.
- 10–25% of patients with diverticulosis will develop diverticulitis during their lifetimes.

- 80% of patients with diverticulitis are 50 years of age or older.
- Risk factors for diverticulosis and subsequent diverticulitis are low dietary fiber intake, obesity, smoking, and lack of physical activity.

Pathophysiology

- Diverticula are most commonly located in the sigmoid colon, where the luminal diameter of the colon is smallest and the intraluminal pressure is highest.
- A fecolith obstructs a diverticulum.
- Microperforations are common.

Clinical and Laboratory Features

- Typical symptoms include left lower quadrant abdominal pain, fever, and nausea. Minor hematochezia may occur.
- The presence of diffuse tenderness or rebound tenderness on physical examination may indicate perforation and requires urgent surgical intervention.
- Leukocytosis is common.

Complications

- Abscess.
- Fistulas.
- Colonic stricture.
- Peritonitis.
- Perforation.

Diagnosis

- CT with intravenous, oral, and rectal contrast.

Treatment

- Antibiotic therapy with coverage for Gram-negative rods and anaerobes; no advantage to intravenous route over oral administration.
- If peritoneal signs are present, urgent surgical intervention is needed. Complicated diverticulitis may also require surgical resection, if the patient fails to improve with conservative measures.
- Repeated bouts of uncomplicated diverticulitis do not mandate surgical intervention; however, in immunocompromised patients, a lower threshold for surgical intervention applies.
- A preoperative colonoscopy is not mandatory but should be considered to rule out malignancy.
- Elective colonic resection is generally scheduled 6 weeks after the acute attack of diverticulitis.

Intestinal Obstruction

General

- Intestinal obstruction accounts for 15% of all cases of acute abdominal pain presenting to an emergency department, and for >300 000 hospitalizations per year in the US.

Classification

- Small-bowel obstruction (SBO) or large-bowel obstruction (LBO).
- Partial or complete.

Etiology

- SBO in children:
  - Meconium ileus.
  - Intussusception.
  - Intestinal atresia.
- SBO in adults:
  - Postoperative adhesions (70–75% of cases).
  - Incarcerated hernia.
  - Tumors.
  - Crohn's disease.
- LBO:
  - Colon cancer (60% of cases).
  - Strictures from chronic diverticular disease (20%).
  - Colonic volvulus (5%).
  - Intussusception.
  - Extrinsic compression.
  - Fecal impaction.

Clinical and Laboratory Features

- Symptoms common to both SBO and LBO:
  - Acute onset of cramping abdominal pain with progressive obstipation.
  - Dehydration resulting in tachycardia, hypotension, and dry mucous membranes.
- Symptoms present predominantly in SBO:
  - Nausea and vomiting.
- Physical examination may reveal abdominal distention with tympany. Bowel sounds are initially hyperactive and become progressively hypoactive.

- Laboratory tests are usually nonspecific; leukocytosis and electrolyte abnormalities may be present.

Complications

- Bowel wall ischemia, necrosis, perforation, and peritonitis.

Delayed diagnosis increases mortality, especially in the elderly and in patients with comorbidities.

Diagnosis

- Plain abdominal X-ray in the supine and upright position (see Chapter 27).
  - Diagnostic in 50–70% of cases.
    - ○ SBO: dilated proximal small-bowel loops and collapsed, gasless distal small-bowel loops; air-fluid levels at different levels depending on the site of obstruction.
    - ○ LBO: dilated large bowel without air in the rectum, a volvulus, (sigmoid or cecal), or dilatation proximal to the obstruction. A paralytic LBO may show a massively dilated colon with a cecal diameter >10 cm.
- CT: 'gold standard'; sensitivity 92% and specificity 95% for diagnosing bowel obstruction.

Treatment

- Partial SBO:
  - Conservative therapy with rehydration, antiemetics, bowel rest and a nasogastric tube for decompression. Avoidance of narcotics is encouraged.
  - Surgical intervention is recommended if the patient fails to improve with conservative measures or if mesenteric ischemia is suspected.
- Complete SBO or LBO:
  - Surgical intervention is almost always needed.
  - Rarely, a colonic stent may be used for LBO due to obstructing colon cancer.

Gastrointestinal Tract Perforation

General

- The incidence of gastrointestinal tract perforations in the US is 100 per 100 000 population per year.
- The mortality rate is 30–50%.

Etiology

- Penetrating foreign body: gunshot, foreign body ingestion, iatrogenic with endoscopy (primarily dilation or colonic polypectomy).
- Extrinsic compression of the lumen: tumor, hernia, adhesions, volvulus.
- Intrinsic compression of the lumen: tumor.
- Damage to the gastrointestinal wall: peptic ulcer, diverticulitis, Crohn's disease
- Gastrointestinal ischemia.
- Infection: cytomegalovirus, *Salmonella typhi* infection.

Clinical and Laboratory Features

- Sudden onset of severe abdominal pain. Peritoneal signs (guarding and rebound tenderness) are typically present on physical examination but may be absent in the elderly, ill, or immunocompromised patient. Bowel sounds may be absent.
- Marked leukocytosis, thrombocytosis, elevated serum lactate levels; serum amylase may be elevated, and serum electrolytes may be abnormal.

Diagnosis

- Imaging with chest and abdominal X-rays or helical CT (sensitivity 95%, specificity 97%) to assess for free air.

Treatment

- Broad-spectrum antibiotics and fluid resuscitation should begin immediately. No oral intake is allowed.
- Emergent surgical consultation and operative planning.

Acute Mesenteric Ischemia

Classification and Etiology

- Superior mesenteric artery embolus (SMAE) accounts for 40–50% of patients with acute mesenteric ischemia: most common source is cardiac arrhythmia.
- Superior mesenteric artery thrombus (SMAT) is the source in 25% of patients, and may be caused by atherosclerosis, a hypercoagulable state, vasculitis, or prolonged hypotension.
- Nonocclusive mesenteric ischemia (NOMI): no identifiable occlusive lesion, usually due to a 'low-flow' state, such as hypotension, sepsis, or severe heart failure.

- Mesenteric vein thrombosis (MVT) makes up 10–15% of patients with acute mesenteric ischemia, usually affects the superior mesenteric vein, and is caused by a hypercoagulable state (infection, malignancy, estrogen therapy), portal hypertension, or pancreatitis.

> Ischemic colitis is not classified as acute mesenteric ischemia. Acute mesenteric ischemia occurs in the distribution of the celiac axis and superior mesenteric artery, whereas ischemic colitis occurs in the distribution of the inferior mesenteric artery. Patients with ischemic colitis are older and present mainly with hematochezia. Angiography is not indicated in the evaluation of patients with ischemic colitis.

Clinical Features

- Persistent, poorly localized pain out of proportion to findings on physical examination.
- Hypovolemic shock may be present in up to 25% of patients.

Diagnosis

- Abdominal X-ray: 'thumbprinting,' pneumatosis cystoides intestinalis, portal venous gas bubbles.
- SMAE, SMAT: conventional angiography or CT angiography.
- NOMI: angiography with papaverine.
- MVT: abdominal CT.

Treatment

- Most patients should be volume resuscitated and anticoagulated with heparin. Angiography may permit the intra-arterial infusion of papaverine therapeutically for SAME or NOMI. Once peritoneal signs appear, surgical intervention with embolectomy or thrombectomy and resection of infarcted bowel is mandatory.

Ruptured Abdominal Aortic Aneurysm

General

- An abdominal aortic aneurysm (AAA) is a localized dilatation of the aorta beyond 3 cm in diameter (normal <2.4 cm). An AAA may rupture once the diameter is >4 cm. The prevalence increases with age, and men are more frequently affected than women (5:1). Ruptured AAAs are responsible for 15 000 deaths annually in the US. The most important risk factor is smoking.

- More than 90% of AAAs are located below the renal arteries.

Pathophysiology

- The basic mechanism underlying the development and rupture of an AAA is thought to be degradation of the tunica media (smooth muscle wall layer) by proteolytic enzymes, mainly matrix metalloproteinases.

Clinical Features

- Abrupt onset of acute abdominal (mid-abdominal, paravertebral, or flank) pain.
- Hypovolemic shock is usually encountered.
- A palpable pulsatile mass may be present, but the sensitivity of this finding ranges from 44% to 97%.

Diagnosis

- Bedside ultrasonography in the emergency department.
- Abdominal CT should not delay surgical intervention.

Treatment

- Rapid fluid resuscitation and immediate surgery. The mortality rate still remains over 50%.

Pearls

- Evaluation of acute abdominal pain at the extremes of age (infants and the elderly) may present a challenge due to difficulty in obtaining the history and potentially misleading laboratory data. Therefore, a carefully obtained history, thorough physical examination, and high index of suspicion are needed to make a diagnosis and institute appropriate treatment.
- During evaluation of acute abdominal pain, conditions of the abdominal wall, such as muscle strain or herpes zoster infection, should be considered. Serum amylase and lipase levels should be obtained in patients with acute abdominal pain. These tests are not included in a comprehensive metabolic panel in most laboratories. Surgical consultation should be obtained early, especially in patients who have peritoneal signs and those who are hemodynamically unstable (with tachycardia and hypotension).

Questions

Questions 1 and 2 relate to Clinical Vignette 1.

1 Which of the following is the most appropriate next diagnostic test?
   A Doppler ultrasonography of the portal, splenic, and superior mesenteric vein.
   B Doppler ultrasonography of the celiac, superior mesenteric, and inferior mesenteric arteries.
   C Computed tomography (CT).
   D Mesenteric arteriography.
   E Exploratory laparotomy.

2 Which of the following is the most likely diagnosis?
   A Mesenteric ischemia.
   B Small-bowel obstruction.
   C Appendicitis.
   D Cholecystitis.
   E Perforated peptic ulcer.

Questions 3 and 4 relate to Clinical Vignette 2.

3 Which of the following is the most likely diagnosis?
   A Bowel obstruction.
   B Perforated peptic ulcer.
   C Choledocholithiasis.
   D Acute myocardial infarction.
   E Renal colic.

4 Which of the following tests should be done next?
   A Magnetic resonance imaging.
   B Abdominal ultrasonography.
   C Plain x-ray of the abdomen.
   D Mesenteric angiography.
   E Exploratory laparoscopy.

5 A 47-year-old man presents to the emergency department with a 2-day history of progressive left lower quadrant abdominal pain. The pain is constant and associated with low-grade fever, nausea, and constipation. His past medical history is unremarkable. Physical examination is remarkable for a temperature of 101.5 °F (38.6 °C), blood pressure 110/70 mmHg, and pulse rate 112 per minute. The abdominal examination reveals guarding in the left lower quadrant and tenderness to palpation. There is no rebound

tenderness, and bowel sounds are present. Laboratory test results are remarkable for a white blood cell count of 15 000 mm^{-3}. Which of the following is the next best step in the management of this patient?

A Colonoscopy.

B Abdominal ultrasonography.

C Plain X-ray of the abdomen.

D Barium enema.

E Intravenous antibiotics.

Answers

1 C

CT should be the next examination. Doppler ultrasonography of the splanchnic vessels (arteries or veins) is generally unreliable due to overlying bowel gas. Mesenteric arteriography may be diagnostic (and potentially therapeutic) in mesenteric ischemia, but not in any of the other causes of acute abdominal pain. The patient does not have peritoneal signs, and exploratory laparotomy is not immediately indicated.

2 A

The patient's severe, persistent periumbilical pain in the face of minimal findings on physical examination and normal laboratory test results and a history of coronary artery disease are concerning for mesenteric ischemia. All other diagnoses listed are possible, but mesenteric ischemia must be ruled out because it is a life-threatening emergency.

3 B

Physical examination in this patient (peritoneal signs, absent bowel sounds) is most concerning for a perforated viscous. Given the use of nonsteroidal anti-inflammatory drugs, a perforated peptic ulcer is a likely possibility. Bowel obstruction causes colicky pain and bowel sounds are generally present, although they may be high pitched or absent in prolonged obstruction. Abdominal pain associated with choledocholithiasis, acute myocardial infarction, and renal colic do not cause peritonitis.

4 C

A plain X-ray of the abdomen with an upright chest X-ray would be the appropriate next examination to evaluate for free air. If these conventional X-rays are inconclusive, a CT would be necessary, since it has a high sensitivity and specificity. However, X-rays may be obtained at the bedside and generally are more expeditious. All the other diagnostic tests listed are not indicated in this patient.

5 E

This patient's clinical presentation is suspicious for diverticulitis. Because he is febrile and has an elevated white blood cell count, it is reasonable to administer antibiotics immediately. CT, not ultrasonography, is the diagnostic test of choice. Colonoscopy and barium enema are contraindicated when acute diverticulitis is suspected because of the increased risk of perforation. A plain X-ray of the abdomen has a poor diagnostic yield in this scenario.

Further Reading

Bhangu, A., Soreide, K., DiSaverio, S., *et al.* (2015) Acute appendicitis: modern understanding of pathogenesis, diagnosis, and management. *Lancet,* **386,** 1278–1287.

Hayden, G.E. and Sprouse, K.L. (2011) Bowel obstruction and hernia. *Emergency Medical Clinics of North America,* **29,** 319–345.

Lewiss, R.E., Egan, D.J., and Shreves, A. (2011) Vascular abdominal emergencies. *Emergency Medical Clinics of North America,* **29,** 253–272.

McNamara, R. and Dean, A.J. (2011) Approach to acute abdominal pain. *Emergency Medical Clinics of North America,* **29,** 159–173.

Morris, A.M., Regenbogen, S.E., Hardiman, K.M., *et al.* (2014) Sigmoid diverticulitis: a systematic review. *Journal of the American Medical Association,* **311,** 287–297.

Panebianco, N.L., Jahnes, K., and Mills, A.M. (2011) Imaging and laboratory testing in acute abdominal pain. *Emergency Medical Clinics of North America,* **29,** 175–193.

Weblink

http://www.ncbi.nlm.nih.gov/pmc/articles/PMC3468117/

Picture Gallery

Sonali S. Sakaria and Saurabh Chawla

26

Classic Skin Manifestations

Melanie S. Harrison, Robert A. Swerlick, and Zakiya P. Rice

Clinical Vignette 1

A 20-year-old man presents with a 3-month history of intermittent bright red blood per rectum. He denies constipation, abdominal pain, weight loss, or melena. His past medical history is unremarkable. Family history is notable for colonic polyps in his father, paternal uncle, and several cousins. Physical examination shows faded hyperpigmented macules concentrated around the lips and buccal mucosa. Abdominal examination reveals a soft, nontender, nondistended abdomen with no palpable masses and no hepatosplenomegaly. Bowel sounds are normal. Rectal examination reveals brown stool that is positive for occult blood. Laboratory testing shows a hemoglobin level of $8\,g\,dl^{-1}$, iron $20\,\mu g\,dl^{-1}$, ferritin $10\,ng\,ml^{-1}$, total iron binding capacity $394\,\mu g\,dl^{-1}$, and iron saturation 4.9%. Colonoscopy reveals numerous polyps ranging in size from 2 mm to 2 cm throughout the colon. Some of the polyps are ulcerated. Esophagogastroduodenoscopy (EGD) shows multiple gastric and duodenal polyps. Polypectomy of several large polyps is performed. Histologic examination of polyps from the colon, stomach, and duodenum reveal disorganization and proliferation of the muscularis mucosa with normal overlying epithelium, suggestive of hamartomas.

Clinical Vignette 2

A 35-year-old woman presents with a 6-week history of bloody diarrhea and fatigue. She reports rectal pain with bowel movements and fecal urgency. Approximately 1 week ago, she noticed tender red lesions on both anterior shins. She denies trauma to the areas. Physical examination is remarkable for

Sitaraman and Friedman's Essentials of Gastroenterology, Second Edition.
Edited by Shanthi Srinivasan and Lawrence S. Friedman.
© 2018 John Wiley & Sons Ltd. Published 2018 by John Wiley & Sons Ltd.

raised, tender, erythematous nodules on the anterior shins. Abdominal examination is significant for mild left lower quadrant tenderness without rebound tenderness or guarding. Rectal examination reveals bloody stools. Routine laboratory tests including a complete blood count and comprehensive metabolic panel are normal with the exception of a hemoglobin level of $10\,g\,dl^{-1}$. Stool examination is positive for fecal leukocytes, but bacterial cultures, examination for ova and parasites, and a test for *Clostridium difficile* toxin are negative. Colonoscopy reveals friable mucosa with exudates involving the rectum and sigmoid colon. The remaining colonic mucosa and terminal ileum appear normal. Colonic mucosal biopsies of the affected areas reveal crypt abscesses and crypt architectural distortion as well as inflammatory infiltrates in the lamina propria.

Erythema Nodosum

- Erythema nodosum (EN) is an inflammatory condition of the subcutaneous fat.
- Typical lesions measure 1–10 cm in size, and are shiny, tender, red, nonulcerating nodules on the anterior shins (Figure 26.1). They may also be seen on the arms, face, thighs, and neck. Associated symptoms include arthralgias, fever, and malaise.

Figure 26.1 Erythema nodosum.

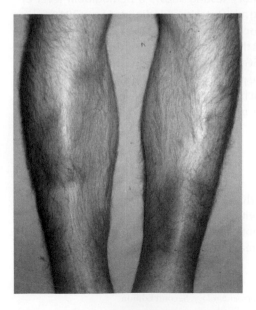

- The cause of EN is unknown in 30–50% of patients. In the remainder, EN may be associated with a wide variety of conditions such as inflammatory and autoimmune disorders (inflammatory bowel disease [IBD], Behçet's disease), infections (most commonly streptococcal, systemic fungal, and tuberculosis), pregnancy, medications (sulfonamides, oral contraceptives), and malignancy.
- EN affects 4–7% of persons with IBD, and has a predilection for females. It is the most common cutaneous finding of IBD. EN parallels the activity of the underlying IBD and improves with treatment of the IBD.
- EN may also be associated with infectious colitis caused by *Yersinia enterocolitica*, *Shigella flexneri*, and *Campylobacter jejuni*.
- The diagnosis of EN is made by recognition of its classic appearance. Biopsy of a lesion may be performed when the diagnosis is unclear. Histologic examination reveals panniculitis with acute and chronic inflammation localized to the fibrous septae between the fat lobules of the dermis. Once a diagnosis of EN is made, a thorough work-up to elucidate the underlying cause should be performed.
- Therapy includes treatment of the underlying disease, bed rest, elevation of the legs, nonsteroidal anti-inflammatory drugs (NSAIDs), glucocorticoids, and topical potassium iodide.

Pyoderma Gangrenosum

- Pyoderma gangrenosum (PG) is an ulcerative cutaneous disorder.
- Lesions begin as pustules or nodules that rapidly ulcerate.
- Lesions are tender and painful, with an elevated dusky purple border (Figure 26.2).
- Confirming PG is a diagnosis of exclusion, as the clinical findings are nonspecific.

Figure 26.2 **Pyoderma gangrenosum.**

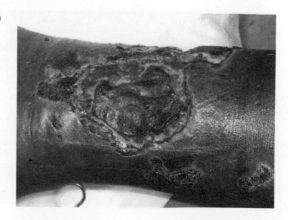

- PG affects up to 5% of persons with ulcerative colitis, and 1% of those with Crohn's disease.
- Some 50% of patients with PG will eventually have an associated systemic disease, which is most commonly ulcerative colitis or Crohn's disease (20–30%). A colonoscopy should be performed in all patients with PG.
- Other systemic conditions associated with PG include hematologic malignancies and some forms of arthritis.
- Management includes treatment of underlying IBD, gentle local wound care and dressings, topical and/or systemic glucocorticoids, topical tacrolimus, and other immunosuppressive drugs. Tumor necrosis factor-alpha inhibitors have been shown to benefit some patients, with infliximab being the most studied.
- Debridement or surgery should be avoided because of pathergy, a condition in which minor trauma leads to worsening of lesions, which may be resistant to healing.

Henoch–Schonlein Purpura

- Henoch–Schonlein purpura (HSP) is a systemic vasculitis characterized by palpable purpura, arthralgias, abdominal pain, and renal disease.
- Palpable purpura typically occurs on the buttocks and legs and may have vesicles or ulcerations (Figure 26.3).
- Gastrointestinal symptoms include abdominal pain, gastrointestinal hemorrhage, intussusception, and perforation. These symptoms can precede the rash in about 20% of cases.
- The diagnosis of HSP is made by identifying characteristic findings. Biopsy of a lesion shows a leukocytoclastic vasculitis with immunoglobulin A (IgA) deposits in the superficial capillaries.

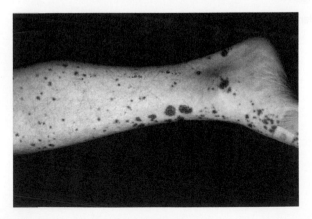

Figure 26.3 Henoch–Schonlein purpura.

- Most cases of HSP are self-limiting and require no treatment other than symptom control with analgesics for arthralgias and abdominal pain.

Hereditary Hemorrhagic Telangiectasia (Osler–Weber–Rendu Disease)

- Hereditary hemorrhagic telangiectasia is an autosomal dominant vascular disorder characterized by telangiectasias, arteriovenous malformations, and aneurysms of the skin, lung, brain, and gastrointestinal tract (see Chapter 22).
- Epistaxis, gastrointestinal hemorrhage, and iron-deficiency anemia are common complications of the disease.
- Skin lesions are 1–3 mm macular telangiectasias of the face, lips, tongue, conjunctivae, chest, fingers, and feet (Figure 26.4).
- The diagnosis is based on four criteria: (1) spontaneous recurrent epistaxis; (2) mucocutaneous telangiectasias; (3) visceral involvement; and (4) a first-degree family member with the disease. The diagnosis may be confirmed by genetic testing for the endoglin or the activin receptor-like kinase type I (ALK-1) gene mutation.
- Treatment is supportive with iron supplements and/or periodic blood transfusions for anemia, as well as ablation of telangiectasias using laser for the skin lesions and argon plasma coagulation for lesions in the gastrointestinal tract. Systemic therapy such as estrogen and progesterone may also be used.

Peutz–Jeghers Syndrome

- Peutz–Jeghers syndrome (PJS) is an autosomal dominant hereditary intestinal polyposis syndrome characterized by the development of benign hamartomatous polyps (see Chapter 10). Typical cutaneous lesions in PJS

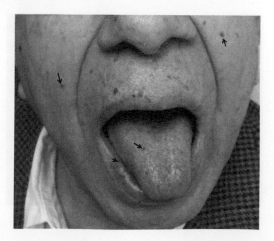

Figure 26.4 Hereditary hemorrhagic telangiectasia. The arrows point to telangiectasias. Photograph courtesy of Dr Elise Brantley, Emory University, Atlanta, GA, USA.

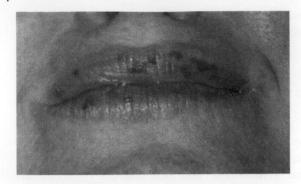

Figure 26.5 Peutz–Jeghers syndrome. Hyperpigmented papules on the lips are shown.

include hyperpigmented papules 1–5 mm in size that occur on the lips, buccal mucosa, palms, soles, and digits, as well as around the eyes, anus, and mouth (Figure 26.5).

- Patients with PJS have a germline mutation in the *STK11(LKB1)* gene, which encodes a serine threonine kinase.
- Hamartomatous polyps have only a small malignant potential; however, patients with PJS have an increased risk of developing carcinomas of the pancreas, liver, lungs, breast, ovaries, uterus, testicles, and other organs. Close surveillance for malignancies is recommended in patients with PJS.

Acanthosis Nigricans

- Acanthosis nigricans (AN) is characterized by hyperpigmented, velvety, thickened skin typically in areas of body folds such as the neck, axilla, groin, and umbilicus (Figure 26.6). Multiple skin tags may be present.

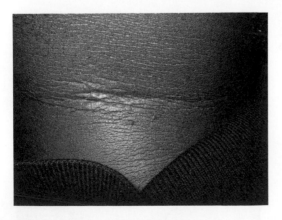

Figure 26.6 Acanthosis nigricans. Hyperpigmented, thickened skin in the neck is shown.

- AN may be inherited or associated with metabolic or endocrine disorders that are typically associated with insulin resistance such as obesity, type 2 diabetes mellitus, and polycystic ovary syndrome.
- AN may rarely occur as a paraneoplastic syndrome associated with visceral adenocarcinomas, most commonly gastric adenocarcinoma.
- The diagnosis is made by the classic appearance of the lesion; a skin biopsy is rarely needed unless the diagnosis is uncertain.
- Persons with AN should be screened for diabetes mellitus and, if appropriate, malignancy.
- AN may resolve when the underlying cause is treated.

Dermatitis Herpetiformis

- Dermatitis herpetiformis (DH) is a chronic, blistering skin condition. It is characterized by small, intensely pruritic, papulovesicular lesions located in a symmetrical manner most commonly on the scalp and extensor surfaces of the elbows, forearms, knees, back, and buttocks (Figure 26.7).
- DH is associated with celiac disease, and occurs in up to 25% of persons with celiac disease.
- The diagnosis of DH with celiac disease is confirmed by the detection of tissue transglutaminase antibodies in serum and characteristic findings on small-intestinal biopsy (see Chapter 6). The diagnosis of DH may also be made by skin biopsy and direct immunofluorescence for IgA deposits in the dermal papillae.
- Definitive treatment is a gluten-free diet for celiac disease. Resolution of skin lesions on a gluten-free diet takes an average of 2 years. Therefore, dapsone is commonly used as a bridge therapy, as lesions typically resolve within days on this medication.

Figure 26.7 Dermatitis herpetiformis.

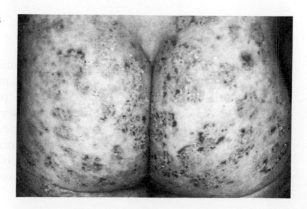

Figure 26.8 Lichen planus.

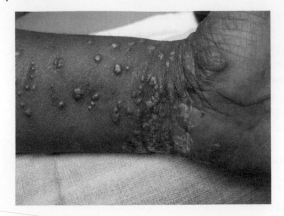

Lichen Planus

- Lichen planus (LP) is a chronic inflammatory disorder involving the oral mucosa and skin.
- Lesions are polygonal, purple, flat-topped papules with white plaques, and affect the flexures of the wrist, arms, and legs (Figure 26.8).
- Oral lesions may present as asymptomatic lacelike lesions on the buccal mucosa or painful erosive lesions on the tongue, buccal mucosa, or gingiva.
- LP is typically found in adulthood and is more common in women than in men.
- LP is associated with chronic hepatitis C and primary biliary cholangitis.
- The diagnosis of LP is made by skin biopsy. Direct immunofluorescence shows deposits of immunoglobulins and complement. Deposits of fibrin and fibrinogen are present in the basement membrane.
- Treatment is with topical gluococorticoids. Systemic glucocorticoids, phototherapy, or acitretin are alternatives in patients with widespread disease.

Mixed Cryoglobulinemia

- Mixed cryoglobulinemia (MC) occurs when immune complexes deposit in blood vessels, resulting in vasculitis of small and medium-sized vessels.
- Skin manifestations of MC include palpable purpura or erythematous macules, commonly seen on the lower extremities (Figure 26.9).
- Other findings include arthralgias, peripheral neuropathy, lymphadenopathy, hepatosplenomegaly, renal disease, and hypocomplementemia.
- MC is most closely associated with hepatitis C. It is less commonly associated with other chronic infections and connective tissue diseases.

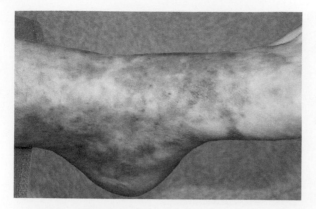

Figure 26.9 Mixed cryoglobulinemia. Palpable purpura associated with mixed cryoglobulinemia is shown.

- The diagnosis of MC is made by the detection of purpura, circulating cryoglobulins, and low complement levels.
- Skin biopsy reveals a leukoclastic vasculitis. Deposits of IgM, IgG, and complement C3 may be seen with direct immunofluorescence.
- Treatment includes therapy of the underlying disorder, including antiviral therapy for chronic hepatitis C (or B). Immunosuppressive therapy may be used in patients with a more severe course of cryoglobulinemia. Rarely, plasma exchange may be needed.

Porphyria Cutanea Tarda

- Porphyria cutanea tarda (PCT) is a metabolic disorder caused by the deficiency of urobilinogen decarboxylase, an enzyme in the heme synthesis pathway.
- PCT is characterized by increased skin fragility, facial hypertrichosis, blistering, milia, and skin hyperpigmentation, typically of sun-exposed areas (Figure 26.10).
- PCT is associated with chronic hepatitis C and hemochromatosis.
- Multiple factors can exacerbate PCT, including alcohol, iron, sunlight, and estrogens.
- The diagnosis of PCT is made by the measurement of total plasma, serum, or spot urine porphyrins, followed by more specific testing if positive.
- Treatment includes avoidance of exacerbating factors and treatment of underlying hepatitis C or hemochromatosis. In addition, phlebotomy and low-dose hydroxychloroquine are highly effective.

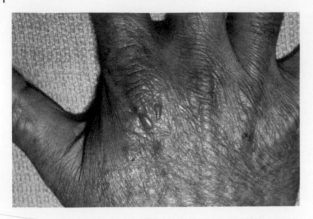

Figure 26.10 Porphyria cutanea tarda.

Polyarteritis Nodosa

- Polyarteritis nodosa (PN) is a systemic vasculitis of small and medium-sized arteries.
- Cutaneous involvement in PN occurs in 25% of cases.
- Cutaneous lesions are characterized by tender nodules 0.5–1 cm in size along the distribution of the superficial arteries (Figure 26.11).
- Most cases of PN are idiopathic, but PN can be commonly associated with chronic hepatitis B and, in some cases, hepatitis C virus infection or hairy cell leukemia.
- The diagnosis of PN is made by tissue biopsy, which reveals arteritis, or angiography, which shows microaneurysms.
- Treatment is with glucocorticoids, with the addition of cyclophosphamide in moderate to severe disease.

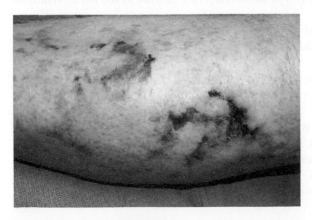

Figure 26.11 Polyarteritis nodosa.

Further Reading

Mirowski, G.W., Leblanc, J. and Mark, L.A. (2016) Oral disease and oral-cutaneous manifestations of gastrointestinal and liver disease, in *Sleisenger and Fordtran's Gastrointestinal and Liver Disease: Pathophysiology/Diagnosis/ Management*, 10th edition (eds M. Feldman, L.S. Friedman, and L.J. Brandt), Saunders Elsevier, Philadelphia, pp. 377–396.

Shah, K.R., Boland, C.R., Patel, M., *et al.* (2013) Cutaneous manifestations of gastrointestinal disease, Part I. *Journal of the American Academy of Dermatology*, **68**, 1–21.

Thrash, B., Patel, M., Shah, K.R., *et al.* (2013) Cutaneous manifestations of gastrointestinal disease, Part II. *Journal of the American Academy of Dermatology*, **68**, 1–33.

Weblinks

http://dermatlas.net
http://www.dermis.net/dermisroot/en/home/index.htm

27

Classic Images

Pardeep K. Mittal, Courtney C. Moreno, William C. Small, and Saurabh Chawla

Achalasia

Achalasia is an esophageal motor disorder characterized by the absence of esophageal peristalsis and failure of the lower esophageal sphincter to relax with swallowing (see Chapter 2). The radiologic study of choice in the diagnosis of achalasia is a barium swallow (barium esophagogram) performed under fluoroscopic guidance. Radiographic signs of esophageal achalasia on fluoroscopic barium swallow (Figure 27.1) include:

- Marked dilatation of the esophagus, often with an air-fluid level.
- Multiple uncoordinated tertiary contractions in early stages and absence of peristalsis in late stages.
- Smooth, tapered, conical narrowing of the distal esophagus ('bird's beak' sign) at the lower esophageal sphincter.
- Narrowed segment of <3.5 cm in length and proximal dilatation (>4 cm).

A normal barium swallow does not exclude achalasia. The diagnosis of achalasia should be confirmed by esophageal manometry. Endoscopy is generally performed to exclude secondary causes of achalasia such as an infiltrating carcinoma at the gastroesophageal junction.

Esophageal Ulcer

Esophagitis and esophageal ulcers may be caused by gastroesophageal reflux disease, viral infections (human immunodeficiency virus, cytomegalovirus, herpes simplex virus), and medications (see Chapter 2). Fluoroscopic studies

Sitaraman and Friedman's Essentials of Gastroenterology, Second Edition.
Edited by Shanthi Srinivasan and Lawrence S. Friedman.
© 2018 John Wiley & Sons Ltd. Published 2018 by John Wiley & Sons Ltd.

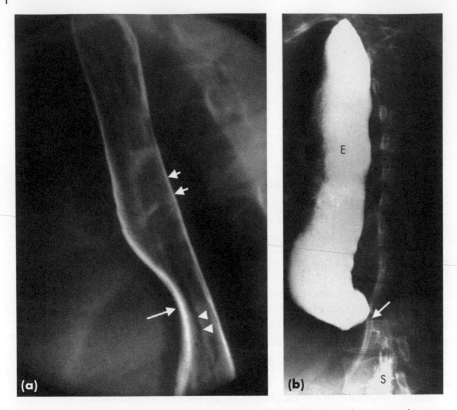

Figure 27.1 Barium swallow of achalasia. (a) A normal esophagogram shows smooth mucosal lining (short arrows), normal fold thickness (arrowheads) and retrocardiac impression (long arrow). (b) In achalasia there is uniform dilatation of the esophagus (E) to the level of the gastroesophageal (GE) junction (arrow). Note the tapered appearance of the GE junction with the column of barium above. S, stomach.

using barium are inexpensive and simple to perform, and provide critical assessment of the esophagus. Barium studies are often used as an initial step in the diagnostic work-up of dysphagia and serve as a complementary test to endoscopy. The radiographic signs of esophageal ulcer or esophagitis (Figure 27.2) include:

- Thickened esophageal folds (>3 mm).
- Limited esophageal distensibility (asymmetric flattening).
- Abnormal motility.
- Mucosal plaques and nodules.
- Erosions and ulcerations.
- Localized stricture(s).

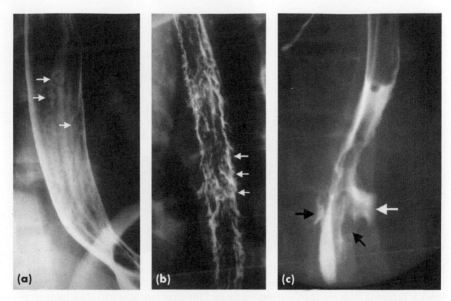

Figure 27.2 Barium swallow of esophageal ulcers. (a) Herpetic esophagitis is seen as multiple small, esophageal ulcers (arrows) in the midesophagus. Note the radiolucent mound of edema surrounding the ulcers. The remainder of the mucosa is normal. (b) Esophageal candidiasis is seen as a grossly irregular esophageal contour due to innumerable plaques and pseudo-membranes (arrows), with trapping of barium between lesions. (c) Cytomegalovirus esophagitis is seen as a large, flat ulcer in the mid-esophagus (white arrow) with multiple satellite ulcers (black arrows).

Gastric Ulcer (Benign versus Malignant)

Gastric ulcers can be benign (peptic ulcer disease) or malignant (gastric adeno-carcinoma, lymphoma, metastasis). Endoscopy is the diagnostic procedure of choice in patients suspected of gastric ulcer. Nevertheless, a double-contrast barium study has a sensitivity of 95% for detecting malignant gastric ulcer, and may be used as an alternative to endoscopy in selected patients for either detection or follow-up of a gastric ulcer. The radiographic signs consistent with a **benign** ulcer (Figure 27.3; Table 27.1) include the following:

- Smooth ulcer mound with tapering edges.
- Edematous ulcer collar with an overhanging mucosal edge.
- Ulcer projecting beyond the expected lumen.
- Radiating folds extending into the ulcer crater.
- Depth of ulcer greater than width.
- Sharply marginated contour.
- Hampton line (a thin, sharp, lucent line that traverses the orifice of the ulcer).

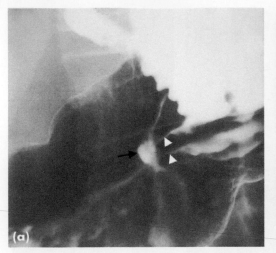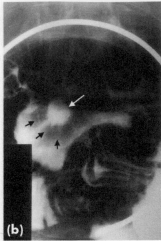

Figure 27.3 Double-contrast barium radiograph of benign gastric ulcers. (a) A benign (en face) barium-filled ulcer is seen in the posterior wall of the gastric body (arrow). Thin, regular radiating folds are seen converging toward the ulcer (arrowheads). (b) A large ulcer (white arrow) is seen on the lesser curvature; its projection from the lumen of the stomach is consistent with a benign lesion. This ulcer is surrounded by a prominent ring of edema represented by the lucent area around the crater (black arrows).

Table 27.1 Radiographic findings of benign and malignant gastric ulcers.

Radiographic finding	Benign	Malignant
Hampton line*	Present	Absent
Extension beyond gastric wall	Yes	No
Folds	Smooth, even	Irregular, nodular
Ulcer shape	Round, oval, or linear	Irregular
Associated mass	Absent	Present
Carmen meniscus sign†	Absent	Present
Healing	Complete	Usually incomplete

*A Hampton line is a thin, sharp lucent line that traverses the orifice of the ulcer.
†A Carmen meniscus sign indicates a large, flat-based, inwardly folded ulcer with heaped-up edges.

The radiographic signs of a **malignant** gastric ulcer (Figure 27.4) include the following:

- Eccentric location of the ulcer within the tumor mound.
- Width greater than depth.

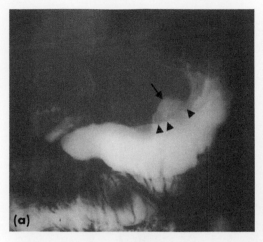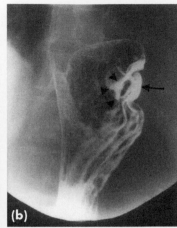

Figure 27.4 Double-contrast barium radiograph of malignant gastric ulcer. (a) A malignant ulcerated mass is seen along the lesser curvature of the gastric body (arrow) with a sharply demarcated shelf (arrowheads). (b) A malignant polypoid ulcer (arrow) is seen along the greater curvature of the gastric fundus and body junction projecting into the lumen. Note the associated distorted gastric folds (arrowheads).

- Nodular, rolled, irregular, or shouldered edges.
- Carmen meniscus sign (a large, flat-based, inwardly folded ulcer with heaped-up edges).

The Normal Plain Abdominal Film

A plain abdominal film (Figure 27.5) is most often used to assess for bowel obstruction or perforation in patients who present with acute abdominal pain (see Chapters 23 and 25). Relatively large amounts of gas are normally present in the stomach and colon, but only a small amount of air is seen in the small intestine. The presence of bowel gas is helpful in assessing the position and diameter of the bowel. Air and fluid represent normal bowel contents, and the presence of three to five air–fluid levels <2.5 cm in length is considered normal on an upright film.

The amount of air present in a normal colon is quite variable, but sufficient gas is usually present for the colonic haustra to be identified readily. The colonic diameter is also variable, with the transverse colon measuring up to 5.5 cm in diameter. A colonic diameter >9 cm is considered abnormal, and indicates obstruction or ileus. The borders of the kidneys and the posterior borders of the liver and spleen can often be identified by the fat that surrounds them. The fat lines may be displaced due to enlargement of these organs or effaced by inflammation or fluid.

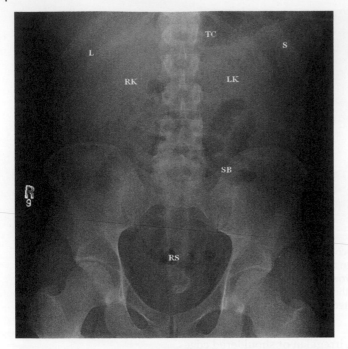

Figure 27.5 A normal plain abdominal film. L, liver; S, spleen; RK, right kidney; LK, left kidney; TC, transverse colon; SB, small bowel; RS, rectosigmoid colon.

Small Intestinal Obstruction

On a plain abdominal film, the normal small-intestinal lumen diameter is ≤2.5 cm for jejunum and 3.0 cm for ileum. A small-bowel diameter measuring >3.0 cm should raise the suspicion of obstruction (mechanical or functional) in the appropriate clinical setting (Table 27.2). The hallmark of mechanical bowel obstruction is a point of transition between dilated and nondilated bowel (Figure 27.6). Functional bowel obstruction (called **pseudo-obstruction** or **ileus**) causes diffuse bowel dilatation with no transition point.

Intestinal Perforation

The presence of free intraperitoneal air (**pneumoperitoneum**) almost always indicates the perforation of a viscus, most commonly a perforated duodenal or gastric ulcer. Additional causes of pneumoperitoneum include trauma, inflammatory bowel disease, recent surgery, and infection of the peritoneal cavity with gas-producing organisms.

Table 27.2 Causes of dilated small intestine (>3 cm).

Mechanical obstruction	Functional obstruction (pseudo-obstruction)
Adhesions (75% of small-bowel obstructions)	Adynamic ileus:
Incarcerated hernia	After surgery
Volvulus	After trauma
Extrinsic tumor	Drugs (e.g., opiates, barbiturates)
Congenital stenosis	Electrolyte imbalance
Intraluminal lesions:	Ischemia
Bezoar	Peritoneal inflammation
Foreign body	Vagotomy
Gallstone ileus	Collagen vascular disorders:
Intussusception	Dermatomyositis
Meconium	Scleroderma
Tumor	Malabsorption syndromes
	Chronic idiopathic pseudo-obstruction

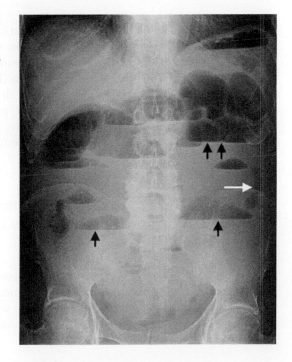

Figure 27.6 Upright abdominal film showing small-intestinal obstruction. Note the dilated small-bowel loops with multiple air–fluid levels (black arrows), a tell-tale sign of bowel obstruction. Note the decompressed loop of descending colon (white arrow) distal to the obstruction.

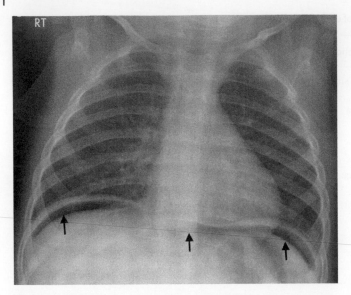

Figure 27.7 Chest radiograph showing intestinal perforation. Free intraperitoneal air (arrows) along the undersurface of the diaphragm indicates a perforated viscus.

A plain film is valuable in the acute setting to exclude pneumoperitoneum. As little as 1 ml of free air can be detected on an erect chest X-ray or left lateral decubitus abdominal film. A small amount of free air can be detected under the right hemi-diaphragm on erect films (Figure 27.7). It may be difficult, however, to differentiate free air under the left hemidiaphragm from normal air in the stomach or colon. Free air is typically seen between the liver and the abdominal wall on a lateral decubitus film. Abdominal computed tomography (CT) is usually performed to confirm perforation noted on a plain abdominal film.

Normal Cross-Sectional Anatomy of the Abdomen on Computed tomography and Magnetic Resonance Imaging

Computed tomography (CT) and magnetic resonance imaging (MRI), with and without contrast, are commonly used diagnostic tests. CT and MRI allow precise visualization of organs and structures within the abdominal and/or pelvic cavity. Figure 27.8 outlines intra-abdominal organs and structures seen on CT and MRI.

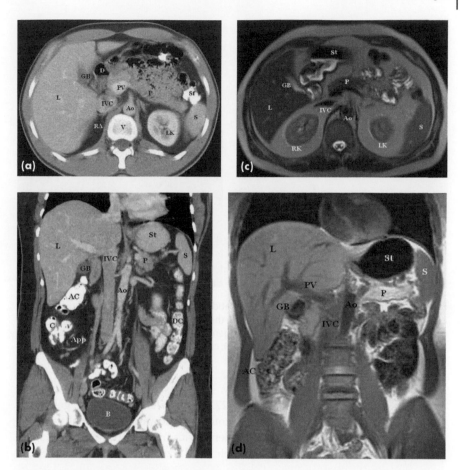

Figure 27.8 Normal cross-sectional anatomy of the abdomen CT (a,b) and MRI (c,d). AC, ascending colon; Ao, aorta; App, appendix; B, bladder; D, duodenum; DC, descending colon; GB, gallbladder; IVC, inferior vena cava; L, liver; LK, left kidney; RA, right adrenal; RK, right kidney; P, pancreas; PV, portal vein; S, spleen; St, stomach; Sf, splenic flexure of the colon; V, vertebral body.

Cholelithiasis

Gallstones can be visualized on abdominal plain films, ultrasonography, and CT. As outlined below, ultrasonography is the test of choice to detect gallstones. On plain films, only 10–15% of gallstones are readily visible (Figure 27.9a). Small radiopaque gallstones tend to be uniform in attenuation, while larger stones typically show a peripheral or laminated pattern of calcification.

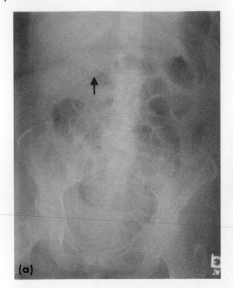
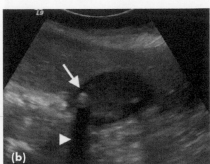

Figure 27.9 Imaging of gallstones. (a) A plain abdominal film shows a round, radiopaque calculus (arrow) in the right upper quadrant, in the typical location for gallstones. (b) An ultrasonographic image shows an echogenic focus in the gallbladder lumen (arrow) with posterior acoustic shadowing (arrowhead), characteristic of a gallstone.

By comparison, with ultrasonography, the sensitivity and specificity for detection of gallstones is >95% (Figure 27.9b). On ultrasonography, gallstones appear as echogenic foci that produce acoustic shadows and are usually mobile. On CT, up to 20% of gallstones are isodense with bile and not detected; some gallstones may be missed because of their small size.

Choledocholithiasis

Ultrasonography has varying degree of sensitivity (50–80%) but high specificity (approximately 95%) for detecting bile duct stones. Magnetic resonance cholangiopancreatography (MRCP) (Figure 27.10a) is highly accurate in the diagnosis of choledocholithiasis, with a sensitivity of 92–94% and specificity of 99%.

Signs of biliary dilatation on MRCP include the following (Figure 27.10b):

- Multiple branching tubular or round structures coursing toward the porta hepatitis.
- Diameter of intrahepatic bile ducts larger than that of adjacent portal vein diameter.
- Dilatation of bile duct >6 mm.
- Gallbladder diameter >5 cm.

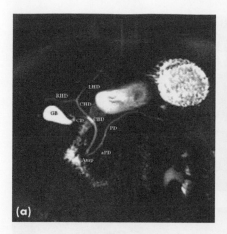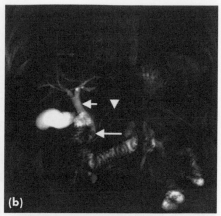

Figure 27.10 Magnetic resonance cholangiopancreatography (MRCP) of choledocholithiasis. (a) Normal MRCP shows biliary system anatomy Including bile duct (BD), cystic duct (CD), gallbladder (GB), common hepatic duct (CHD), right hepatic duct (RHD) and left hepatic duct (LHD), pancreatic duct (PD), accessory pancreatic duct (aPD), and duodenal ampulla (Amp). (b) Choledocholithiasis as seen on a coronal MRCP image in a patient with obstructive jaundice shows a distal bile duct stone (long arrow) with dilatation of the proximal hepatic and intrahepatic bile ducts (short arrow). Note the normal pancreatic duct (arrowhead).

Acute Cholecystitis

Ultrasonography (Figure 27.11a), along with CT and scintigraphy, is used for the diagnosis of acute cholecystitis and related complications (see Chapter 21). The radiographic features of acute cholecystitis on ultrasonography, CT, or MRI (Figure 27.11b) include the following:

- A distended gallbladder with wall thickening.
- Presence of gallstones.
- Inflammatory stranding in pericholecystic fat.
- Blurring of interface between gallbladder and liver.

Complications of acute cholecystitis include the following:

- **Gangrenous cholecystitis**, defined as gallbladder wall necrosis with a high risk of perforation. Gangrenous cholecystitis is seen as asymmetric gallbladder wall thickening with multiple lucent layers, indicating ulceration and edema.
- **Gallbladder perforation** (Figure 27.11c) is a life-threatening complication that may lead to pericholecystic abscess and/or generalized peritonitis.
- **Emphysematous cholecystitis** is an infection of the gallbladder with gas-forming organisms. It is common in diabetic patients. On CT, emphysematous cholecystitis is seen as intramural gas with an arc-like configuration, intraluminal gas, or both.

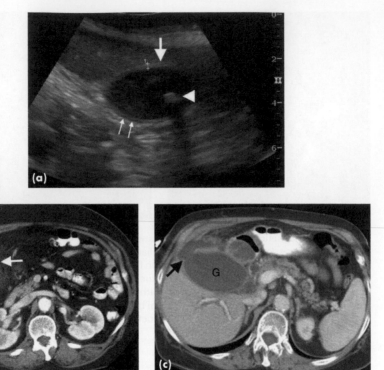

Figure 27.11 Imaging of acute cholecystitis. (a) An ultrasonographic image shows a distended gallbladder lumen with sludge, calculus (arrowhead), wall thickening (arrow), and thin rim of pericholecystic fluid (thin arrows) in a patient with acute calculous cholecystitis. (b) Axial contrast-enhanced CT image shows a dilated gallbladder (G) with a thickened wall (white arrow) and pericholecystic fluid (white arrowhead). (c) CT image shows acute perforated cholecystitis with focal discontinuity in the gallbladder (G) wall (arrow) and expulsion of the bile into the pericholecystic fluid.

- **Mirizzi syndrome** refers to a condition resulting from a cystic duct stone eroding into the adjacent common hepatic duct and causing obstruction. A gallstone may be seen at the junction of the cystic and the common hepatic ducts with associated cholecystitis and biliary obstruction.

Hepatic Masses

Hepatic hemangioma

Hemangioma is the most common benign tumor of the liver, occurring in up to 20% of the general population. It is composed of multiple vascular channels lined by a single layer of endothelial cells that are supported by thin fibrous stroma. Hepatic hemangiomas are most commonly seen in women.

On CT or MRI, hemangiomas demonstrate peripheral nodular enhancement on the arterial phase, with slow progressive centripetal enhancement in more delayed images. The time required for the contrast agent to fill in centrally depends on the size of the hemangioma (Figure 27.12). The term 'giant' hemangioma is used for lesions >10 cm in diameter.

Focal Nodular Hyperplasia

Focal nodular hyperplasia (FNH) is the second most common benign hepatic tumor (after hemangioma). Often discovered incidentally, FNH results from a congenital vascular malformation that induces localized hepatocellular hyperplasia and is composed of normal constituents of liver, such as hepatocytes,

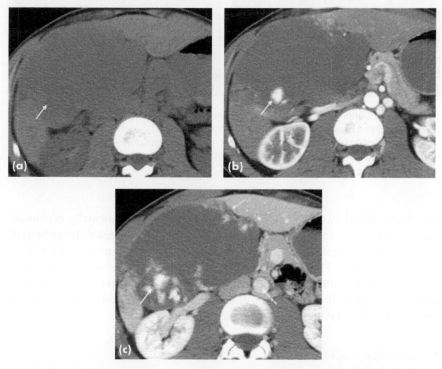

Figure 27.12 Imaging of cavernous hemangioma. (a–c) CT of cavernous hemangioma. (a) An unenhanced CT image shows a mass in the medial segment of the left hepatic lobe that is isoattenuating with blood (arrow). Following contrast administration, the mass shows peripheral nodular enhancement (arrow) in the arterial phase (b) with progressive centripetal enhancement (arrow) in the venous phase (c), similar to a blood vessel (dashed arrow). (d–g) MRI of cavernous hemangioma in the right hepatic lobe.

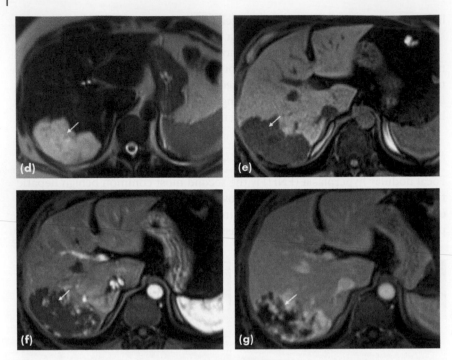

Figure 27.12 (Continued) (d) A T2-weighted image shows a hyperintense lesion. (e) A T1-weighted precontrast image shows a hypointense mass in the right hepatic lobe (arrow). Following contrast administration, the mass shows peripheral nodular enhancement (arrow) in the arterial phase (f) with progressive centripetal enhancement in the venous phase (g), similar to a blood vessel.

bile ducts, blood vessels, and Kupffer cells, but in an abnormally organized pattern. Oral contraceptives do not cause FNH but may increase the growth of FNH. Liver biochemical test results are usually normal in patients with FNH.

On CT or MRI, FNH frequently demonstrates a central scar from which fibrous bands radiate in a spoke-wheel pattern toward the periphery. On post-contrast dynamic imaging, FNH demonstrates avid arterial phase enhancement with delayed enhancement of the scar (Figure 27.13).

Hepatocellular Adenoma

Hepatocellular adenoma (HCA) is a rare, usually benign, tumor that occurs predominantly in women of childbearing age and is associated with oral contraceptive use. HCA can regress or completely disappear after withdrawal of oral contraceptives. In men, HCA is usually associated with use of anabolic steroids; it may also be associated with glycogen storage disease type 1.

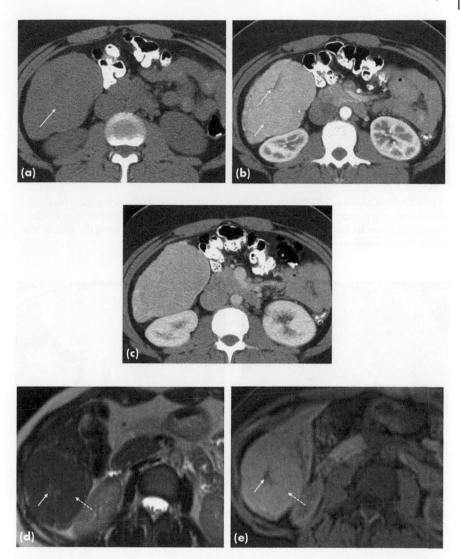

Figure 27.13 Imaging of focal nodular hyperplasia. (a–c) CT of focal nodular hyperplasia. (a) An unenhanced CT image shows an isoattenuating mass involving the right hepatic lobe with a central low attenuation scar (arrow). Following contrast administration, the mass shows avid enhancement (arrow) in the arterial phase (b) and a nonenhancing scar (dashed arrow). (c) In the portal venous phase, the mass becomes isodense with the liver, and the scar shows delayed enhancement. (d–g) MRI of focal nodular hyperplasia. (d) A T2-weighted image shows a slightly hyperintense lesion (dashed arrow) with a hyperintense central scar (arrow). (e) A T1-weighted precontrast image shows the corresponding isointense mass (dashed arrow) and a hypointense central scar (arrow).

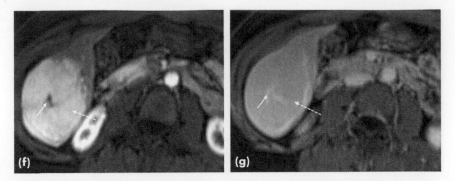

Figure 27.13 (Continued) (f) The arterial phase shows an avidly enhancing mass (dashed arrow) and no enhancement of the central scar (arrow). (g) A delayed postcontrast image shows that the mass becomes isointense with the liver (dashed arrow), and the central scar shows hyperenhancement (arrow).

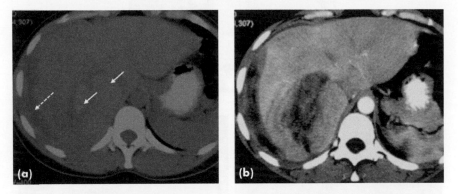

Figure 27.14 CT of hepatocellular adenoma (HCA). (a) An unenhanced CT image shows a heterogeneous mass involving the right hepatic lobe, subcapsular in location, with hyperdense areas due to hemorrhage (arrows) as well as perihepatic high-density fluid (dashed arrow). (b) Following contrast administration, heterogeneous enhancement is consistent with a ruptured HCA.

HCA consists of sheets of normal hepatocytes, and these hepatocytes may be rich in fat or glycogen. Bile ducts are absent, but a few Kupffer cells are present. A pseudocapsule is usually present. HCA has a tendency to undergo hemorrhage. In rare cases, malignant transformation of HCA has also been reported.

On CT or MRI, an HCA appears as a heterogeneous hypervascular mass and may demonstrate internal hemorrhage and/or intra-lesional fat (Figure 27.14).

The comparative features of focal nodular hyperplasia (FNH) and hepatocellular adenoma (HCA) are summarized in Table 27.3.

Table 27.3 Comparative features of focal nodular hyperplasia (FNH) and hepatocellular adenoma (HCA).

	FNH	HCA
Gender	Female	Female
Oral contraceptive use	No	Yes
Imaging features:		
Multiple	Yes	Yes
Central scar	Yes/No	No
Arterial enhancement	Intense homogenous	Inhomogeneous
Washout of contrast agent	No	Yes
Intralesional fat	No	Yes
Internal hemorrhage	No	Yes
Bile ducts on histology	Yes	No
Malignant transformation	No	Yes

Role of Hepatobiliary Agents in Liver Imaging

Gadoxetate disodium (Eovist™, Primovist™) is a relatively recently approved contrast agent that has both extracellular and hepatocyte-specific properties. After injection, approximately 50% of this agent is excreted by the kidneys, and the other 50% is transported into liver cells and then excreted into the biliary system. Enhancement of the normal liver parenchyma on T1-weighted sequences peaks at approximately 20 minutes and persists for up to 2 hours. Therefore, gadoxetate sodium provides a wide time window to image the liver. It is useful for distinguishing FNH from HCA and metastatic lesions, detecting bile leaks and biliary obstruction, and evaluating a hepaticojejunostomy.

Hepatocellular Carcinoma

Hepatocellular carcinoma (HCC) is the most common primary malignant tumor of the liver, and usually occurs in patients with underlying chronic liver disease and cirrhosis due to hepatitis B or C, alcohol, nonalcoholic fatty liver disease, or hemochromatosis. HCC consists of thickened cords of hepatocytes, and typically lacks Kupffer cells. It may be solitary in 50% of cases, multifocal in 40%, and infiltrative in 10%. HCC is a vascular tumor that receives its blood supply from the hepatic artery, and has a tendency to invade vascular structures like the portal vein and hepatic veins. Serum alpha fetoprotein levels are often elevated, especially with large HCCs.

In classic HCC, CT or MRI shows heterogeneous arterial hyperenhancement with rapid washout on the venous or interstitial phase and a persistent pseudo-capsule, whereas imaging of infiltrative HCC reveals involvement of the portal vein and washout of the contrast agent but no pseudocapsule (Figure 27.15).

Cholangiocarcinoma

Cholangiocarcinoma is the second most common primary hepatic tumor after HCC. Cholangiocarcinoma arises from the epithelium of intrahepatic and extrahepatic bile ducts. Predisposing factors include inflammatory bowel disease, primary sclerosing cholangitis, choledochcal cysts, and exposure to Thorotrast (a contrast agent used in the past).

There are two types of cholangiocarcinoma:

- **Intrahepatic cholangiocarcinoma** arises from the peripheral ducts, constitutes 10% of cases, and presents as a mass-like tumor that obstructs the peripheral ducts and causes capsular retraction. These tumors demonstrate progressive delayed enhancement due to abundant fibrous stroma on dynamic contrast imaging (Figure 27.16).
- **Extrahepatic cholangiocarcinoma** is the most common type and occurs in approximately 90% of cases. It is usually small with superficial spreading that results in early obstruction and dilatation of the proximal bile ducts, which is out of proportion to the volume of tumor. The most common location of the tumor stricture is at the confluence of the distal right and left intrahepatic ducts (Klatskin tumor) (Figure 27.17).
- Distal common duct cholangiocarcinoma is similar to a Klatskin tumor and arises in the distal bile duct, often with resulting high-grade bile duct obstruction.

Pancreatitis

CT is used to diagnose and stage pancreatitis. A dedicated CT pancreatic protocol with intravenous contrast administration is used.

Acute Pancreatitis

The pancreas may appear normal in mild acute pancreatitis, but edema of the pancreas and surrounding fat may be seen. In acute pancreatitis (Figure 27.18), the pancreas appears enlarged with patchy high attenuation of the surrounding fat. A small amount of fluid may be seen around the adjacent vessels with associated thickening of the fascial planes.

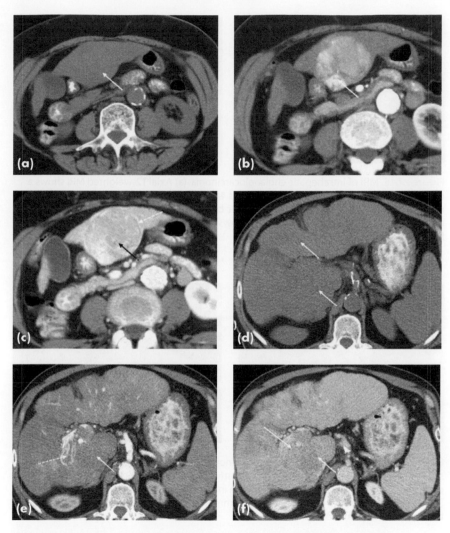

Figure 27.15 Imaging of hepatocellular carcinoma (HCC). (a–c) Classic HCC. (a) An unenhanced CT image shows a hypoattenuating mass in the left hepatic lobe (arrow) in a patient with cirrhosis. Following contrast administration, the mass shows avid heterogeneous enhancement (arrow) on the arterial phase (b) but washout (black arrow) on the portal venous phase (c), with a persistent pseudocapsule (dashed arrow). (d–f) Infiltrative HCC with portal vein involvement. (d) An unenhanced CT image shows a hypoattenuating ill-defined mass involving the right hepatic lobe (arrows) in a patient with cirrhosis. Following contrast administration, the mass shows heterogeneous enhancement (arrow) along with enhancement of the portal vein (dashed arrow) on the arterial phase (e), but shows washout of the mass (arrows) on the portal venous phase (f) tumor thrombus in the portal vein.

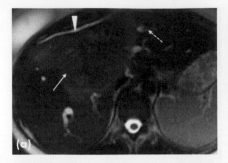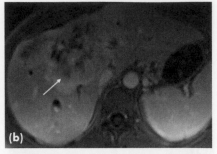

Figure 27.16 MRI of intrahepatic cholangiocarcinoma. (a) Axial T2-weighted MRI shows a mildly hyperintense mass (arrow) in segments 4A and 8 of the liver with associated capsular retraction (arrowhead) and subtle intrahepatic biliary dilatation (dashed arrow) due to a mass effect. (b) Delayed postcontrast MRI shows progressive enhancement (arrow) due to a fibrous stroma.

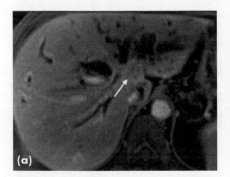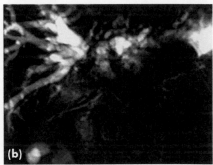

Figure 27.17 Imaging of hilar cholangiocarcinoma (Klatskin tumor). (a) Postcontrast MRI shows an enhancing infiltrative hilar mass relative to the liver parenchyma (arrow) predominantly in segment 4B, with extension into the periductal soft tissues of segment 3. (b) MRCP shows that the mass isolates the common left hepatic duct from the confluence of the anterior and posterior right ducts.

Due to its superior soft-tissue contrast, MRI can provide information regarding pancreatic ducts, pancreatic parenchyma, adjacent soft tissues, and vascular networks in a single session.

- Advantages of MRI in patients with pancreatitis:
  - No radiation hazard.
  - Useful in patients who cannot receive iodinated contrast due to allergy or other contraindications.
  - Superior to CT for detecting choledocholithiasis, pancreatic necrosis, hemorrhage, pseduocysts, or pseudoaneurysm.

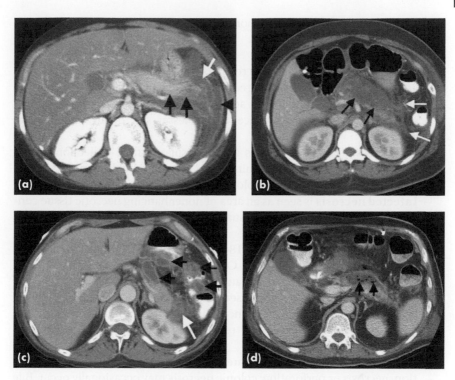

Figure 27.18 CT of acute pancreatitis and its complications. (a) An axial contrast-enhanced CT image of acute pancreatitis shows pancreatic parenchymal thickening predominantly affecting the distal body and tail (black arrows). There is associated inflammation causing blurring of the peripancreatic fat (white arrow) and free fluid (black arrowhead). (b) An axial contrast-enhanced CT image of acute necrotizing pancreatitis shows thickened, poorly enhancing pancreatic parenchyma (black arrows) with surrounding inflammation (white arrows) consistent with pancreatic necrosis. (c) Pancreatic pseudocysts in the same patient after 4 weeks. The image shows multiple fluid collections around the pancreas with peripheral rim enhancement (black arrows) and residual pancreatic inflammation (white arrow). (d) An axial contrast-enhanced CT image of a pancreatic abscess shows liquefaction of the pancreatic tissue with multiple foci of air (arrows) due to superimposed infection.

- More accurate and reliable than CT for early assessment and severity of the pancreatitis.
- MRCP highlights pancreatic ductal strictures, pancreatic duct integrity, and possible communication of the duct with a pseudocyst.
- Limitations:
  - Requires patient cooperation and breath-holding; otherwise, motion artifacts can affect the visualization of the pancreas and its adjacent structures.
  - Time-consuming and relatively expensive in comparison with ultrasonography or CT.

CT and MRI are useful in demonstrating complications associated with acute pancreatitis (see Chapter 18).

- Potential findings:
  - **Liquefactive necrosis** of pancreatic parenchyma (Figure 27.18b) is seen as focal or diffuse lack of pancreatic parenchymal enhancement.
  - **Pancreatic fluid collections**: acute collections may be intrapancreatic, anterior to the pararenal space, in the lesser sac, or anywhere in the abdomen.
  - **Pseudocyst** (Figure 27.18c) is an encapsulated fluid collection with a distinct fibrous capsule. It requires at least 4 weeks to develop. Up to 50% of pseudocysts may need radiologic, endoscopic, or surgical drainage.
  - **Infected necrosis** is seen as an area of nonenhancing necrotic tissue containing gas. Infected necrosis usually requires surgical or per-endoscopic debridement.
  - **Pancreatic abscess** (Figure 27.18d) is a circumscribed collection of pus with little or no necrotic tissue. On CT, a pancreatic abscess is seen as a fluid collection with a thick enhancing wall.
  - **Vascular involvement** may be seen as thrombosis or erosion of a blood vessel due to a direct effect of pancreatic enzymes on peripancreatic blood vessels. Erosion of a vessel may result in acute hemorrhage or pseudoaneurysm formation.
  - **Gastrointestinal tract involvement**: most common is duodenal obstruction, necrosis or perforation; colonic necrosis may occasionally occur. Bile duct obstruction or stricture may also be seen.

Chronic Pancreatitis

The most common cause of chronic pancreatitis is alcohol abuse (see Chapter 19). The features of chronic pancreatitis on CT (Figure 27.19) include the following:

- Parenchymal atrophy: usually generalized but may be focal.
- Dilated main pancreatic duct >3 mm: the duct appears beaded with alternating areas of dilatation and narrowing.
- Pancreatic calcification is usually associated with alcoholic pancreatitis; calcifications may vary from finely stippled to coarse.
- Fascial thickening and chronic inflammatory changes in the surrounding tissue.

Pancreatic Adenocarcinoma

Pancreatic adenocarcinoma is a malignant tumor that arises from the ductal epithelium of the exocrine pancreatic gland and represents more than 75% of pancreatic malignancies; 60% of the tumors are located in the head, 25% are in

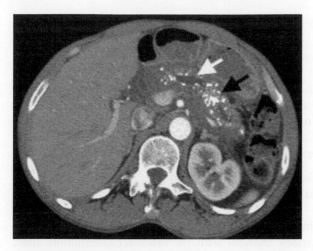

Figure 27.19 CT of chronic pancreatitis. An axial CT image shows multiple foci of coarse pancreatic calcification (black arrow) in a patient with chronic alcoholic pancreatitis. Note the dilated pancreatic duct (white arrow).

the body, 15% are diffuse, and 5% are located in the tail of the pancreas. Pancreatic head masses tend to obstruct the bile duct and present earlier with painless jaundice, even when small in size. By comparison, masses in the tail present later, are larger in size, and may cause pain secondary to local extension.

On CT or MRI, pancreatic adenocarcinoma appears as a heterogeneous, poorly enhancing mass with abrupt obstruction of the pancreatic and bile duct ('double-duct sign') along with pancreatic atrophy distal to tumor (Figure 27.20).

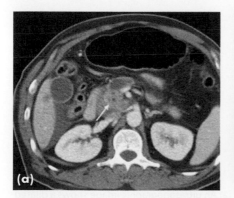
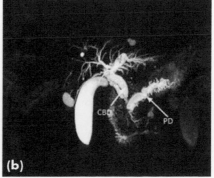

Figure 27.20 CT of pancreatic adenocarcinoma. (a) A postcontrast CT shows a hypoenhancing mass in the head of the pancreas (arrow) causing obstruction of both bile and pancreatic ducts. (b) An MRCP shows a so-called 'double-duct' sign (dilatation of both the bile and pancreatic ducts).

Acute Appendicitis

Ultrasonography is generally used in children with suspected acute appendicitis, and also in patients who have a contraindication to CT (e.g., pregnant woman) (Figure 27.21a). Noncontrast MRI may also be performed in some centers to evaluate for appendicitis in pregnant patients. In general, CT is the preferred imaging method for the diagnosis of acute appendicitis and its complications, with a diagnostic accuracy of 95–98% (see Chapter 25). The imaging signs of appendicitis on CT (Figure 27.21) include the following:

- Appendiceal wall thickening.
- Failure of the appendix to fill with oral contrast or air up to its tip.
- An appendicolith.
- Appendicular wall enhancement with intravenous contrast.
- Surrounding inflammatory changes with increased fat attenuation, fluid, cecal thickening, abscess, and extraluminal gas.

Acute Diverticulitis

Diverticulitis refers to inflammation of colonic diverticula (Figure 27.22), and may be complicated by perforation of a diverticulum and an intramural or localized pericolonic abscess. Other complications of diverticulitis include bowel obstruction, bleeding, peritonitis, sinus tract development, or fistula formation.

CT findings in acute diverticulitis (Figure 27.22b) include the following:

- Diverticular changes with associated inflammation and fat stranding.
- Localized colonic wall thickening.

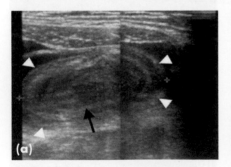 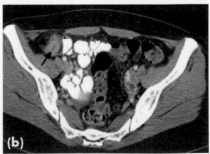

Figure 27.21 Imaging of acute appendicitis. (a) An ultrasonographic image shows a dilated appendix (arrow) with a thickened wall (arrowheads). (b) An axial CT image with oral contrast shows a dilated tubular appendix (arrow) with wall thickening (arrowhead), a typical CT feature of acute appendicitis.

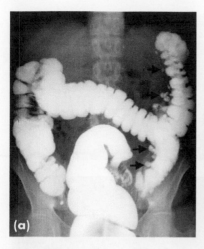 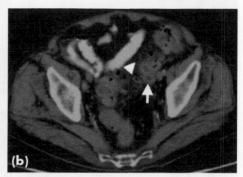

Figure 27.22 Imaging of acute diverticulitis. (a) An anteroposterior film from a barium enema series shows multiple smooth outpouchings from the descending colon (arrows) in a patient with uncomplicated diverticulosis. (b) An axial CT image with oral contrast shows a dilated, thickened colonic diverticulum (arrow) with surrounding mesenteric inflammation (arrowhead), indicating acute diverticulitis.

- A pericolonic abscess.
- Associated fluid that may track down to the root of the sigmoid mesentery.

Crohn's Disease

The diagnosis of Crohn's disease is made by a combination of clinical features, imaging, endoscopy, pathology, laboratory tests, and stool studies (see Chapter 8). Contrast-enhanced imaging studies provide information on the location, extent and severity of disease, as well as complications. The hallmarks of Crohn's disease on imaging studies include aphthous ulcers, confluent deep ulcerations, predominant terminal ileal involvement, discontinuous involvement with intervening regions of normal bowel, asymmetric involvement of the bowel wall, strictures, fistulas, and sinus tract formation.

Small-bowel follow-through radiographic examinations have been largely replaced by video capsule endoscopy, CT, and MRI for the diagnosis of Crohn's disease. A small-bowel series can reveal aphthous ulcers, skip lesions, strictures (string sign), and entero-enteric or enterocolonic fistulas (Figure 27.23a). Enteroclysis, in which contrast material is administered to the duodenum through a nasojejunal tube, is sometimes used to circumvent slow passage of contrast from the stomach into the small intestine.

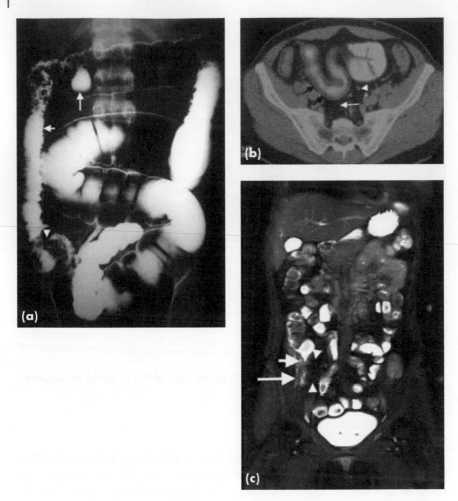

Figure 27.23 Imaging of Crohn's disease. (a) A film from a small-bowel series shows marked ulceration, inflammatory changes, and narrowing of the right colon (short white arrow). Also, note the pseudodiverticulum (long arrow) and severe narrowing of the terminal ileum (arrowhead), consistent with a 'string sign.' (b) An axial CT image with small-bowel thickening (black arrows), fibrofatty proliferation (white arrow), and mesenteric lymphadenopathy (arrowhead) in a patient with Crohn's colitis. (c) Coronal MRI in a patient with Crohn's disease affecting the terminal ileum. There is wall thickening of the terminal ileum (long white arrow) with mesenteric thickening (between arrowheads) and short-segment stricture formation (short white arrow).

CT is not only helpful in the diagnosis of Crohn's disease (Figure 27.23b) and its complications, but it may also be used therapeutically to guide the drainage of an abscess.

Small-bowel MRI (MR enterography) is being used increasingly to diagnose and assess the severity of Crohn's disease and its complications (Figure 27.23c). MRI is helpful in identifying inflammatory processes in the bowel wall and submucosal inflammation and fibrosis. Assessment of submucosal disease on MRI serves as a complement to mucosal assessment using video capsule endoscopy or conventional endoscopy. In conjunction with endoscopic ultra-sonography, MRI is also used to delineate the severity and extent of perianal fistulas. MRI also provides the benefit, as compared with CT, of improved characterization of both acute and chronic soft-tissue inflammatory changes without radiation. This is important in patients who are often young at the time of diagnosis and will need multiple follow-up imaging studies due to the relapsing and episodic nature of the disease.

Ulcerative Colitis

Clinical features, laboratory tests, stool studies, and colonoscopy with biopsies remain the mainstays of the diagnosis of ulcerative colitis (see Chapter 8). **Colonoscopy** is the preferred test to define the extent and severity of colitis and to detect dysplasia and colon cancer. Plain abdominal films may be used to follow colonic dilatation in a patient with toxic megacolon, a complication of ulcerative colitis. Double-contrast barium enema can be helpful in revealing fine mucosal details (Figure 27.24). CT and MRI are of limited use in ulcerative colitis; however, CT plays an important role in the differential diagnosis of ulcerative colitis and in the diagnosis of complications associated with the condition. All imaging modalities lack specificity in this setting. For example, mucosal ulceration or bowel wall thickening depicted on barium studies is nonspecific and encountered in a variety of colitides. Barium enema should be performed cautiously in patients with severe ulcerative colitis because it may cause perforation in a patient with toxic megacolon.

Colorectal Adenocarcinoma

Colorectal cancer commonly appears on imaging as short segmental luminal wall thickening. Clinically, patients may present with hematochezia or iron deficiency anemia (see Chapter 10). The most common site is the rectosigmoid in 25% of cases, followed by the rectum in 20%, ascending colon in 15%, transverse colon in 15%, descending colon in 15%, and cecum in 10% of cases. Once colorectal carcinoma is diagnosed, the entire colon should be surveyed to

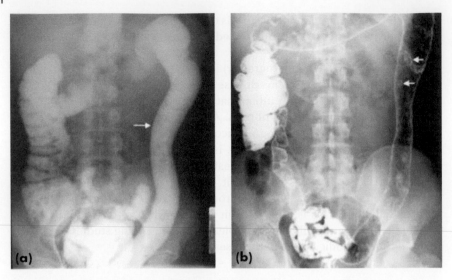

Figure 27.24 Barium enema of ulcerative colitis. Films from a barium enema study show typical features of ulcerative colitis. (a) Contiguous involvement of the distal colon with loss of haustral pattern (arrow). (b) Filiform polyps (arrows).

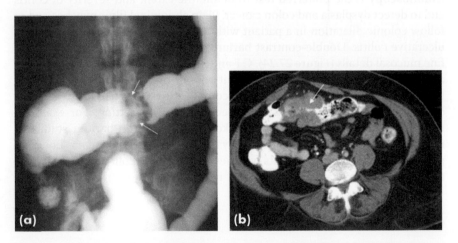

Figure 27.25 Imaging of colorectal adenocarcinoma. (a) A single film from a contrast barium enema shows an apple core lesion involving the transverse colon (arrows). (b) An axial contrast enhanced CT image shows circumferential wall thickening and lumen narrowing of the transverse colon (arrow) consistent with colonic carcinoma.

exclude a synchronous lesion. On imaging, early colorectal carcinoma can appear as a sessile or pedunculated lesion, whereas advanced cancer can appear as an annular, semiannular (saddle-like), polypoid, carpet-like, or apple core lesion (circumferential narrowing of the bowel) (Figure 27.25).

Further Reading

Adam, A. and Dixon, A.K. (2014) Gastrointestinal imaging, in *Grainger & Allison's Diagnostic Radiology*, 6th edition (eds A. Adam, A.K. Dixon, J.H. Gillard, and C.M. Schaefer-Prokop), Churchill-Livingstone, Edinburgh, pp. 591–831.

Brant, W.E. (2012) Gastrointestinal tract, in *Fundamentals of Diagnostic Radiology*, 4th edition (eds W.E. Brant and C. Helms), Lippincott Williams & Wilkins, pp. 670–795.

Sahani, D.V. and Samir, A.E. (2016) Colon, liver and biliary imaging, in *Abdominal Imaging: Expert Radiology Series*, 2nd edition (eds D.V. Sahani and A.E. Samir), Elsevier, Philadelphia. pp. 451–648.

Semelka, R.C., Brown, M.A., and Altun, E. (2016) Liver and biliary imaging, in *Abdominal-Pelvic MRI*, 4th edition. Wiley Blackwell, Oxford, pp. 39–394; 395–460.

Weblink

http://www.radiologyeducation.com/

28

Classic Pathology

Sujaata R. Dwadasi, Mary M. Flynn*, Stephen K. Lau,
and Meena A. Prasad*

Esophageal Squamous Cell Carcinoma

Esophageal squamous cell carcinoma (SSC) is the most common type of esophageal cancer. It typically occurs in adults over age 45, with a peak in the seventh decade of life. The highest incidence rates are in regions of northeast China to the Middle East. It affects men four times as frequently as women, and is nearly sixfold more common in African Americans than Caucasians. Risk factors include alcohol and tobacco use, poverty, caustic esophageal injury, achalasia, and tylosis (genetic hyperkeratosis of the palms and soles). Persons with esophageal squamous cell cancer typically present with progressive dysphagia for solid food and weight loss.

Morphology

- Some 50% of SCCs occur in the middle third of the esophagus.
- Early lesions appear as small, gray–white, plaque-like thickenings. Over time they grow into tumor masses that may be polypoid or exophytic, protruding into and obstructing the lumen.
- Some tumors ulcerate and diffusely infiltrate the esophageal wall, thereby causing thickening, rigidity, and luminal narrowing (Figure 28.1a).

Microscopic Features

- SSC is characterized by irregular nests of infiltrating, atypical squamous cells displaying abundant eosinophilic cytoplasm.

---

* These authors contributed equally to the chapter

Sitaraman and Friedman's Essentials of Gastroenterology, Second Edition.
Edited by Shanthi Srinivasan and Lawrence S. Friedman.
© 2018 John Wiley & Sons Ltd. Published 2018 by John Wiley & Sons Ltd.

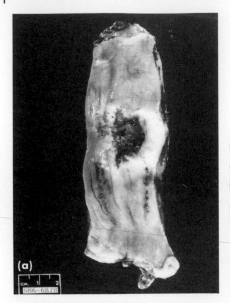
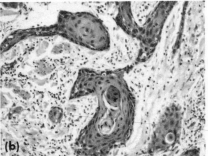

Figure 28.1 Esophageal squamous cell carcinoma. (a) Gross image showing an ulcerated tumor and luminal narrowing in the mid-esophagus. (b) Photomicrograph showing infiltrating nests of atypical epithelial cells with an intraepithelial keratin 'pearl.' Hematoxylin and eosin staining, original magnification × 400.

- A characteristic lesion in SSC is condensation of keratin in the shape of a whorl, known as a keratin 'pearl' (Figure 28.1b).

Barrett's Esophagus and Esophageal Adenocarcinoma

Barrett's esophagus is a complication of chronic gastroesophageal reflux disease (GERD) (see Chapter 1). It is characterized by intestinal metaplasia of the esophageal squamous mucosa. Barrett's esophagus is estimated to occur in approximately 10% of persons with GERD, and is most common in white men aged >50 years. Barrett's esophagus is considered a premalignant lesion. Esophageal adenocarcinoma arises from Barrett's epithelium, and is preceded by dysplasia.

Morphology

- The diagnosis of Barrett's esophagus requires both endoscopic evidence of abnormal mucosa above the gastroesophageal junction and intestinal metaplasia documented by histologic examination.

- Barrett's esophagus can be recognized endoscopically as one or several tongues or patches of salmon-colored mucosa extending proximally from the gastroesophageal junction (Figure 28.2a).
- Esophageal adenocarcinoma usually occurs in the distal third of the esophagus, and may invade the adjacent gastric cardia. It is almost always seen in association with Barrett's esophagus. Esophageal adenocarcinoma may appear as flat or raised patches initially, but over time large masses may develop. Tumors may infiltrate diffusely, ulcerate, and invade deeply (Figure 28.2b).

Microscopic Features

- Intestinal-type columnar epithelium with goblet cells that display distinct mucin vacuoles is generally considered necessary for the diagnosis of Barrett's esophagus (Figure 28.2c).
- When dysplasia is present, the gland architecture is abnormal and shows budding, irregular shape, and cellular crowding. Dysplastic epithelium exhibits irregular stratification, nuclear pleomorphism with hyperchromasia, and an increased nuclear-to-cytoplasmic ratio (Figure 28.2d).
- Invasive esophageal adenocarcinoma shows atypical intestinal-type glandular epithelium with invasion into the underlying lamina propria or deeper layers (Figure 28.2e).

Herpes Virus and Cytomegalovirus Esophagitis

Herpes virus and cytomegalovirus (CMV) infections typically occur in immunocompromised persons, but may occur in healthy persons. Patients with viral esophagitis present with dysphagia and odynophagia and may have superimposed *Candida* esophagitis. The occurrence of these viruses in immunocompetent patients is rare and usually self-limited.

Morphology

- Endoscopy may provide a clue to the type of viral esophagitis. Herpes virus causes vesicles and volcano ulcers in early stages, followed by punched-out (clearly demarcated) ulcers, whereas CMV causes shallow ulcers.

Microscopic Features

- Microscopic features of herpes esophagitis are seen in epithelial cells and include nuclear molding, nuclear chromatin margination, and multinucleated cells (Figure 28.3a). These changes are usually seen at the periphery of an ulcer.

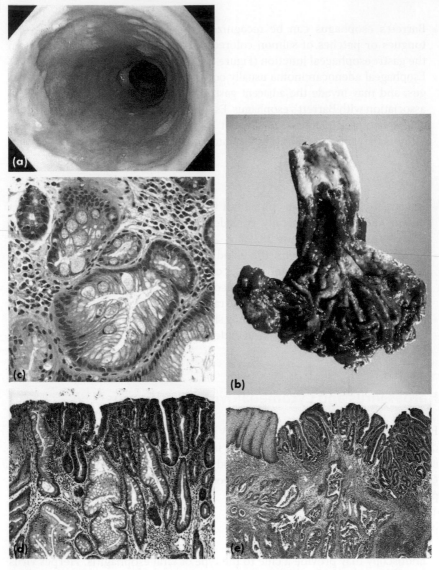

Figure 28.2 Barrett's esophagus and esophageal adenocarcinoma. (a) Endoscopic image of Barrett's esophagus showing salmon-colored mucosa extending superiorly from the gastroesophageal junction. (b) Gross image of an esophageal adenocarcinoma showing an ulcerated lesion in the distal esophagus. (c) Photomicrograph of Barrett's esophagus showing intestinal-type columnar epithelium with goblet cells. Hematoxylin and eosin staining, original magnification × 200. (d) Photomicrograph of Barrett's esophagus showing epithelial dysplasia characterized by cells displaying hyperchromatic nuclei with pleomorphism and increased nuclear-to-cytoplasmic ratio. Hematoxylin and eosin staining, original magnification × 200. (e) Photomicrograph of esophageal adenocarcinoma arising from Barrett's epithelium showing atypical glandular epithelium invading into the lamina propria. Hematoxylin and eosin staining, original magnification × 100.

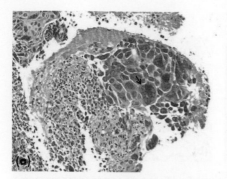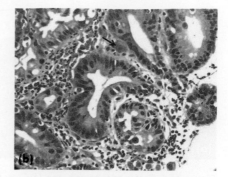

Figure 28.3 Viral esophagitis. (a) Photomicrograph of herpes esophagitis showing squamous epithelial cells at the periphery of an ulcer with characteristic multinucleated giant cell (arrow). Hematoxylin and eosin staining, original magnification × 400. (b) Photomicrograph of cytomegalovirus esophagitis showing intranuclear and intracytoplasmic viral inclusions in the epithelial, stromal (arrow), and endothelial cells. Hematoxylin and eosin staining, original magnification × 400.

- CMV esophagitis is characterized by eosinophilic nuclear and cytoplasmic viral inclusions within epithelial, endothelial, and stromal cells (Figure 28.3b).

Gastric Adenocarcinoma

Gastric cancer is one of the leading causes of cancer-related deaths worldwide. The incidence of gastric adenocarcinoma varies widely with geographic region. The highest incidence is seen in Japan, Chile, Costa Rica, and Eastern Europe. The incidence of gastric adenocarcinoma in the US dropped by 85% during the twentieth century. Common symptoms of gastric adenocarcinoma include weight loss, early satiety, nausea, and vomiting. The most common risk factor for gastric adenocarcinoma is *Helicobacter pylori* infection.

Morphology

- There are two major types of gastric adenocarcinoma: intestinal type and diffuse (infiltrative) type:
  - **Intestinal-type** gastric cancer (54%) tends to form a bulky tumor, exophytic mass, or ulcerated tumor.
  - **Diffuse-type** tumors (32%) grow along the gastric wall. They frequently evoke a desmoplastic reaction that stiffens the gastric wall; such a rigid, thickened wall may impart a leather-bottle appearance to the stomach, termed 'linitis plastica' (Figure 28.4a).

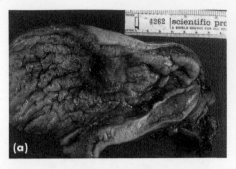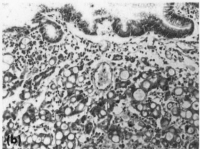

(a)   (b)

Figure 28.4 Gastric adenocarcinoma. (a) Gross image of a diffuse-type gastric adenocarcinoma. Note that the gastric wall is markedly thickened, imparting a leather-bottle appearance to the stomach (linitis plastica), and rugal folds are partially lost. (b) Photomicrograph of diffuse-type gastric adenocarcinoma. Signet-ring cells can be recognized by their large intracytoplasmic mucin vacuoles and peripherally displaced, crescent-shaped nuclei. Hematoxylin and eosin staining, original magnification × 200.

Microscopic Features

- The World Health Organization classification of gastric adenocarcinoma distinguishes four major histologic patterns of gastric cancer, including tubular, papillary, mucinous, and poorly cohesive.
- The neoplastic cells of intestinal-type gastric cancer typically grow in a cohesive fashion to form irregular glands of atypical epithelium that contain apical mucin vacuoles. Abundant mucin may be present in the lumens of the glands.
- The neoplastic cells of diffuse-type gastric cancer are composed of diffusely infiltrating dyshesive cells that generally do not form glands and contain large mucin vacuoles that expand the cytoplasm and displace the nucleus to the periphery, creating a 'signet-ring cell' morphology (Figure 28.4b).

Helicobacter pylori Gastritis

H. pylori is a Gram-negative microaerophilic bacterium that colonizes the surface of epithelial cells of the antrum (see Chapter 3). *H. pylori* is the most common cause of chronic gastritis. In a subset of patients, the gastritis progresses to involve the gastric body and fundus, thereby resulting in pangastritis, which is associated with multifocal mucosal atrophy, reduced acid secretion, intestinal metaplasia, and an increased risk of gastric adenocarcinoma.

Morphology

- When viewed endoscopically, *H. pylori* gastritis appears erythematous (Figure 28.5a) with possible nodularity of the gastric antrum.

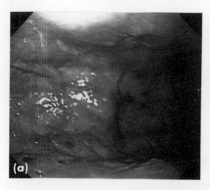 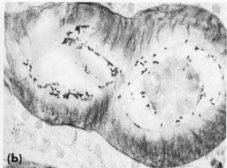

Figure 28.5 *Helicobacter pylori* gastritis. (a) Endoscopic image showing erythema, subepithelial hemorrhages, and erosions of the gastric antrum. (b) Photomicrograph showing abundant spiral-shaped *H. pylori* on the surface of mucous neck cells. Steiner's stain, original magnification ×600.

Microscopic Features

- Due to the patchy distribution of *H. pylori* gastritis, three to five gastric biopsies (according to the Sydney classification system) increases the sensitivity of histologic detection.
- *H. pylori* shows tropism for gastric epithelia, and the bacteria are concentrated within the superficial mucus overlying gastric epithelial cells in the surface and neck regions.
- Organisms are often demonstrated in routine hematoxylin and eosin-stained sections, and can be highlighted with a variety of special stains such as the Steiner stain (Figure 28.5b).
- The characteristic inflammatory infiltrate in *H. pylori* gastritis includes intraepithelial neutrophils that form pit abscesses and an increased number of plasma cells in the lamina propria.

Crohn's Disease

Crohn's disease is a chronic relapsing and remitting inflammatory bowel disease (IBD) that is characterized by transmural inflammation that can occur anywhere in the gastrointestinal tract from the mouth to anus (see Chapter 8).

Morphology

- Transmural inflammation with associated thickening of the bowel wall and constriction of the lumen are characteristic pathologic findings in Crohn's disease (Figure 28.6a).

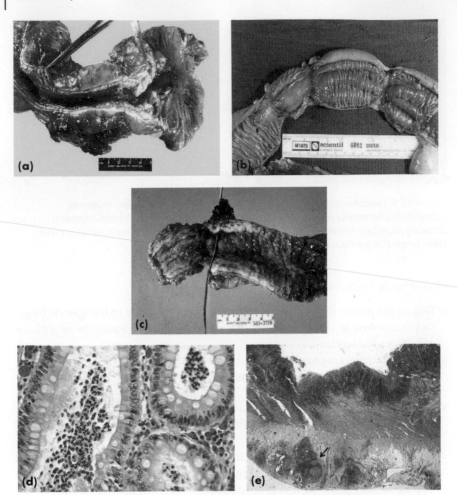

Figure 28.6 Crohn's disease. (a) Gross image of the terminal ileum showing transmural thickening. (b) Gross image of diseased (scarred) segment of the bowel (demarcated by brackets) with normal appearing bowel on either side ('skip lesion'). (c) Gross image of a fistula in the bowel wall. (d) Photomicrograph of a crypt abscess. Hematoxylin and eosin staining, original magnification×400. (e) Photomicrograph showing transmural inflammation, crypt distortion, and a noncaseating granuloma in the serosa (arrow). Hematoxylin and eosin staining, original magnification×40.

- Areas of active disease are sharply demarcated from normal tissue. Multiple distinct areas of affected mucosa with intervening normal mucosa are known as 'skip lesions' (Figure 28.6b).
- Linear mucosal ulceration occurs on the luminal surface, and there is frequently a characteristic 'cobblestone' appearance to the mucosal surface.

- Mesenteric fat extends around the serosal surface, a phenomenon known as 'creeping fat.'
- Fissures may also develop between mucosal folds and form into fistulous tracts (Figure 28.6c) or areas of perforation with abscess formation.

Microscopic Features

- Typically, there is significant destruction and distortion of normal villous and crypt architecture secondary to inflammation.
- Crypt abscesses are frequently present and are characterized by neutrophilic aggregates within the crypts (Figure 28.6d). Crypt abscesses are also seen in other colitides, including infectious colitis and ulcerative colitis.
- In the subserosa, lymphoid aggregates and noncaseating granulomas are typical findings in Crohn's disease (Figure 28.6e).

Celiac Disease

Celiac disease is an autoimmune enteropathy that develops in a genetically predisposed person (see Chapter 6). Over 95% of persons who develop celiac disease carry human leukocyte antigen (HLA) alleles DQ2 or DQ8. The prevalence of celiac disease is 0.5–1% in the US, and the disorder occurs predominantly in Caucasians. Classic symptoms of celiac disease include fatigue, bloating, and chronic diarrhea; however, a majority of patients, especially adults, are asymptomatic. Celiac disease is associated with other autoimmune diseases including autoimmune hypothyroidism, type 1 diabetes mellitus, primary biliary cholangitis, and microscopic colitis. The diagnosis is made by detecting tissue transglutaminase antibodies in serum and characteristic findings on distal duodenal biopsy specimens.

Morphology

- Endoscopy may show 'scalloping' of the small intestinal mucosal folds (Figure 28.7a), a paucity of mucosal folds, mucosal nodularity, or a mosaic pattern, termed 'cracked-mud' appearance.

Microscopic Features

- Microscopic features of celiac disease are categorized according to the Marsh classification:
  - Marsh stage 0: normal mucosa;
  - Marsh stage 1: increased number of intraepithelial lymphocytes, usually exceeding 20 per 100 enterocytes.

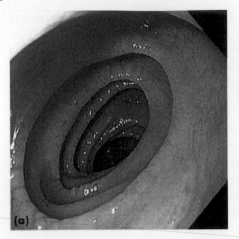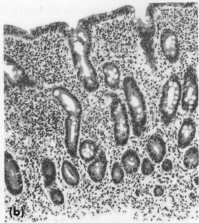

Figure 28.7 Celiac disease. (a) Endoscopic image showing scalloping of the jejunal mucosa. (b) Photomicrograph showing marked villous atrophy. Intraepithelial lymphocytes with dense nuclei are present in the surface epithelium. Hematoxylin and eosin staining, original magnification × 100.

- – Marsh stage 2: proliferation of the crypts of Lieberkühn.
- – Marsh stage 3: partial or complete villous atrophy (Figure 28.7b).
- – Marsh stage 4: hypoplasia of the small bowel architecture.
- • The histologic changes are reversible when the patient is placed on a gluten-free diet.

Colonic Polyps and Adenocarcinoma of the Colon

Colon polyps are growths that occur on the lining of the colon, and can be classified as adenomatous, serrated, hyperplastic, hamartomatous, or inflammatory. Adenomatous polyps, also known as adenomas, are intraepithelial neoplasms that have the propensity to progress to adenocarcinoma (see Chapter 10). Adenomas that are >1 cm, have villous architecture, or have high-grade dysplasia are more likely to progress to adenocarcinoma. Hyperplastic polyps were previously thought to have no malignant potential; however, in 2005, hyperplastic polyps in the proximal colon were reclassified as serrated polyps, which can undergo malignant transformation and account for 10–20% of all colorectal cancers and >30% of 'interval' (between screening colonoscopies) cancers.

Morphology

- • Endoscopically, adenomas appear as polypoid lesions that protrude into the lumen (Figure 28.8a). Adenomas may be sessile (flat) or pedunculated (with a stalk) (Figure 28.8b).

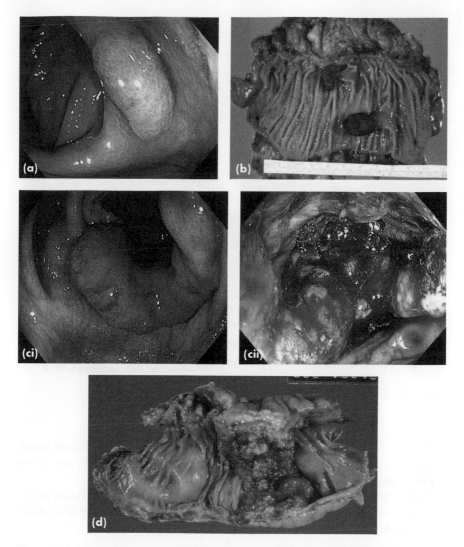

Figure 28.8 Colonic adenoma and adenocarcinoma. (a) Endoscopic view of a tubular adenoma. (b) Gross image of the colon showing two pedunculated adenomas. (c) Endoscopic image of two colonic adenocarcinomas that are semi-circumferential (ci) and ulcerated and obstructing the lumen (cii). (d) Gross image of a colonic adenocarcinoma. Note the elevated, nodular margin surrounding the central area of ulceration. The tumor encircles and infiltrates into the bowel wall. Normal mucosa is seen on either side of the tumor. (e,f) Photomicrographs of a pedunculated tubular adenoma showing well-differentiated glands in a crowded arrangement overlying normal colonic mucosa. The glands of the polyp display increased density with hyperchromatic nuclei and a reduced number of goblet cells. Hematoxylin and eosin staining, original magnification ×40 and ×100, respectively. (g) Photomicrograph of a sessile serrated adenoma. Hematoxylin and eosin staining, original magnification ×4. Note the presence of dilated deeper portions of serrated glands, the so-called 'boot-shaped' glands. (h) Photomicrograph of a moderately differentiated adenocarcinoma displaying glandular morphology with atypical epithelium characterized by pleomorphic, hyperchromatic nuclei, and abnormal mitosis. Hematoxylin and eosin staining, original magnification ×400.

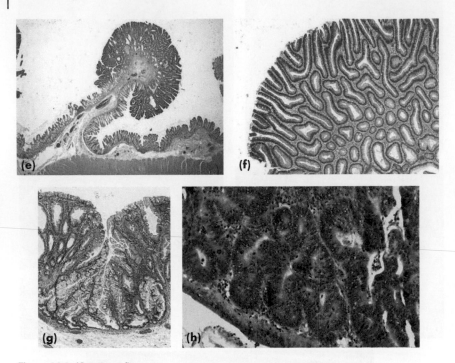

Figure 28.8 (Continued)

- Endoscopically, serrated polyps are typically located in the proximal colon, and have a flat morphology with indistinct borders and a mucus cap. These polyps are pale and often resemble a mucosal fold.
- Endoscopically, adenocarcinoma may appear as a mass lesion that can be circumferential, infiltrate the colon wall, obstruct the lumen, or have ulcerations (Figure 28.8c,d).

Microscopic Features

- Adenomas may be tubular, villous, or tubulovillous. Tubular adenomas have more than 75% tubular architecture, and villous adenomas have more than 50% villous architecture. Tubulovillous adenomas are adenomas with 25–50% villous architecture. The majority of adenomas have tubular morphology.
- Adenomatous epithelium is characterized by hypercellularity of colonic crypts with cells that possess variable amounts of mucin and pleomorphic, hyperchromatic nuclei (Figure 28.8e,f).

- Serrated polyps have mixed hyperplastic epithelium and tubular architecture. They have cellular crowding with serrated papillary infoldings at the edges of the crypts and dilatation or branching at the base of the crypts. These polyps can also have mature goblet cells that secrete mucin, which creates a mucus cap (Figure 28.8 g).
- Most adenocarcinomas are at least moderately differentiated and show atypical, mucin-producing columnar cells. These cells display palisaded, large, oval nuclei that exhibit hyperchromasia, pleomorphism, and excessive mitosis (Figure 28.8 h).

Lynch Syndrome

Lynch syndrome is the most common hereditary cause of colorectal cancer (CRC). It accounts for about 3% of all CRCs. This autosomal dominant syndrome occurs due to genetic mutations of DNA mismatch repair genes (*MLH1, MSH2, MSH6, PMS2*) or the *EPCAM* (epithelial cell adhesion molecule) gene. The adenoma-to-carcinoma sequence progresses more much quickly in patients with Lynch syndrome (35 months) in the general population of patients in whom CRC develops (10–15 years).

Morphology

- The morphology of CRC and adenomatous polyps in Lynch syndrome is indistinguishable from that in sporadic CRC.
- CRC and adenomas in Lynch syndrome are more likely to occur in the proximal than distal colon.
- Patients with Lynch syndrome may also have synchronous or metachronous tumors.

Microscopic Features

- On polymerase chain reaction microsatellite instability testing of tumor specimens, Lynch syndrome tumors have a high microsatellite instability (MSI-H).
- Tumors in Lynch syndrome are usually poorly differentiated and can have signet cells, mucinous features, medullary features, infiltrating lymphocytes, or a Crohn's-like lymphoid reaction (Figure 28.9a,b).
- Immunohistochemistry (IHC) staining for mismatch proteins in Lynch syndrome tumors can identify defective mismatch repair gene products. Negative staining (loss of staining) of MLH1, MSH2, MSH6, or PMS2 can be seen in Lynch syndrome. IHC for mismatch repair proteins in polyps is less sensitive.

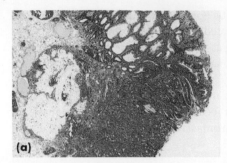 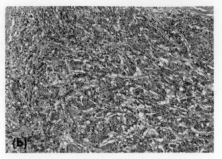

Figure 28.9 Adenocarcinoma in Lynch syndrome. (a) Photomicrograph showing poorly differentiated adenocarcinoma with solid and mucinous features arising in background of sessile serrated adenoma. Hematoxylin and eosin staining, original magnification×2.
(b) Photomicrograph showing poorly differentiated solid adenocarcinoma with lymphocytic infiltrate, the so-called medullary carcinoma. Hematoxylin and eosin staining, original magnification×10. Such morphology has been associated with MSI.

Carcinoid Tumor

The majority of carcinoid tumors are found in the gastrointestinal tract; approximately 40% occur in the small intestine, 25% in the colon, 25% in the appendix, and less than 10% in the stomach. These tumors are typically well differentiated and have a slow, indolent course.

Morphology

- Carcinoid tumors are nodular or polypoid in appearance (Figure 28.10a) and yellow or tan in color. Endoscopically they appear as submucosal nodules.

Microscopic Features

- Carcinoid tumors are characterized by relatively uniform trabecula or gland-like nests of cells with eosinophilic cytoplasm and a central round-to-oval, stippled nucleus (Figure 28.10b).
- The microscopic appearance of the nucleus is often described as a 'salt-and-pepper' pattern due to the fine and coarse clumps of chromatin present.

Pseudomembranous Colitis

The most common cause of pseudomembranous colitis is *Clostridium difficile* infection (see Chapter 5). Risk factors for developing *C. difficile* colitis include recent antibiotic use, recent hospitalization, inflammatory bowel disease,

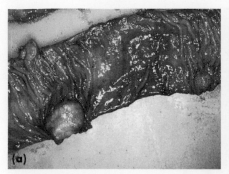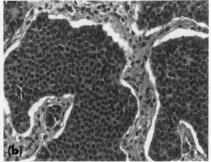

Figure 28.10 Carcinoid tumor. (a) Gross image of the ileum showing a submucosal, tan-colored polypoid tumor. (b) Photomicrograph showing an irregular nest of relatively uniform, small neuroendocrine cells with round nuclei and eosinophilic cytoplasm. Hematoxylin and eosin staining, original magnification × 40.

chemotherapy, and older age. Clinical symptoms include watery diarrhea, leukocytosis, fever, abdominal pain, and dehydration. The diagnosis is made by detecting *C. difficile* toxins or genes in the stool. Flexible sigmoidoscopy or colonoscopy is usually not required to make the diagnosis but, when performed, may reveal characteristic 'pseudomembranes' that appear as yellow, gray, or white plaques 2–5 mm in diameter.

Morphology

- Tan-colored pseudomembranes are present at sites of mucosal injury. An adherent layer of inflammatory cells and debris forms the superficial pseudomembrane layer.

Microscopic Features

- The characteristic histopathologic finding resembles a 'volcano-like eruption' in the mucosal epithelium (Figure 28.11). This 'eruption' is characterized by damaged crypts that are distended by neutrophils, and mucopurulent exudates that cover the mucosal surfaces as the pseudomembranous layer.

Acute Liver Failure Caused by Acetaminophen Toxicity

Acetaminophen is the leading cause of acute liver failure in the US. Approximately half of all cases of acute liver failure in the US are secondary to acetaminophen toxicity. Acetaminophen is metabolized by hepatocytes,

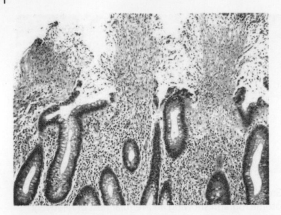

Figure 28.11 Pseudomembranous colitis. Photomicrograph showing the classic 'volcano-like' eruption' of mucopurulent exudates extending from the damaged crypts. A predominantly neutrophilic inflammatory infiltrate is seen in the lamina propria. Hematoxylin and eosin staining, original magnification × 200.

largely by conjugation with sulfate and glucuronide derivatives, and is excreted renally. The remainder is converted to a toxic intermediate by the cytochrome P-450 system. The toxic intermediate subsequently undergoes reduction by glutathione into a nontoxic metabolite. Most acetaminophen ingestions leading to acute liver failure exceed 15 g per day. When toxic levels of acetaminophen are ingested, its metabolism by the cytochrome P-450 pathway is increased. In the settings of alcohol use, malnourishment, fasting, viral illness with dehydration, or ingestion of other substances or medications that are known to induce the activity of the cytochrome P-450 oxidative enzymes, glutathione levels are depleted, resulting in hepatocyte injury and cell death, with subsequent liver failure. High serum aminotransferase levels, often in the thousands, are typically seen. N-acetylcysteine is an antidote for acetaminophen toxicity.

Microscopic Features

- The classic histologic feature of acetaminophen toxicity is hepatocyte necrosis in a centrilobular pattern (zone 3 of the hepatic acinus) (Figure 28.12). Severe toxicity causes massive necrosis. The zone 3 necrosis can also result from ischemic hepatitis and several other toxin mediated injuries.
- Inflammatory infiltration is usually minimal. This is in contrast to other etiologies (e.g., viral hepatitis) in which marked inflammation and massive necrosis are common.

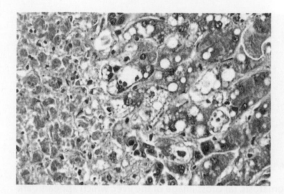

Figure 28.12 Acute liver failure caused by acetaminophen toxicity. Photomicrograph of a liver biopsy specimen showing necrotic hepatocytes on the left and early stages of cell injury and death, including ballooning, steatosis, and apoptosis, on the right. Note the relative absence of an inflammatory infiltrate. Hematoxylin and eosin staining, original magnification × 100.

Hereditary Hemochromatosis

Hereditary hemochromatosis (HH) comprises several inherited disorders of iron homeostasis characterized by increased intestinal absorption of iron that results in deposition of iron in the liver, pancreas, heart, and other organs (see Chapter 15). It most commonly affects populations of northern European origin. HH is caused most often by a gene mutation in the *HFE* gene that results in unregulated intestinal iron absorption. This leads to increased hepatic iron content, which is reflected in elevated serum ferritin levels. Treatment consists of therapeutic phlebotomy to reduce iron stores.

Morphology

- In hemochromatosis, the liver is typically enlarged due to iron accumulation.
- The dark brown color of the liver is due to extensive iron deposition (Figure 28.13a).

Microscopic Features

- The extensive iron deposition within the liver in HH is highlighted by staining with Perls' Prussian blue (Figure 28.13b). The intense blue granules correspond to ferritin and hemosiderin deposition within the siderosomes (iron-laden lysosomes).

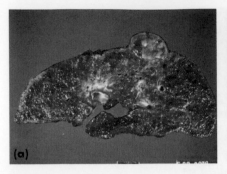
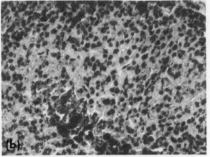

Figure 28.13 Hereditary hemochromatosis. (a) Gross image of the liver, which appears dark brown due to extensive iron deposition. Hepatocellular carcinoma is seen protruding above the capsule. (b) Photomicrograph showing extensive hemosiderin deposition highlighted with Perls' Prussian blue stain. Hematoxylin and eosin staining, original magnification × 200.

Alcoholic Liver Disease

Alcoholic liver disease consists of an overlapping spectrum of three entities: hepatic steatosis (fatty liver); alcoholic hepatitis; and cirrhosis (see Chapter 14). Alcoholic steatosis is reversible with cessation of alcohol. Although alcoholic hepatitis is reversible with abstinence, repeated episodes lead to irreversible fibrosis and cirrhosis.

Morphology

- If concurrent hepatic steatosis is present, the gross liver specimen may be enlarged, yellow, and greasy-appearing (Figure 28.14a).
- Alcoholic cirrhosis is typically micronodular in appearance (Figure 28.14b).

Microscopic Features

- Steatosis is typically macrovesicular, in which lipid accumulation compresses and displaces the hepatocyte nucleus to the periphery of the cell (Figure 28.14c).
- The histologic features of alcoholic hepatitis include a neutrophilic infiltrate with hepatocyte swelling and necrosis (Figure 28.14d) and Mallory bodies (or Mallory hyaline). Mallory (or Mallory–Denk) bodies (Figure 28.14e) are eosinophilic intracytoplasmic inclusions of keratin filaments that are characteristic of alcoholic liver disease. However, Mallory bodies are not specific for alcoholic liver disease, and may be present in Wilson disease, primary biliary cholangitis, and nonalcoholic fatty liver disease.

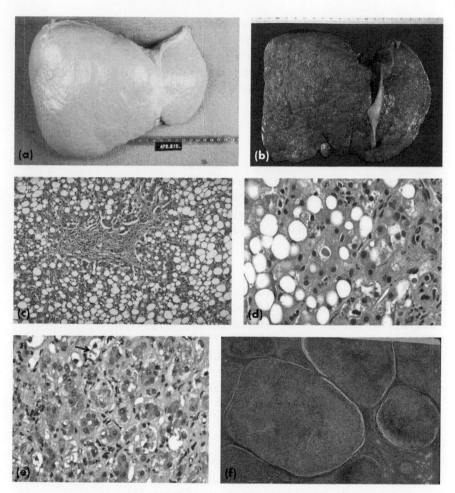

Figure 28.14 Alcoholic liver disease. (a) Gross image of hepatic steatosis (fatty liver). Note the yellowish shiny appearance of the liver. (b) Gross image of a liver with predominantly micronodular cirrhosis. (c) Photomicrograph of hepatic steatosis showing lipid vacuoles compressing and displacing the hepatocyte nucleus to the periphery of the cell. Hematoxylin and eosin staining, original magnification × 100. (d) Photomicrograph of alcoholic hepatitis showing hepatocyte swelling and necrosis with a surrounding inflammatory infiltrate containing neutrophils. Hematoxylin and eosin staining, original magnification × 400. (e) Photomicrograph of alcoholic hepatitis showing a Mallory body, with the characteristic twisted-rope appearance (arrow) seen within a degenerating hepatocyte. Hematoxylin and eosin staining, original magnification × 200.
(f) Photomicrograph of a cirrhotic liver showing regenerative nodules of hepatocytes surrounded by dense fibrous connective tissue. Masson's trichrome staining, original magnification × 40.

- With repeated bouts of alcoholic hepatitis, sinusoidal stellate cells and portal tract fibroblasts may be activated, resulting in fibrosis and cirrhosis. Alcohol-associated cirrhosis is typically micronodular and characterized by regenerative nodules with surrounding fibrous tissue that bridges portal tracts (Figure 28.14f). Steatosis and Mallory bodies in some remaining hepatocytes may be a clue to the etiology.

Cholestasis

Cholestasis occurs secondary to impaired bile flow, causing accumulation of bile salts within hepatocytes. Causes of cholestasis include bile duct obstruction (e.g., gallstones, primary sclerosing cholangitis, cholangiocarcinoma, primary biliary cholangitis) and medications (see Chapters 20 and 21).

Microscopic Features

- Brown bile pigments collect in the cytoplasm of hepatocytes and result in a fine, foamy appearance, termed feathery degeneration (Figure 28.15).
- Hepatocytes become enlarged and edematous in appearance.
- There may be associated proliferation of bile duct epithelial cells, edema of the portal tracts, and neutrophilic infiltration. Bile plugs may develop in dilated bile canaliculi.
- Unrelieved obstruction can lead to portal tract fibrosis and eventually to cirrhosis.

Wilson Disease

Wilson disease is an autosomal recessive disorder that results in the accumulation of copper in the liver, brain, and eye (see Chapter 15).

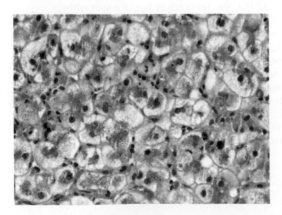

Figure 28.15 Cholestasis. Photomicrograph showing brown bile pigment in the cytoplasm of hepatocytes. Feathery degeneration of hepatocytes is present. Hematoxylin and eosin staining, original magnification × 200.

Figure 28.16 Wilson disease. Photomicrograph showing accumulation of copper (reddish granules) within hepatocytes. Orceine stain, original magnification × 200. Illustration courtesy of Matthew Lim, MD, Department of Pathology, Emory University, Atlanta, GA, USA.

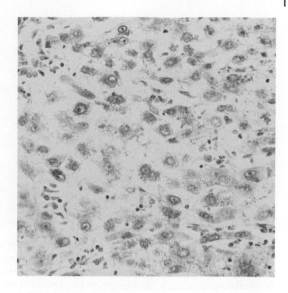

Microscopic Features

- Hepatic damage in Wilson disease can range from mild changes such as steatosis to massive necrosis.
- Histologic features include vacuolated nuclei, mild to moderate fatty changes, and focal hepatocyte necrosis (Figure 28.16). Biopsy may show classic histologic features of autoimmune hepatitis. Cytochemical staining for copper and copper binding protein may be helpful in establishing the diagnosis.

Primary Biliary Cholangitis

Primary biliary cholangitis (formerly primary biliary cirrhosis) is a cholestatic liver disease that predominantly affects middle-aged women and results in the destruction of intrahepatic bile ducts by an autoimmune-mediated inflammatory process (see Chapter 15).

Morphology

- In primary biliary cholangitis the severity of disease varies in different areas of the liver.
- Early in the course of the disease the liver appears normal; however, as the disease progresses the liver appears green due to bile stasis (Figure 28.17a).

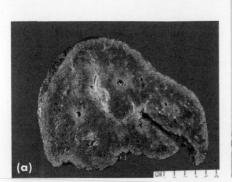
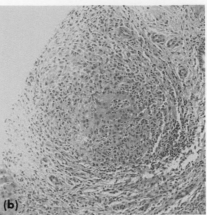

Figure 28.17 Primary biliary cholangitis. (a) Gross image showing a cirrhotic liver with cholestasis. (b) Photomicrograph showing a dense chronic inflammatory infiltrate with a granuloma in the portal tract and loss of bile ductules. Hematoxylin and eosin staining, original magnification × 200. Illustration courtesy of Matthew Lim, MD, Department of Pathology, Emory University, Atlanta, GA, USA.

Microscopic Features

- Primary biliary cholangitis primarily affects interlobular and septal bile ducts.
- Early in the disease, lymphocytes, macrophages, and plasma cells infiltrate the portal tracts (Figure 28.17b). Inflammatory cells accumulate around the bile ducts.
- Loss of interlobular bile ducts is a cardinal feature. Noncaseating granulomas, called 'the florid duct lesion' (Figure 28.17b), and lymphocytic infiltration are seen in the portal tracts.
- As the disease progresses there is an increase in periportal lesions with extension into the hepatic parenchyma. This is referred to as 'interface hepatitis', and is characterized by either lymphocytic piecemeal necrosis or biliary piecemeal necrosis, the latter marked by ductular proliferation and neutrophilic infiltration.
- End-stage primary biliary cholangitis is histologically indistinguishable from other causes of cirrhosis.

Alpha-1 Antitrypsin Deficiency

Alpha-1 antitrypsin deficiency is an autosomal recessive disorder that results in precocious emphysema and liver disease (see Chapter 15). Liver disease occurs in persons who are ZZ homozygotes as a result of accumulation of

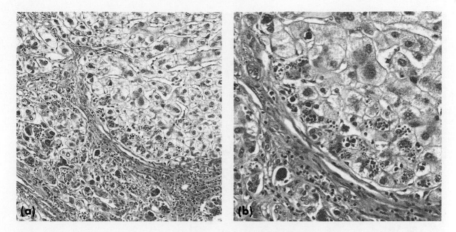

Figure 28.18 Alpha-1 antitrypsin deficiency. Photomicrographs showing eosinophilic hyaline intracytoplasmic inclusions in periportal hepatocytes. Periodic acid Schiff staining, original magnifications (a) × 200; (b) × 400.

abnormal alpha-1 antitrypsin in hepatocytes, leading to an autophagocytic response, mitochondrial dysfunction, and an inflammatory response with hepatocyte damage.

Morphology

- The liver may exhibit a variety of findings, ranging from cholestasis to fibrosis to cirrhosis.

Microscopic Features

- The hallmark of alpha-1 antitrypsin deficiency is the presence of eosinophilic cytoplasmic globules in hepatocytes that are highlighted by periodic acid–Schiff stain (Figure 28.18a,b).
- End-stage cirrhosis in alpha-1 antitrypsin deficiency is indistinguishable from that associated with other causes of cirrhosis.

Autoimmune Hepatitis

Autoimmune hepatitis is a chronic necroinflammatory disorder that is characterized by circulating serum autoantibodies, hypergammaglobulinemia, and interface hepatitis on histologic examination of the liver (see Chapter 15).

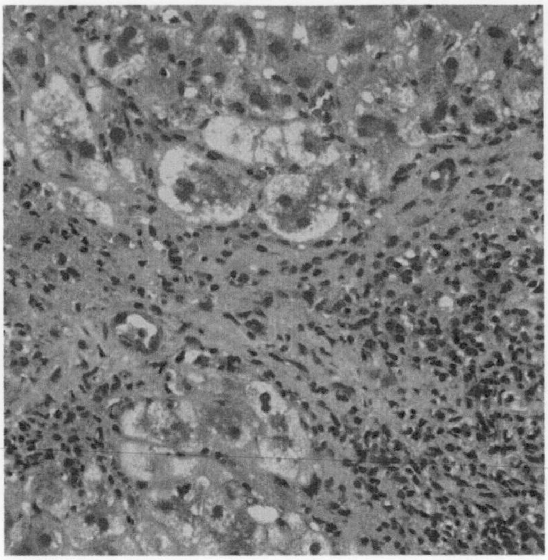

Figure 28.19 Autoimmune hepatitis. Photomicrograph showing interface hepatitis. Note the dense inflammatory infiltrate with plasma cells and lymphocytes and degeneration of hepatocytes in the periportal area. Hematoxylin and eosin staining, original magnification × 400. Illustration courtesy of Matthew Lim, MD, Department of Pathology, Emory University, Atlanta, GA, USA.

Microscopic Features

- Autoimmune hepatitis is characterized by interface hepatitis seen as marked portal and periportal inflammation with lymphocytes and macrophages that spill through the limiting plates encircling periportal hepatocytes, a pattern termed 'rosetting.'
- Autoimmune hepatitis typically displays a marked plasma cell infiltrate (Figure 28.19), which is uncommon in other forms of hepatitis.
- Bridging necrosis and cirrhosis are similar to that seen in other chronic liver diseases.

Primary Sclerosing Cholangitis

Primary sclerosing cholangitis is a cholestatic liver disease characterized by inflammation of both intrahepatic and extrahepatic bile ducts, leading to multifocal bile duct strictures. Small duct primary sclerosing cholangitis is a variant with characteristic histologic features but normal cholangiography.

Microscopic Features

- Early in the disease process histologic findings are often nonspecific.
- Primary sclerosing cholangitis is histologically characterized by progressive periductal fibrosis. The classic histopathologic finding is periductal concentric fibrosis, called 'onion skin' fibrosis (Figure 28.20a).

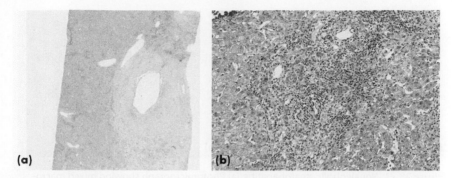

Figure 28.20 Primary sclerosing cholangitis. (a) Photomicrograph showing a dilated bile duct with a thickened fibrotic wall. Hematoxylin and eosin staining, original magnification × 0.5. (b) Photomicrograph showing ductular proliferation. Hematoxylin and eosin staining, original magnification × 10.

Nonalcoholic Steatohepatitis

Nonalcoholic steatohepatitis (NASH) is characterized by the presence of both hepatic steatosis as well as evidence of hepatocellular injury (see Chapter 14). It is seen most frequently in people with features of metabolic syndrome, and is a severe form of nonalcoholic fatty liver disease.

Microscopic Features

- Histologic features of NASH include macrovesicular steatosis, hepatocyte ballooning, and lobular inflammation. Inflammatory cells are primarily lymphocytes and Kupffer cells (Figure 28.21b).
- Hepatocyte ballooning is characterized by loss of normal hepatocyte shape, with swelling and enlargement of the hepatocytes.
- Histologically, NASH is indistinguishable from alcoholic steatohepatitis.

Intraductal Papillary Mucinous Neoplasm of the Pancreas

Intraductal papillary mucinous neoplasms (IPMN) are a subtype of pancreatic cystic neoplasms. These are neoplasms of the pancreatic ductal system that are characterized by dilated main pancreatic duct or side branches. Main-duct IPMNs have a high malignant potential, and are treated with surgical resection. Side-branch IPMNs have a low to moderate malignant potential, and can often be monitored with cross-sectional imaging.

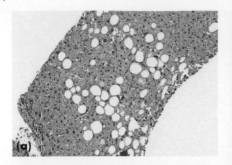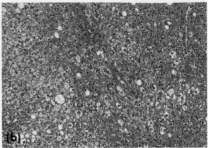

Figure 28.21 Nonalcoholic steatohepatitis. (a) Photomicrograph showing mixed macro- and microsteatosis. Hematoxylin and eosin staining, original magnification × 10. No Mallory bodies are identified. (b) Photomicrograph showing steatosis and balloon degeneration of hepatocytes. Hematoxylin and eosin staining, original magnification × 10.

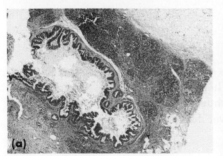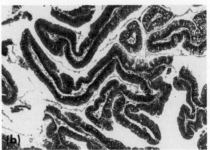

Figure 28.22 Intraductal papillary mucinous neoplasm (IPMN) of the pancreas. (a) Photomicrograph showing dilated duct lined by papillary epithelium with adjacent relatively spared pancreatic parenchyma. Hematoxylin and eosin staining, original magnification × 2. (b) Photomicrograph showing an IPMN with high grade dysplasia. Hematoxylin and eosin staining, original magnification × 5. Note the papillary epithelial lining with hyperchromatic nuclei, loss of polarization, and prominent nucleoli.

Microscopic Features

- Typical findings on cytology include mucinous columnar cells that stain positive for mucin.
- They can be hyperplastic or dysplastic (Figure 28.22b).

Mucinous Cystic Neoplasm of the Pancreas

Mucinous cystic neoplasms are a subtype of pancreatic cystic neoplasm that are almost exclusively seen in females and often present as an incidental finding on imaging. These have a moderate malignant potential and are treated with surgical resection.

Microscopic Features

- Typical cytology findings include columnar cells that stain positive for mucin.

Serous Cystic Tumors of the Pancreas

Serous cystic tumors are a subtype of pancreatic cystic neoplasms. The majority of serous cystic tumors are serous cystadenomas. Unless symptomatic, these are benign tumors that can be managed conservatively. They are most commonly seen in older women in the fifth to seventh decade of life.

Microscopic Features

- Typical cytology findings include cuboidal cells that stain positive for glycogen (Figure 28.23).

Solid Pseudopapillary Tumors of the Pancreas

Solid pseudopapillary tumors are a rare subtype of pancreatic cystic neoplasms. These are typically seen in young women in the second to third decade of life. They have moderate to high malignant potential and are treated with surgical resection.

Microscopic Features

- Typical cytology includes branching papillae with myxoid stroma.

Figure 28.23 Serous cystadenoma. Photomicrograph showing a high-power view of a serous cystadenoma with variably sized cysts lined by compressed tumor cells and more solid areas comprised of bland tumor cells with round nuclei and clear cytoplasm. Hematoxylin and eosin staining, original magnification × 20.

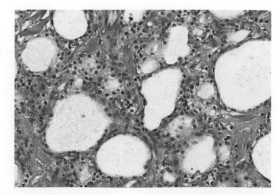

Pancreatic Pseudocyst

A pancreatic pseudocyst is a type of pancreatic cystic lesion. It is a mature collection of fluid around the pancreas that typically develops as a complication of pancreatitis. Pancreatic pseudocysts have no malignant potential.

Microscopic Features

- Typical cytologic features include the presence of neutrophils, macrophages, and histiocytes with negative staining for mucin.

Further Reading

Kumar, V., Abbas, A., and Fausto, N. (eds) (2010) *Robbins and Cotran Pathologic Basis of Disease*, 8th edition, Saunders Elsevier, Philadelphia.
Odze, R.D. and Goldblum, J.R. (eds) (2015) *Odze and Goldblum Surgical Pathology of the GI Tract, Liver Biliary Tract and Pancreas*, 3rd edition, Elsevier, Philadelphia.

Weblinks

http://www.humpath.com/
http://library.med.utah.edu/WebPath/GIHTML/GIIDX.html

Index

Note: Page numbers in *italic* denote figures, those in **bold** denote tables.

Sitaraman and Friedman's Essentials of Gastroenterology, Second Edition.
Edited by Shanthi Srinivasan and Lawrence S. Friedman.
© 2018 John Wiley & Sons Ltd. Published 2018 by John Wiley & Sons Ltd.

Printed and bound by CPI Group (UK) Ltd, Croydon, CR0 4YY

09/10/2024

14571429-0005